International perspectives on women, health and culture:
A world-wide anthology

Editorial consultants

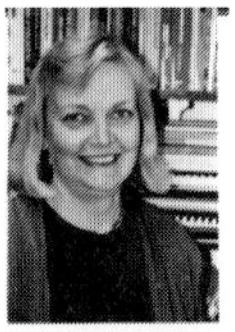

Lorraine Cathro, BEd, MEd, PhD: consultant for the Americas; chair, Advisory Council to the President, Status of Women, University of Saskatchewan, Saskatoon, Saskatchewan, Canada; Cathro Educational Consulting

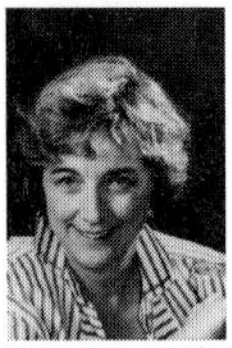

Marian Crook, PhD(in progress), MA, BScN: consultant, Women's Issues; author and writer; Canadian Research Institute for the Advancement of Women, Vancouver, British Columbia, Canada

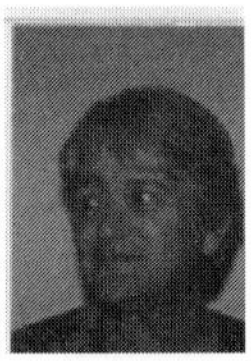

Carol Jackson, PhD(c), FRCNA, MN: co-ordinator, Child and Parent Health Nursing, RMIT, Faculty of Nursing, Bundoora, Australia

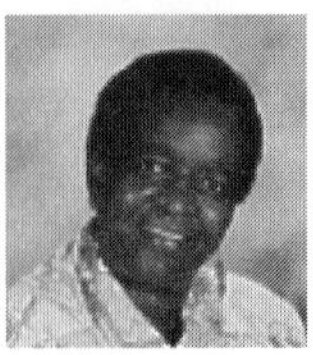

Joyce C Kadandara, BA(Hons), Sociology: PGDip, Social Administration: nurse/midwife; member of Women's Health and Development Projects, member of the Global Commission on Women, World Health Organisation; Zimbabwe

International perspectives on women, health and culture: *A world-wide anthology*

Edited by

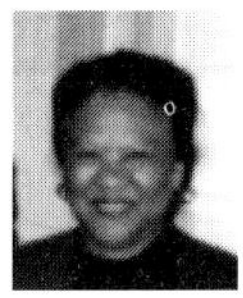

Lourdes Fernandez-Heber, EdD, PhD
and Theresa George, MS, PhD

Quay Books

Quay Books Division
Mark Allen Publishing Ltd, Jesses Farm
Snow Hill, Dinton, Nr Salisbury, Wilts, SP3 5HN

British Library Cataloguing in Publication Data
A catalogue record for this book is available from the British Library

ISBN 1 85642 108 2

Printed and bound in the United Kingdom by Redwood Books, Trowbridge, Wiltshire

Contents

Contributors

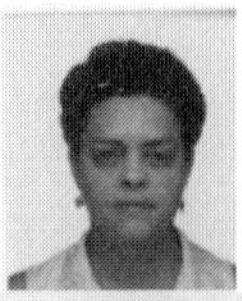

Mariza Silva Almeida, MN: assistant professor, Department of Community Nursing, Federal University of Bahia, Salvador, Bahia, Brazil

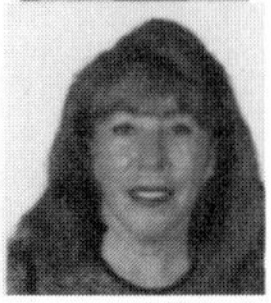

Delvair de Brito Alves, MEd, PhD: teacher (retired), Nursing School, Federal University of Bahia, Bahia, Brazil; visiting teacher, Federal University of Sargipe

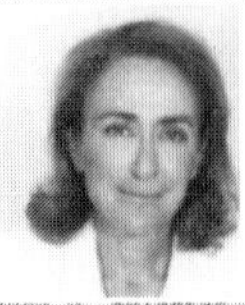

Thalia Attié, PhD: psychologist and psychoanalyst; independent practice in Lebanon, France and Mexico

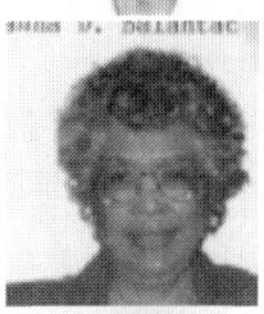

Deanna D Balantac, MS, RN: professor of nursing, California State University, Sacramento, California, United States of America

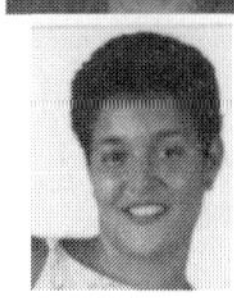

Ailema Cardoso Barbosa: graduate student, Nursing School, Federal University of Bahia, Bahia, Brazil

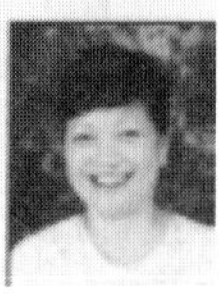

Mollyn V Bohnen, EdD, RN: professor of nursing, California State University, Sacramento, California, United States of America

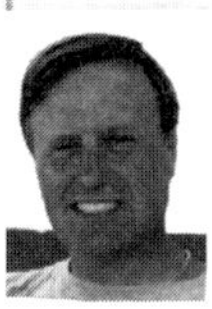

David Bullivent, MA, BSc, DipH&SW, DMS: general manager, Oncology Services, Plymouth Hospital NHS Trust, United Kingdom

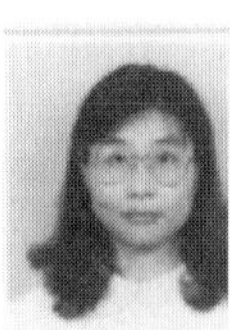

Shu-Yuan Chao, DNSc, RN: associate professor, Chong-Gung Institute of Nursing, Republic of China

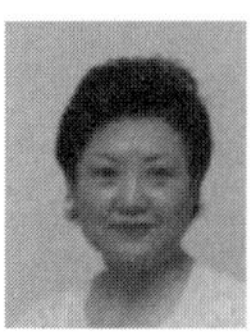

Sang Soon Choi, RN., PhD: professor and chair, Department of Nursing, Yonsei University, Wonju College of Medicine, Republic of Korea

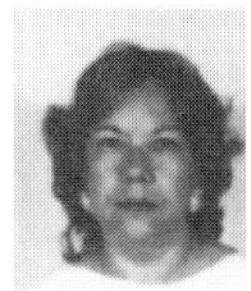

María Elena Colomé, BEd: acting professor, Health Polytechnic Institute, Santiago de Cuba, Cuba

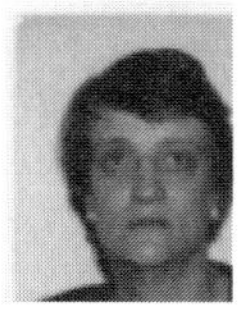

Valerie Ehlers, DLittPhil, RGN, RM, RT, RNA., RPN: senior lecturer, Department of Advanced Nursing Science, University of South Africa, Republic of South Africa

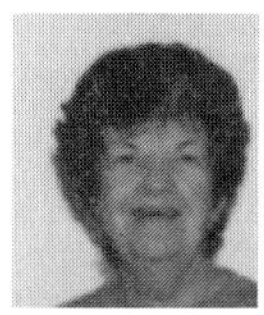

Gloria Geller, PhD: Faculty of Social Work, University of Regina, Saskatchewan, Canada

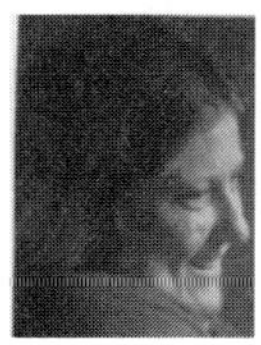

Dale Gietzelt, PhD: post-doctoral research fellow, Faculty of Nursing, University of Technology, Sydney, Australia

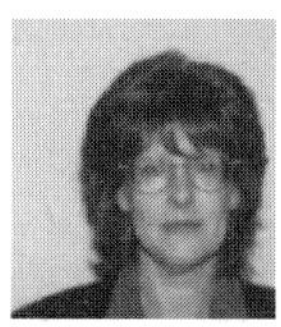

Mary Ruckles Hampton, EdD: Department of Psychology, Luther College, University of Regina, Saskatchewan, Canada

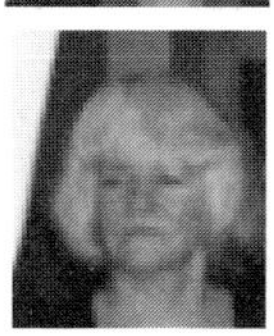

Joellen W Hawkins, RNC, PhD, FAAN: Boston College School of Nursing, Chestnut Hill, Massachusetts, United States of America

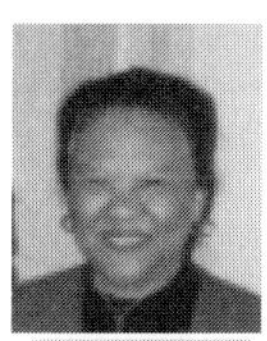

Lourdes Fernandez-Heber, BScN, MEd, EdD, PhD: professor, Nursing, University of Saskatchewan, Saskatoon, Saskatchewan, Canada

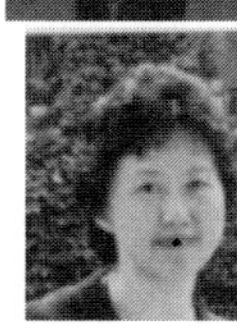

Yow-Hwey Hu, PhD: associate professor, Institute of Health and Welfare Policy, National Yang-Ming University, Taipei, Republic of China

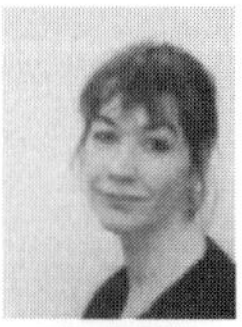

Abbey Hyde, PhD: lecturer, Department of Nursing, University College, Dublin, Republic of Ireland

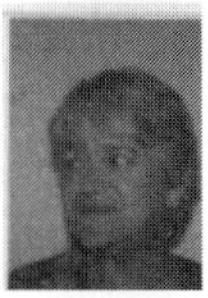

Carol Jackson, PhD(c), , MN: co-ordinator, Child and Parent Health Nursing, RMIT, Faculty of Nursing, Bundoora, Australia

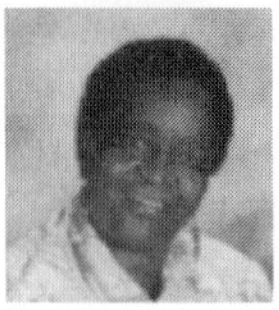

Joyce C Kadandara, BA(Hons) Sociology; PG Dip, Social Administration: nurse/midwife; member of Women's Health Global Commission on Women, World Health Organization; Zimbabwe

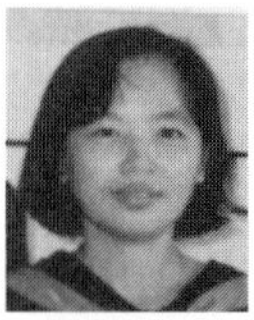

Shu-Chen Kuo: research assistant, Institute of Health and Welfare Policy, National Yang-Ming University, Taipei, Republic of China

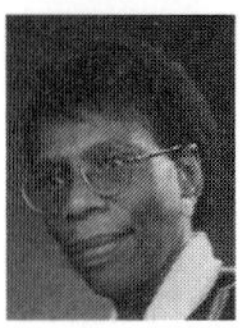

Maureen G G Laryea, RN, DPhil: School of Nursing, Memorial University, St. John's, Newfoundland

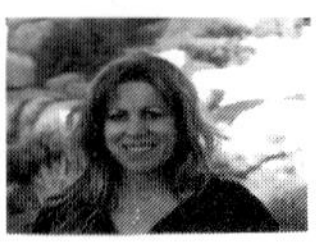

Janna Lesser, PhD, RN, CS: post-doctoral research fellow, School of Nursing, University of California at Los Angeles, California, United States of America

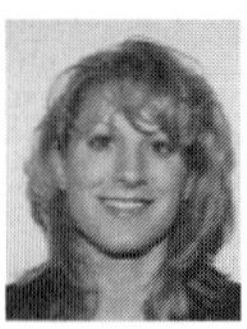

Martha Marie Lywak, BA(Hons), MPA: Auditor, Winnipeg, Manitoba, Canada

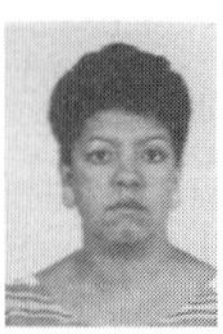

Marilyn Maturell, BEd: acting professor, Higher Institute of Medical Sciences, Santiago de Cuba, Cuba

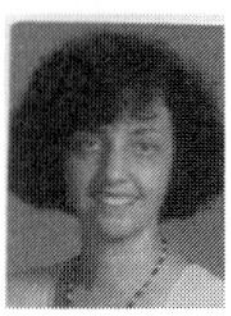

Ana Márcia Spanó Nakano, RN, PhD: Universidad de Sao Paulo, Escola de Enfermagem de Ribeirao Preto, Sao Paulo, Brazil

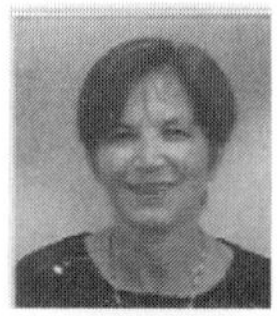

Zohar Nir, PhD(c), MA, RN: senior teacher, Recanati School for Community Health Professions, Ben-Gurion University of the Negev, Beer-Sheva, Israel

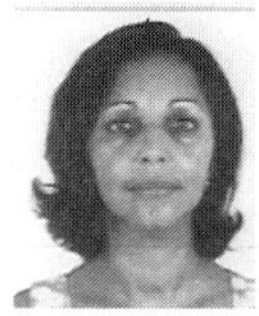

Elizete Passos, DEd: professor of philosophy, Federal University of Bahia, Salvador, Bahia, Brazil

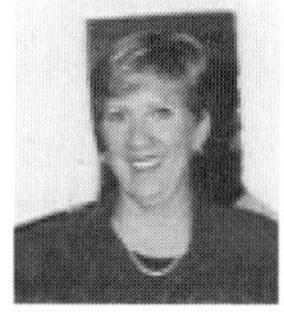

Carole W Pearce, RNC, PhD: University of Massachusetts, Lwell, Massachusetts, United States of America

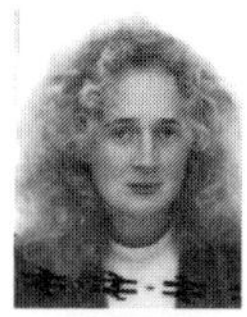

Jacqueline Reeve, RGN, RNT. BA, MSc,.PGDipAE, PhD(s): senior lecturer, Nursing, University of Plymouth, United Kingdom

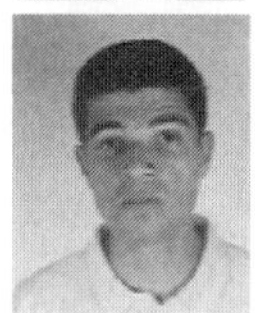

Valdemar de Almeida Rodrigues: graduate student, Nursing School, Federal University of Bahia, Bahia, Brazil

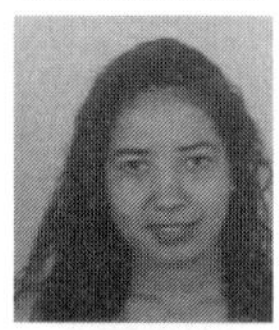

Jussilene Jesus Souza: graduate student, Nursing School, Federal University of Bahia, Bahia, Brazil

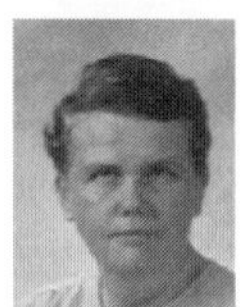

Margaret Storey, RN, PhD: professor, College of Nursing, Yonsei University, Republic of Korea

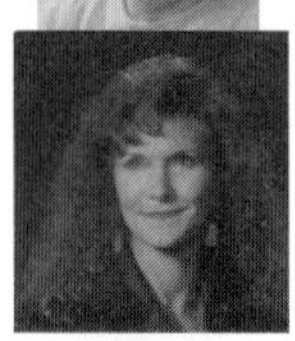

Vicki L Torsch, RN, MSN, MA, PhD: adjunct affiliate, Women's Studies Program, University of Oklahoma, Oklahoma, United States of America

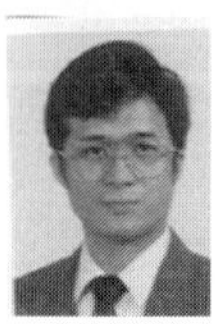

Jeffrey J H Tsai: visiting staff, Emerging Medicine, Department of Emergency, Veterans General Hospital, Taipei, Republic of China

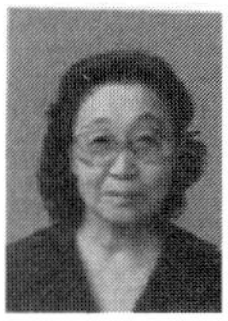

Yoshiko Susanna Uchiyama, RN, Professor, Department of Nursing, School of Health Sciences, Tokai University, Kanagawa, Japan

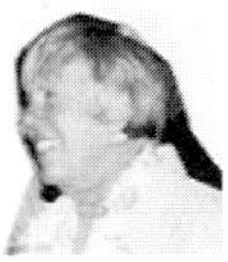

Nancy W Veeder, PhD, MBA, LICSW: Boston College Graduate School of Social Work, Chestnut Hill, Massachusetts, United States of America

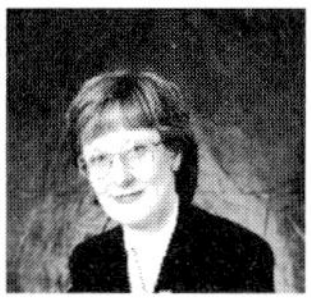

Joan Wagner, BScN, DHSA, MEd, RN: executive director, Victorian Order of Nurses (Edmonton), Edmonton, Alberta, Canada

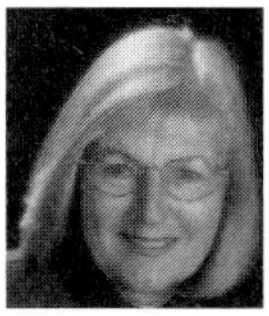

Shirley Yakimishyn, BScN, MEd, RN: co-ordinator, Victorian Order of Nurses, Edmonton, Alberta, Canada

Inger Frombach, BA: Department of Psychology, Luther College, University of Regina, Saskatchewan, Canada

David Galisky, PhD: University of the Negev, Israel

Theresa George, BSc, MS, PhD: former Faculty of Nursing, University of Manitoba, Winnipeg, Manitoba, Canada

Valerie A Hamel, RNC, MS: Women's Health Practitioner, and Founder, Four Women Inc, 450 Read Street, Attleboro MA,

Marli Villela Mamede, RN, PhD: Universidad de Sao Paulo, Escola de Enfermagem de Ribeirao Preto, Sao Paulo, Brazil

Peggy S Matteson, RNC, PhD: Northeastern University College of Nursing, Boston, Massachusetts, United States of America

Tessa Merry, , RN: PIC nurse, VON, Edmonton Branch, Edmonton, Alberta, Canada

Carol J McMahon-Morin, RN, CS-FNP, MS: family nurse practitioner in private collaborative practice, Newbury Port, MA, USA

Patricia Roth, EdD, RN: professor, University of San Diego, San Diego, California, USA

Ellen Trabka, RN, CS-FNP, MS: family nurse practitioner, Teaque, New Mexico, USA

Susan L Williams, RN, MSW, LICSW: supervisor, Community Social Work Services, UNA Health Services, Franklin Medical Center, Greenfield, MA, USA

Sharlene Wolbeck, BScN, RN: PIC nurse, VON, Edmonton Branch, Edmonton, Alberta, Canada

Donna Zachariah, , RN: PIC nurse, VON, Edmonton Branch, Edmonton, Alberta Canada

Acknowledgements

This compendium of readings on women's health issues is an outcome of the conference presentations at the 8th International Congress on Women's Health Issues, held at the University of Saskatchewan, Canada, in June 1997. The editors gratefully acknowledge the contribution to this international effort from 13 countries, including Japan, Mexico, Australia, Brazil, Korea, the United States, Canada, Ireland, Britain, South Africa, Israel, Zimbabwe and the Republic of China (Taiwan). The international nature gives this work a cross-cultural perspective on women's health issues.

We are also grateful to Research Services, University of Saskatchewan, for awards that made the project viable: the Publication Grant Award and the Innovation Fund Award. Thanks are also due to Carol Jackson, a Fellow of the Royal College of Nursing in Australia, who assisted as editorial consultant for Australia and Asia. She gave us the great idea of the book title. Marion Crook, advisor to the British Columbia Health Minister on Women's Issues, gave us her editorial expertise. Lorraine Cathro, former adviser on Women's Issues to the President, University of Saskatchewan, assisted as editorial consultant for the Americas. Joyce Kadandara, officer for women's issues for economic and political development, with the World Health Organization, gave us specific advice on issues affecting women in Africa, and also gave us the incentive to pursue the moral issues of special concern to women in developing countries. Vicki Torsch, University of Oklahoma, Women's Studies, provided critical comments on this project.

The editors hope to continue the international research and dialogue on women's health, economic, political, social and cultural issues around the globe.

Thanks go to Professor Barbara Cardenas for providing English interpretation of Portugese material. We are all grateful to Lou's family — Dr Wes Heber, their daughter Jackie and son Wally — for their continued support in this project, while Lou continued to do other community development in the Philippines.

We thank Valery Marston, editor and publisher of Quay Books, who recognized this book project as vital to women around the world, to share and learn from each other's diversity of perception and learning through research.

Lourdes Fernandez-Heber, EdD, PhD
Theresa George, MS, PhD

Foreword

Phyllis Noerager Stern, DNS, FAAN, NAP,
Professor, Indiana University & Council General,
International Council on Women's Health Issues

Like most good ideas, the International Council on Women's Health Issues started with a conversation between colleagues in the hall. The hall was in the School of Nursing at Dalhousie University in Halifax, Nova Scotia, Canada; the colleagues were Lynette Mensah, Brenda Montgomery and me; and the theme was an international congress on women's health issues. We had in mind a small conference with 20 or 30 research papers, mostly presented by North Americans. Our motives were to offer a showcase for exchange of knowledge on women's health. We wanted a world-wide perspective, but expected less, thinking to start small and just proceed according to response. We had no funding, relying instead on volunteers from the School of Nursing.

The response to the call for abstracts caught us by surprise: we received over 200 applications for presentations. We were unprepared. In the months preceding the October 1984 congress, we sorted out the paper presentations, shopped for a venue and applied everywhere for funds — from the mayor of Halifax, the commissioner of health and the provincial and federal governments.

We invited keynote speakers. Nancy Woods, now Director of the Center for Research on Women' Health Issues at the University of Washington, was one; Margarethe Lorensen, who heads the School of Nursing at the University of Oslo was another.

A heart specialist from Johns Hopkins University was on the programme. His research results over 20 years had convinced him that, through hormone replacement therapy, women could protect themselves from heart attacks. Radical feminists in the audience, opposed to the 'medicalization of menopause', snarled in response.

The big surprise, however, was the quality of the research abstracts we received — we only had room for 100 — and the overall enthusiastic response of the audience. Added to this, we had representation from every continent of the world. Word travelled around the convention halls that this was an important innovation that must continue. Thus we formed the International Council on Women's Health Issues as an organizing body for future congresses.

At the second congress in 1986, again in Halifax, we elected a slate of officers and a board of directors. We went international in 1988 when the first president, Jeannette Sasmor, hosted the third congress in Tampa, Florida, United States. By that time, we were able to persuade the president-elect, Marion Pybus, to hold the fourth congress in New Zealand in 1990. By 1991, demand was such that we were forced to produce yearly congresses, which took place in such places as Phoenix, Arizona, US; Copenhagen, Denmark; Toronto, Ontario, Canada; Gaberone, Botswana; Galveston, Texas, US; Kong Kaen, Thailand; and Saskatoon, Saskatchewan, Canada.

Although most presenters at international congresses went on to publish their work in refereed journals, the Saskatoon papers represent the first collection of congress papers in a single volume. We owe Lou Heber and Theresa George a debt of gratitude for bringing together a remarkable group of research, and then editing this exciting work. I feel certain that the writings contained here will add, in a meaningful and international way, to our knowledge of women's health.

Introduction

Lourdes Fernandez-Heber
Theresa George

The book is a collection of selected peer-reviewed articles chosen from the papers presented during the Eighth International Congress on Women's Health Issues, held in Saskatoon, Saskatchewan, Canada, in June 1997.

The content of the book is diverse — as diverse as the people who wrote it, the cultures from which they come and the research they have done. The uniqueness of the book is that the voices are from women scholars from diverse cultures, political persuasions and economic situations presenting the health conditions of their people from their own vantage points, without being filtered through the minds of western scholars from a western ideological vantage point. The anthology examines a range of health issues currently confronting women around the world, be they western or non-western. In spite of the diversity of the papers in this book, there is a sense of coherence and connectedness shared by all authors, as women all over the world share the common burden of oppression within the world culture of patriarchy. The connectedness of women everywhere with their families, their environments, their cultures, their spiritual heritages — in short, the context consciences of women — make them more vulnerable to experiencing difficulties when any of these areas are affected. Women in all these countries carry the primary responsibility for the health of their families and themselves, and in most countries the majority of indigenous health workers who care for the health of men, women and children are women.

The articles in this book cover a vast area of the globe, presenting the economic and political situations of women and their health needs from several vantage points, such as cultural, spiritual, personal and familial viewpoints. Although the book is not a comprehensive analysis of women's health situation around the globe, it does provide an initial understanding of the diversity and connectedness of women's issues and health needs across a wide area of the world.

We, as editors, hope that the articles, carefully chosen for this book from more than 100 papers presented at the conference, will enlighten readers about the diversity of women's situations around the world. We also hope that the papers will carry the message to the reader that, in this diversity, women of the world in many ways are similar and have similar core needs that are often unmet in a world still permeated by patriarchal ideology and western neo-colonialism.

Both of us had the privilege of being born and spending the formative years in what today we call developing countries, in essence colonized or neo-colonized countries. We also had the privilege of living, working and researching in Africa, Asia and North America, which we hope has made us much more attuned to the nuances of diversity and connectedness.

It is with a sense of satisfaction and a sense of urgency that we present this book to academics, activists and all women who are concerned about the total health of women of the world.

Section I:

Theoretical and practical issues

The social ideology that portrays women as weak, incapable of rational judgement, morally defective and in many ways in need of being watched over, puts women world-wide into a situation of powerlessness and dependency. This condition has prompted women of the world, led by the United Nations, to form an international forum for women to develop strategies to improve the conditions of women world-wide. The United Nations Decade of Women and several international forums held during the last decade brought to the forefront women's situation of oppression, but in actuality little has changed for many women around the world, and in many cases oppressive regimes have made women's conditions worse. At the close of the twentieth century, the condition of women world-wide leaves much to be desired, as shown in a recent United Nations report, stating that women still do 75% of the world's work but own just 1% of the property and 10% of the wealth (United Nations International Women's Conference reports, Nairobi, 1985 and Beijing, 1995).

With this backdrop, the authors in this section look at where women are and why their work is devalued in spite of its importance. **Dr. Attié**, a psychologist and activist from Mexico, discusses women's situation at the end of the twentieth century and argues that, even though open repression of women appears to have disappeared, an insidious type of repression exists at many levels throughout women's lives. Equal rights on paper do not always carry over into action, and some women are more equal than others. She further discusses the three roles women have to play in society: to be a good wife, a good mother and a good woman. This presents the dilemma that both society and women face by posing the questions 'What is a woman nowadays?' and 'Why can't a woman be like a man?'

Joyce Kadandara, from Africa, foresees a new era of peace, hope and development for women in developing countries, especially Africa. She discusses the Chivi Women's Project in Zimbabwe, which was directed to help women in income-generating activities, to improve women's literacy and to thus promote women's health. Investing in women's health and economic and literacy development, she argues, is the basis for the development of post-colonial Africa.

Theresa George's chapter presents the women fish sellers in two fishing villages along the southern coast of India, which will lead us to question whether theories of wife abuse developed within the western value system can be transposed to different ethnic and cultural groups.

Lou Heber's chapter deals with self-awareness, which is essential in theorizing healthcare professionals' action during client care. The healthcare provider counsellor examines philosophical issues, and ethical values are used as the foundation of professional healthcare practice. The healthcare giver and educator has to be more meaningful and realistic to her commitment in 'caring'. It is through a holistic healthcare approach to caring that the application of self-theory can be made effective. 'Valuing' is a nursing theory that will evolve, enhancing creativity and innovation to human caring in professional nursing practice and providing experience in self-reflective work.

Maria Elena Colomé and **Marilyn Maturell** present the enviable (compared to other Caribbean islands) health conditions in Cuba. They point out the role women play as community health workers in bringing better health to the common people of Cuba. Data collected from the city of Santiago de Cuba is presented to show that women's work in preventive medicine, child care, nutrition, sex and family planning education, and improvement of sanitary conditions are variables that have created a better level of health in this city and other similar cities in Cuba.

1

Women's discomfort at the end of the twentieth century

Thalia Attié

Introduction

I do not pretend to know everything about women, but what enables me to write about the subject is that I am a woman myself. After focussing on this point, I will talk like a man: 'What do they want?' he might ask. 'They've got everything. They are liberated' — we can ask from what — 'they can vote, have access to university, organize congresses, talk in public', and so forth. Being a woman myself, I can ask: 'They are liberated, but are they free?' I will leave this question open, and perhaps an answer will be found at this conference.

Before addressing the subject, I would like to give a brief overview of women's history in Europe, prior to the twentieth century, so we can note that (1) since time began, women's image and fate have been surrounded by contradictions; and (2) their rights diminished during periods of political hardening.

In the most ancient civilizations, women's status was that of a minor, little different from their children's. A change might have been expected with the advent of Christianity, but with the apostles' transmission, the role of a woman receded from being a supposed companion of her husband to submission to him. During the Middle Ages, the image of women fluctuated between the witch and the pure lady. However, at that time they could administer property and take their husbands place in cases of absence or illness. From the thirteenth century, their rights began to weaken: heritage and name could no longer be transmitted through them. Only in the fifteenth century was a husband forbidden to beat his wife. From the sixteenth century, he was responsible for her behaviour and from the sixteenth to the eighteenth centuries, the position of the Middle Ages theologians was restated: women were told to value their conjugal duties over their maternal ones. As for the Christian moralists, they reproached mothers for their 'culpable tenderness' towards their children, while at the same time blaming those who sent their babies out to nurse. At this time, doctors started to recommend that mothers breastfeed their children.

By the seventeenth century, 'a new woman appeared': neither courtesan nor good woman, she was a townswoman who dedicated herself to being a woman within literary circles, social circles, etc. During the eighteenth century, women became responsible for their own behaviour, and could even oppose their husbands' decisions about their children. Breastfeeding was highly recommended by medical authorities, even though it was not in favour socially. At the end of this century, the feminist press appeared. The Napoleonic Code in the nineteenth century commanded wives to obey their husbands. To not love their own children became a crime. Nonetheless, at the end of the century, women obtained the right to vote in some countries.

We must remember that until the end of the nineteenth century and the early part of the twentieth, most societies were agricultural rather than industrial, and men and women had specific roles with respect to work as well as family.

So why do women feel some discomfort at the end of the twentieth century, when they have almost got it all?

While open repression may have disap- peared, there is still an insidious type that affects women at different stages in their lives. Erickson (1972) identified it as women going through a crisis in the sense that they had reached a 'crucial moment', or a 'turning point' in the history of people when they have to choose between different possibilities. Dowling (1982) defines this crisis as a period in which people question themselves about their capacities and their identities.

This chapter analyses three main factors that contribute to the discomfort women feel today: social factors, educational and work factors, and the different roles women must assume.

What has changed?

To see what has changed in our societies so that women must redefine themselves at the end of the twentieth century, we must keep in mind three turning points in women's history during this century: social changes before the 1960s, the 1960s and the 1980s and after.

Before the 1960s

The **longevity** of human beings has been extended by approximately 40 years since the last century. This means women cannot define themselves solely in terms of their maternal role, which occupies only a quarter of their lives. Furthermore, as Livi-Bacci (1978) pointed out, while we could suppose that, during the last century and the early part of this one, pregnancy and lactation occupied 13 years of a woman's life, nowadays they account for only one year and nine months. In other words, longevity and the reduction of fecundity changed the cycle and meaning of the different stages of women's lives.

The **industrialization** of society affects family life. From the extended family, where everyone had a role to fulfil, we passed to the nuclear family — or even the mononuclear family — where each member accumulates more than one role or has to deal with the lack of specific ones.

As for **housekeeping tasks**, new machines and products were invented to help make women's daily work easier, leaving them with much more time for other pursuits. Further, before the 1960s, mending clothes, preparing jellies or canning food contributed to the family economy, while after the 1960s these were no longer economically or socially justified contributions to family welfare.

The 1960s

The 1960s marked a turning point in other terms as well. The ideology of the 1960s, even if now forgotten, left internalized traces in people's minds, and still contributes to some discomfort in women. The three slogans of this period were: equality, communication and orgasm at any price.

- **Equality** was often confounded with interchangeability. Women soon discovered that some were more equal than others. It is no longer a mystery that, at the end of this century, we are still far from equality, in terms of education, work, sharing household tasks or taking care of children.
- **Communication**. Women and men do not share either the same world or terms of reference, neither do they communicate in the same way. This can cause many misunderstandings that contribute to some discomfort. For instance, as Frischer (1997) states, 'Women are more interested in responsibilities than in power, in the matter for itself than in its social signification . . . Men seem incapable of imagining that a desire for self-realisation could register in a logic other than that of dominating the other.' Moreover, even among women themselves, communication became less evident, whether they were working or not.
- **Orgasm at any price**. As we can see, this slogan must have weighed as much on men as on women. It was another subtle way to gain dominion over women's bodies. Fortunately, it was men who were first to trigger the alarm, so it was taken seriously (Farrell, 1975; Goldberg, 1976). However, this helped women free themselves from reducing their bodies to mere copies of men's (Nadaud, 1980). From lechery to psychoanalysis, 'the words of sex' are men's words that carry hidden virile values of power and domination. This is why we welcome the fact that women need no longer be ashamed of their sex, suffering neither 'penis envy' nor patiently accepting having their orgasms' exact nature analysed in terms of men's functions (Bruckner and Finkielkraut, 1977). There is nothing to report about a woman's pleasure; voluptuousness is not something that can be measured visually or externally; pleasure is not a matter of quantity; women do not use their bodies to break records as some men apparently try to do.

Finally, in the 1960s, girls invaded **universities** and went into the **work market**.

The 1980s and after

The feminist movement was almost forgotten. Split between extremes, with the quiet women proclaiming their difference, the majority of women let the movement down: those over 40 years because they thought that what had been gained could not be lost, and the younger women because they considered as natural all that had been gained. What remained of the movement concentrated on matters concerning women's bodies — abortion, violation, sexual harassment — as they realised that their petitions for equality were not really being answered. In the 1990s, women's matters are not so important, and researchers and the media have turned their interests to the relationships between men and women.

Are women right or wrong to feel discomfort, to be bewildered, today, almost at the beginning of the twenty-first century? Let us analyse the question in terms of the body, and in terms of education and work.

The body

1. **The aspect**. In less than five years, high heels have returned, together with straight skirts that restrain movement. This was accompanied by a change in women's ideal figure. Plain, natural women are out of fashion. Thanks to plastic surgery and silicone, women are expected to have curvaceous breasts, bottoms and even lips.

2. **Reproduction**. Women have the pill, so they are under stress, feeling a pressure to reproduce before they reach 40 years of age (this occurred before the 1980s), and if possible before their 30s (this is today's view), just when their jobs are taking off.

   Infertility is considered to be the woman's fault because she did not want to bear a child earlier; many women go through needless consultations over infertility, and through painful examinations before the doctor realises that the infertility is due to the man.

   Once they are **pregnant**, women must go for regular medical check-ups.

   Women are really infantilised: I was more than astonished when I found a 200-page American book, translated into Spanish, all about how to **breastfeed** a baby.

   One must be blind and deaf nowadays to fail to notice the fuss over women's **menopause**, a subject on which I will not comment, as well as the attacks or even the repeal of the **abortion** law and its practice at the end of the twentieth century in what is called the Occidental Society or the First World.

In view of what we have stated here, can we really claim that because they have the pill, women must feel liberated, and ignore the insidious social mechanisms operating to reapply constraints to women's bodies.

Education

Although inestimable benefits have been realized for women's education and work possibilities, their 'liberation, in this respect is also illusory.

- Even if they are as welcome at **birth** as boys, baby girls are not going to perpetuate the family name in most cases
- Educated **to please** more than to demonstrate what they are able to achieve, little girls can play with boys as long as they are always careful not to be **tomboys**, too rough or too aggressive. These silent precepts will not help them in their future lives, especially if they undertake a career
- The advantages they have in primary school over boys begin to disappear at **secondary** school as teachers pay less attention to them, especially in scientific subjects
- **Adolescents** can go out at night, with some **restrictions** on their hours and their choice of friends. In most cases, it will be the boys who will **pay** for them. This will have consequences for the way they deal with money in the future.
- If they go to **university**, they will be wary of excelling in their careers. Many believe that excellence in education will scare away the boys, so they must make a choice about whether or not they should study while finding a husband.

Girls and then women receive contradictory messages during their education, contributing to their development into persons who will have to adapt to the people around them, who will not make too many claims for themselves, who will have a great deal of dependency and insecurity about their actual and future image — in short, about their identity.

Messages from the media and the facts about career women

The feminine press and the mixed press in the 1970s used to encourage women to have a career and to work in the media — to be 'liberated' —, but this began to reverse around the mid-1980s. A hidden agenda focussed on a frame of reference that career women would find themselves alone at around the age 30 or 40 years, and they would regret it. At the end of the

1990s, this insidious movement is placing special emphasis on the importance, the well-being and the joys of women remaining at home to take care of the family.

Apparently, there is no alternative for women: it must be either a career or marriage. In *Fortune and Misfortune of the Married Woman*, de Singly (1997) shows that the higher a woman's scholarly dowry, the more she is favoured in the work market, but the more she is disadvantaged in the marriage market.

Without mentioning the inequality of wages and the 'glass ceiling' of working women, I would like to point out that women suffer similar inequalities in the scholarly work market. Single women have less chances than bachelors of gaining employment, although they have better prospects than married women.

- If a woman wants a career, she must postpone having a child
- Her career will be considered to be secondary to her husband's. For instance, if he is transferred to another town or country, she leaves her job more readily than he does
- Her career develops less smoothly than his. Many women leave their jobs after the birth of a child. In general, many go back to work after the last child goes to school. However, they have to choose between being mothers, then workers; workers, then mothers; or workers and mothers
- Nowadays, many women have gone or want to go back to work after a divorce or when children are grown. They are surely disadvantaged if they stopped or never worked
- As a profession becomes more feminine, or is 'invaded' by women, it loses some of its social and economic prestige.

All these facts allow Frischer (*The Misogynist's Revenge*, 1997) to write, 'If the professional implication of women over forty years old seems to be an irreversible phenomenon, the prognosis seems much more eventual for those in age to procreate, including the 15–20 years old on the edge of choosing an orientation.'

As we can see, equality in working conditions for women and men is far from a reality, although it exists in the texts. What will be the aim of the new women in the twenty-first century? As de Singly (1997) notes, a good marriage with a low level of scholarship could be a good investment for women, but marriage would have to last for the whole life, which is not the direction in which it seems to be going.

Let us examine what happens if women get married.

Married with children

Whether married women with children stay at home or choose to work, they feel uneasy. In the first case, they could feel like parasites on society in general or on their family; in the second case, they may feel that they are neglecting their husbands and children. Feelings of guilt are generated by both situations

Apart from this, married women with children may find themselves 'relative and tri-dimensional', as Elizabeth Badinter (1980) states: 'Relative because they only conceive themselves in relation to the father and to the child. Tri-dimensional because, on top of this double relation, the mother is also a woman, which means a specific being endowed with its own specific aspirations that have often nothing to do with those of the husband or the child's desire.'

Indeed, women have at least three roles to fulfil: woman, wife and mother. We shall see that these three roles often conflict with each other.

What does it mean to be a wife, in the present political climate? For centuries, women have been defined as someone's daughter or wife. Being a wife within the nuclear family, has implications of being a housekeeper, a hostess, a promoter of the husband's career, a representative of his social success; his escort, companion, friend and lover. To fulfil this multivaried role is too much for one person; even fulfilling one of these demanding roles can prove difficult for some women. We can see how these subroles may conflict with each other, provoking discomfort in women.

Being a mother. Since women can choose whether or not to be a mother, this role at the end of the twentieth century carries the most conflict. It is no longer just caring about a child's physical, intellectual or emotional well-being. Physical care includes alimentary expertise, such as dietetic care; health expertise with expectations of skilled paramedic and hygiene care; and clothing a child to meet modern aesthetic standards. Intellectual care ranges from stimulating the child's interests and intelligence, to cultural care and even to making up for the deficiencies of the local educational system. To ensure a child's emotional well-being, mothers must also acquire the professional skills of eminent psychologists, and continually read and update themselves on the, often contradictory, theories of childcare, which are currently being promulgated.

Many mothers feel defrauded of their role: day nurseries, schools and physical or mental health institutions not only counsel them, but also provide them with a role model, often designed to make them feel guilty for not being the perfect mother. Dispossessed, but made to feel responsible and culpable for their children, modern mothers — unless they hold very clear ideas about their role, and an environment that supports these conceptions and beliefs about raising a child — find themselves submerged in endless doubts.

That brings us to the main question: **What does it mean to be a woman at the end of the twentieth century?** Is she still the Almighty Mother of ancient cultures, or the abnegated Virgin of occidental religions? Is she a human being endowed with reason or is she, like Le Bon's crowd, irrational, whimsical and unstable? Is she still a kind of man without a penis as the classical psychoanalysis theory portrayed?

She could be a kind of Marilyn Monroe combined with Ursula Andress, with a touch of the Madonna for the old ones; a kind of Cindy Crawford mixed with Claudia Schiffer, Naomi Campbell or other stars for the young ones. Will she choose to be the loving wife and mother or the successful single bachelor, turned into the lonely single woman by the media since the mid 1990s, when the Super Woman passed out of fashion?

Bewildered by all the images and myths about her, and reflected back to her, a woman does not know which role to choose, and if she chooses she then doubts her choice.

As we discussed, there are conflicts within each role. The following are some of the main areas of conflict.

Conflicts between the three roles

In general, being a mother and wife does not appear to be a problem. A woman can give preference to one or the other, depending on her personality, current circumstances, surroundings and the era in which she lives. Nevertheless, conflicts can occur between these roles during periods of crisis; for example, illness.

On top of this, if women pretend to be Women (with a capital w), who also want to consider their own needs, are they then guilty of neglecting their roles of Wife and Mother (with capitals)? For example, can they be the superbly dressed hostess, she is trying to emulate, while changing the baby's diaper, or when preparing a meal?

If, a woman also works outside the home, when could she find time to perfectly fulfil these different roles?

Conclusion

Having now obtained some of the benefits they have sought over the years, women have now dropped some of their illusions. The Super Women of the 1970s and 1980s discovered their positions were untenable: from being sufferers of men's oppression they became their own oppressors. And found that they were still different from men.

Feeling somewhat trapped, and even defrauded, women, at the end of the twentieth century, are seeking a new definition or a new identity from among the contradictory messages they receive, and the roles they have sought to fulfil. For the women who went through all or part of the turmoil of the twentieth century, it is not surprising that they are anxious or feel some discomfort about where their future path is heading.

References

Badinter E (1980) *L'amour en plus*. Flammarion, Paris

Bruckner P, Finkielkraut A (1977) *Le nouveau désordre amoureux*. Deuil, Paris

Dowling C (1982) *Le complexe de Cendrillon*. Grasset, Paris

Erickson E (1972) *Adolescence et crise*. Flammarion, Paris

Farrell W (1975) *The liberated man*. Bantam, London

Frischer D (1997) *La revanche des mysogines*. Albin Michel, Paris

Goldberg H (1976) *The hazards of being male*. Signet, New York

Livi-Bacci M (1978) Le changement démographique et le cycle de view des femmes. In: Sullerot E (ed.). *Le fait féminin*. Fayard, Paris

Nadaud J (1980) Couples 'libertins,' tricycles our tandem. In: *Couples, Autrement, Points*. Paris

de Singly F (1997) *Fortune et infortune de la femme mariée*. PUF, Paris

2

Empowering women in poverty

Joyce C Kadandara

Introduction

Zimbabwe is a country of 10.4 million people (1992 census), politically divided into eight administrative provinces. The health status is fairly typical of that of other developing countries with similar per capita incomes. Life expectancy is 64 years, and maternal mortality stands at 283 per 100,000 live births (Zimbabwe Demographic and Health Survey Report, 1994).

Zimbabwe is a relatively young country, gaining political independence in 1980. However, as a country it belongs to one of the largest continents, one endowed with a wealth of natural resources, but also a sad history of colonization and plunder of those resources.

It has been noted that the footprints of a family leading a child across an African mud flat more than a million years ago are the oldest known fossil footprints. What better testimony could there be of the universal and timeless recognition of the special needs of the family, women and children for care and attention?

The challenge of African women and the issues that need to be addressed to free them from the chains of illiteracy, poor health and poverty are many. Like their counterparts the world over, they have raised their voices at the major women's conferences — Mexico City, Copenhagen, Nairobi, Cairo and Beijing — where they carried a burning torch to symbolize their determination to acquire equality, peace and development in the land of their birth.

Africa's political, economic and social structures continue to be fragile, and, in spite of some improvements in health indicators, such as maternal and infant mortality rates, the quality of life of the African woman remains as low as that of her counterparts in the Third World and in inner-city neighbourhoods. Women's rights and women's health and developmental issues are now slowly moving from the sidelines into the mainstream of development.

Women's roles have long been discussed, but in my part of the world, belts have to be tightened and women's voices heard loud and clear across the land to proclaim the needs and aspirations of that 51% of the Zimbabwean population who are women, and to mirror the plight of their counterparts in other parts of Africa and the world at large.

Women are born poor and die poor. Poverty is the world's deadliest disease. It wields its destructive influence at every stage of its victim's life; the only escape is an early grave. This is a common feature in the developing world.

The 'feminisation section' of poverty is a world-wide phenomenon. Various factors con- tribute to the predominance of women among the ranks of the poorest of the poor. The growing numbers of woman-headed households, the perennial problems of male migration into cities and neighbouring countries looking for employment and the scourge of HIV/AIDS have left many women behind, unable to plan their lives and those of their children meaningfully. Older women are now being burdened with additional responsibilities, caring for orphaned children.

Poverty should not only be understood in terms of economic factors. Poverty of the mind, which is starved of information and due to illiteracy, has kept women in the dark, unable to 'read their world' for centuries.

However, let us salute the women from the developing world because of their inherent strength and excellent management of meagre resources. They have produced and nurtured brilliant sons and daughters who may take Africa to the promised land.

Empowering women in poverty to escape from poverty requires a clear vision to map the tortuous road ahead. The widening gaps not just between the rich and the poor, but between the poor and the poorest of all, pose risks in overall socioeconomic development and human resource development targeted at women and girl children.

What can we do as concerned women to put across our concerns and to act as lead agencies by articulating the needs of the poor? Governments now need to invest in women's health and development. They need to focus attention on the diversity of women's needs 'from the womb to the tomb', ie. over a woman's whole life-cycle. They can only do so if women articulate their needs clearly and, where possible, backed by research findings.

Zimbabwe's Ministry of Health and Child Welfare published its policy document on health, 'Planning for Equity in Health', in 1984. The policy laid the foundation for all Zimbabweans to access health services. Health is the cornerstone of all development activities. In Zimbabwe, great emphasis is placed on promoting prevention and rehabilitation services, with a strong curative services back-up.

In 1987, a project was launched concentrating on health, functional literacy and income generation in a small population of vulnerable women in one province. 'Promoting Women's Health, Functional Literacy and Income-Generating Activities through Intersectoral Action' (1987 to date), or the 'Chivi Women's Project', was started by the Ministry of Health and Child Welfare, supported by the World Health Organization. The study targeted four areas: women's health; functional literacy; income-generating activities; and leadership development.

Studies undertaken by four African countries (Ghana, Nigeria, Zambia and Zimbabwe) had laid the foundations for the Accra declaration of December 1991. The declaration and action agenda were submitted to the World Health Assembly and to the General Assembly of the United Nations. The approach to health and development pioneered in the four African countries inspired two important resolutions. Resolution WHA 45.24 called for setting up a task force on health and development policies, while Resolution WHA 45.25 called for setting up the WHO Global Commission on Women's Health, an advocacy and policy analysis group looking at the various factors that have a bearing on women's health and development.

In a quest to give hope to the vulnerable women in the Chivi area, Zimbabwe agreed to participate, the result being the Chivi Women's Project. The project was to empower women by providing support and skills through community extension officers from relevant line ministries, the private sector and interested agencies. Seed money to set up a revolving fund for projects identified by the women was also provided by WHO and was to be managed by the women themselves with the support of the provincial health management team.

Empowering women out of poverty: The 'Chivi Women's Project'

The Chivi district was chosen as a test case for health promotion and relevant factors as they affect family well-being, and to work as a catalyst to promote better health habits and additional income for a better quality of life. Chivi is one of the least developed districts of Zimbabwe.

The district falls in ecological regions 4 and 5; it has poor rainfall and has suffered persistent droughts for the last 15 years. It has a poor communication networks in terms of roads and telecommunications. Six wards of the Chivi district were selected for the project.

Criteria used to select the vulnerable women

A descriptive cross-sectional study of a qualitative and quantitative nature was carried out using a structured questionnaire and focus group discussions with the women and other rural community leaders. The questionnaire was developed by a small team and pre-tested in another district. This process resulted in some alterations to the questionnaire.

The characteristics of the 855 women selected from the six wards in the project area were:

- the women had to be of child-bearing age (15 to 49 years old) who had lost a child under age five due to preventable disease or because of ignorance
- they were illiterate (unable to read and write)
- they had poor income (below the poverty line of that community)
- they were the heads of their households because their husbands had died or abandoned them. (This point was only discovered when the pilot project had already been launched)

- they had poor housing, sanitation and water supply.

Implementation of the project

The project had its teething problems. Problems encountered at various levels will be highlighted later in this chapter. The implementation consisted of the following:

- a multisectoral baseline survey carried out by a small team established a profile of the population — health status, health risk factors, economic and education levels, and availability of health and other community services
- strategies for implementation were agreed to by the women and the intersectoral committee, with a built-in mechanism for monitoring and evaluation
- there were ongoing reviews of project's progress through local and intercountry meetings of the four countries involved in the women's project
- project results were disseminated to policy and decision makers (a Zimbabwe intercountry meeting was held in December 1995). A video on the Chivi women's project was also produced.

Observed outcomes

Education is now recognised as the key to women's advancement and improved quality of life. Since the inception of the Chivi women's project in 1987, despite the severe drought of 1992/93, literacy primers covering various social, economic and health aspects were printed and distributed to the project centres. Additional literacy primers, learning aids and teaching aids were developed. The primers cover the following health issues:

- acute respiratory infections
- diarrhoeal disease
- immunisation
- personal and environmental hygiene
- nutrition.

To date, 73% of the vulnerable women have graduated to basic literacy. Women in the project have won national literacy competitions. They are now able to make their own teaching/learning aids, have developed a high degree of confidence and self-worth, and are now empowered to assume positions of leadership in their communities. The women are also able to make independent decisions.

Health status

The internal evaluation and management information system carried out in 1992/93 revealed marked achievements in the following health indicators (90–100% coverage):

- access to health care
- receiving post-natal care and delivery of health facilities or being attended by a trained midwife
- knowledge of health matters and positive health behaviour
- immunisation coverage
- nutritional status of children under age five years
- knowledge of salt and sugar solutions and utilisation of the formula
- use of family planning methods. This was found to be high and showing an upward trend; 62% of respondents used a modern method of family planning, compared to the national average of 36%.

On the negative side, water and sanitation programmes were not well-developed and needed additional support.

Income-generating activities

A sound economic base was seen as important in providing the women of Chivi with additional income to help break the ever-increasing cycle of deprivation. Most of the women in rural Zimbabwe are subsistence farmers. They toil long hours trying to eke a living from the fields. Women work longer hours than men. In my part of the world, women work on average 18 to 20 hours per day. They wake at dawn to walk several miles to fetch water and firewood for bathing and preparing family meals. This type of work continues all day in addition to other household chores, field work and farm work, on top of which they are also caring for the children and husband.

Most women in the project did not have a sound in-depth economic base. Almost everybody was involved in running a small vegetable garden. The produce is used mainly for family consumption and for selling at give-away prices to neighbours. Support was solicited from other extension workers involved in agriculture, small business enterprises and donor agencies. Feasibility market studies were carried out by relevant experts from line ministries and other experts identified. For Zimbabwe, starting and sustaining viable economic activities has been a struggle in empowering women out of poverty. This area has not been easy and still needs much support.

WHO gave some seed money and this was lent to women to start income-generating activities, such as a viable gardening project in the village of Masinire. An irrigation dam was built and it is hoped that the garden project will become a more viable economic concern. The money lent is paid back and goes into a revolving fund for future borrowing. A grinding mill was also purchased, a material tie-and-dye group seems to have great potential and a cattle fattening project has been started. These are some of the small beginnings to a brighter and independent future for the women of Chivi and their families.

Management information systems

At the beginning of the women's health project, there were no guidelines on the reporting system for projects by the four participating countries. In May 1990, at a two-day meeting held in WHO's Geneva offices, a framework for the management information system (MIS) was agreed upon. The baseline survey and main components of the project would include health, functional literacy, economic activities and leadership development. Countries were to adapt the MIS to suit their own country's conditions.

Conclusion and general observations

- communities in the six wards have supported the women because the women's project was planned and agreed to by the community members themselves
- the levels of awareness about basic health in the communities increased substantially. Health services are now more accessible and rural health services are provided free
- major successes have been scored in the fields of family planning and immunisation coverage, which currently stands at 80% (Zimbabwe Health and Demographic Survey Report, 1994). The project women featured very highly in this area
- intersectoral collaboration can be useful if all people involved work in unison. Once hopes are raised for any communities, especially the vulnerable groups, promises have to be kept and a high degree of trust and transparency demonstrated. Frustrations can occur among those co-ordinating and spearheading activities if other members of the intersectoral team do not attend scheduled meetings and do not produce required reports
- functional literacy did make a difference in the project women's social lives and performance of tasks. Having one's eyes and mind opened by being able to 'read one's world' is a great adventure and milestone. Availability of information to empower women is one of the major undertakings needed in the project district and others where the project will be replicated if resources become available
- the district, provincial and national staff working on the Chivi women's project developed analytic skills, diplomacy, patience and a culture of listening to other people's views. The planned replication of the projects in other areas will rely heavily on the Chivi team to work as facilitators in supporting others who will be interested in the project
- meetings were held to sensitise policy and decision-makers about the approach used to give vulnerable women and their families good health, ability to read and write, and develop mechanisms to earn additional funds through identified income-generating activities. More still needs to be done in this area
- there is a need to mobilise political and management support to review existing policies and laws that hinder women's development and participation in the decision-making processes at all levels of community structures
- financing projects of vulnerable groups needs a great deal of marketing and support. Identifying and forming partnerships with financial institutions and donor agencies is an ongoing and taxing exercise. Women work in the informal sector, ie. markets, cottage industries and subsistence farming, where their contributions have not been counted in official statistics. Requests for loans for these women are often rejected, although 'soft windows' are now being opened by financial institutions. This will be a long road in the process of empowering women out of poverty

- resource back-up for women's projects is still a difficult area. Lack of funds and technical expertise has caused many promising projects to close
- like most countries, Zimbabwe has established national mechanisms to develop, implement and monitor policies focussed on women's rights. However, these programmes often lack adequate financial and human resources to spearhead the activities needed to create understanding and support
- although women of the world, like the Chivi project women, perform 66% of the world's work, they earn only 10% of the world's income and own only 1% of the world's property (Zero Population Growth: The Invisible Women March 1990).

Women need to be agents of change and support each other. Women are producers of humanity. Let us redirect the energy expended by our products in negative pursuits to better and progressive use. In many regions of the world, women are frequently invisible or relatively insignificant. At the individual level, tradition and culture have conditioned women to suffer low self-esteem and to accept an inferior status as natural. Women, after a long history of living in abject poverty, poor health conditions, illiteracy and unemployment, have now become an 'endangered species' due to the harsh socio-economic conditions being experienced, the increase of diseases like HIV/AIDS, higher mortality and morbidity rates as a result of their reproductive roles, or violence against women.

Investment in women's health, such as the Chivi women's project is the key ingredient in the formation of human capital and the sustainability of socio-economic development.

In conclusion, investing in women's health and development is a gilt-edged investment for any country. Initiatives taken will empower women out of poverty and accelerate countries to a better future and a better quality of life.

References

Promoting Health through Women's Literacy and Intersectoral Action (1993–94) Final report of the intercountry meeting, Geneva, Switzerland, November 15–19, 1993, and Makundi Benue State, Nigeria, November 21–24, 1994

Promoting Women's Health, Functional Literacy and Income-Generating Activities through Intersectoral Action. Unpublisher Report (1990)

Zero Population Growth: The Invisible Women, March. Unpublished Report (1990)

Zimbabwe Demographic and Health Survey Report (1994)

3

Theoretical limitations of current explanatory models of wife abuse: A discourse

Theresa George

Introduction

Violence against women has been recognised as a significant health and social problem (Campbell, 1995; American Academy of Nursing, 1993; Bachman and Saltzman, 1995). Bohn (1990) states that as long as history has been recorded, women have been physically abused by their intimate male partners. However, it is only since the 1970s that any serious attempt has been made to acknowledge, label, understand and deal with wife abuse as a social problem impacting women's health. Because violence against women is rooted in the accepted norms and traditions of patriarchal culture (note the history of the 'Rule of Thumb'), women often do not perceive the control and oppression they experience in marital relationship as violence, but as a fact of married life. They think they should cope with the violence and make the best of the situation. Alford (1979) argues that 'people come to accept as inevitable that which exists and even believe that it is right'. Alternatives are possible only if they are conceivable. If our definitions of reality do not include other realities and possibilities, we tend to accept what is there as the norm (Alford 1979). Whether or not wife abuse is acknowledged, Reichert (1991) points out, it is a commonplace practice in countries and cultures throughout the world. The United Nations Decade for Women and several national and international meetings on women's global situation have thrust the issue of wife abuse into the forefront. However, our understanding of how women, whose lifestyles may be quite different from the white middle-class norm, deal with the abuse in their lives is still very meagre. This chapter reviews the theories currently being presented in the literature and show the non-fit of these theories for women fish sellers and their situation in the southern coastal villages of Kerala. It also describes how the historical and current lifestyles of the women in the fishing villages affect their conceptualisation of wife abuse in their lives.

Current literature on wife abuse

Many American and Canadian studies on domestic violence show the ubiquitous nature of wife abuse in all levels of society. Pressman (1984) and others argue that, in order to understand wife abuse and why it is so prevalent in society, it is essential to study the social institutions that sanction and define acceptable behaviours for men and women. Accurate statistics on the prevalence of wife abuse are often difficult to come by, since wife abuse often goes unreported for various societal reasons. Since women are still reluctant to break family privacy and talk about what they consider a failure of their marriages, we know about only a proportion of the actual incidents (Staff, 1992; Burris, 1984). A Statistics Canada survey (1993) and a Health and Welfare Canada report (1993) found the following:

1. Ninety-five percent of victims of domestic violence are women;
2. One-quarter of Canadian married women have been assaulted by their spouses; and
3. Abused women wait an average of 35 episodes before turning to the police for assistance.

In spite of these appalling statistics and the more than 300 shelters and counselling programmes for women in Canada, 80 to 90% of women receiving such help return to their partners more than once (Health and Welfare Canada, 1993). The extent of wife abuse in the United States is comparable to that in Canada. Pagelow (1992) reports that, in the United States, some sort of domestic violence occurs in 30% of all marriages and, according to Copeland (1987), more than 2 million American women each year are victimised by their husbands, ex-husbands or boyfriends.

Brown and Williams (1989) report that a little over half of all women murdered in the United States during the first half of the 1980s were murdered by their partners. It is also estimated that 21% of all women, admitted to an urban emergency room in the United States in a one year-period, presented with injuries resulting from partner abuse (Stark *et al*, 1981). The impact of wife abuse on women's physical and mental health has been examined in various studies (Campbell *et al*, 1995). This cursory look at the situation of wife abuse both in the United States and Canada shows the significance of the problem for women, socially and healthwise. Although no attempt was made to collect any overall statistics or epidemiological data regarding wife abuse in the two villages in southern India, the study is valuable as an account of these women's lived experience of wife abuse and their way of conceptualising and dealing with such abuse in their community.

The study population

The women who participated in the study are from two fishing villages in the southern coastal region of Kerala. Kerala lies on the southwest coast of India. It is one of the smallest states, with mountains on its eastern side, separating it from other states in India, and with sea on its west side. Kerala is unique in its culture and lifestyle. It has some of the most fertile land and, traditionally, the people have been either agriculturalists or seafaring fishermen. On its 560km of straight coastline there are many villages where both men and women earn their living catching and selling fish. Kerala is the only state in India where there are proportionately more girls than boys, 1030 to 1000. The systemic destruction of female fetuses and female infanticide, which are prevalent in other parts of India, are not practised here (Gopalan, 1984). Kerala has one of the highest proportions of Christians — 33% (Nayer, 1984).

In the two villages studied, 96% of the people are Christians, their Christian roots going back to the sixteenth century. The lifestyle of the community is well established and routinised. There are no cultural and social activities other than those organised by the church and the local community. The lives of both men and women centre around their church and their work; fishing and selling fish. The women are as involved in their work as the men. No sizeable capital investment is needed to sell fish, yet this work is very important to the economic survival of the women's family and the community as a whole. There are ups and downs in the men's work situation; sometimes the sea is very hostile. The capital investment in boats and fishing equipment is so high that the men seem to have no money for themselves, and are often in debt. Although the women's income is very small, it is their income that puts food on the table every day and it is their income that is stable and dependable. The women know not only their economic value but also their self-worth. Thirty-three of these women fish sellers were interviewed about their lifestyle, their perception of women's value in their community and family, their definition of wife abuse, and their means of dealing with it.

Methodology

There was no attempt to quantify or to study the epidemiological nature of wife abuse in these two villages. Since the main purpose of the inquiry was to learn about the lived experience of wife abuse among the women fish sellers, their strategies for dealing with such abuse, and their conceptions of themselves as wives and women, a qualitative approach was used to collect data. The three different and complementary means that were used to secure data were as comprehensive and accurate as possible. First, since George was living near the community, participant observation was a tool in collecting data about the women's lifestyle and daily activities. She was already well known by the women in the two villages because she was researching mid-life transition among them. Second, in-depth interviews were done with 12 of the women in the community about their experience with abuse and their perception of self in relation to wife abuse. Third, four focus-group discussions were conducted with 33 of the women in the community to collect data on the community's (community of women) experience with wife abuse and their collective perception of what a women and wife should be. The women's stories of their life situation, and their feelings and perceptions of their community's and other women's concept of self in relation to men/husbands were important in understanding the unique nature of wife abuse and the unique way the women deal with wife abuse.

Since George was living near the community and interviewing women about their mid-life transition, rapport with the women had already been established by the time she started to investigate their experience of wife abuse systematically. The fact that she could talk to them in their own language, that her research assistant was from their community, and that all the women in the village knew each other and were involved in each other's lives contributed to the depth and relevance of the data collected. Wife abuse, or what the women call the 'vagaries' of their menfolk, were a common topic of conversation among them.

Daily routine of the women fish sellers

To understand the ease with which these women talked about themselves and the menfolk in their lives, it is important to know something about their everyday routine.

The lives of the women in these two villages did not change much from day to day. To an outsider their routine appears monotonous, and lacking in all the excitement of city life. But a deeper look at the women's daily lives shows that there is a tremendous amount of zest, hilarity and entertainment in them. The woman fish seller starts her day very early. By 5 am. she has made breakfast for her children and her husband, and is out of the house to buy fish at the dock for her business for that day. She may or may not see her husband in the morning, who will be returning from the sea after the night catch, but will see him in him in the evening when she returns home from the market. The camaraderie with other women fish sellers and their get-togethers in the market in the afternoon are not taken as just another chore, but as part of both their livelihood and recreation.

As soon as the women either collect their fish from their husbands or buy them from other fishermen, the women trek to nearby suburban homes carrying their baskets of fish on their heads. Each woman has a regular suburban route, often inherited from her mother, and which she in turn will give to her daughter. Thus, their customers, the suburban housewives, and the sellers know each other well and openly talk about their problems to each other. There is a sort of mutual understanding and recognition between the two groups of women. Although the one is economically well off and the other is poor, the relationship problems they face are a common ground for conversation.

As soon as the women finish their route, usually by about 11am., the women take the remaining fish to the local market. There they meet up with their women friends from the villages. They usually have an allocated place in the market, where they spend the afternoon selling the rest of their fish as well as socialising, joking and having fun. Their work is not easy: the heat, dirt, and the long trek from the seacoast to the suburban villages, and then to the market and back home, are trying. But, rather than complaining, the women appear to enjoy the freedom of these outings, despite the meagre money their work brings them. On returning home from the market, the women buy groceries, usually the rice and vegetables for that day. Fish is a staple, and women keep some aside for their families' supper.

By this time their menfolk, who will have gone to bed after their night at sea, are awake and ready to visit or congregate in some central point to socialise. An integral part of this socialising is alcohol, usually locally brewed alcohol. Since the woman has been selling fish all day, the man knows that his wife has some money. The woman is very frugal with the money she makes, and sets it aside to buy fish at the dock the next morning and to cover household expenses. So when the man asks for money for alcohol, the woman refuses to give him any, claiming that she has no money on her. This is the beginning of a fight. The man, refusing to believe that his wife has no money left, begins to taunt her, launching an argument. The wife seldom gives in, and the husband eventually either gives up or begins striking her. For the man at this stage, proving that he has control over his wife is more important than getting the money. However, rather than giving him money or submitting to his control, the wife just walks out. In the process she may receive more blows, but she does not passively submit to further battering. The woman will go to a friend's house and on her way she will let anyone she encounters know that she is taking off because her husband is acting childishly.

According the parish priest (personal communication), at one time 80% of the men in this village had a drinking problem, and so the above-described scenario is a common one in the village.

The fishing village women's conceptualisation of wife abuse

Verbal taunting, arguments and sometimes physical battering are a regular fact of life for women in the fishing villages. How they deal with it, where they put the blame for such actions and how they perceive themselves in this battering relationship are quite different from what is presented in the literature. The women put the blame squarely on the men for their actions. As one woman said,

> *'My husband still thinks he's his mummy's boy. He hasn't grown up yet. He thinks he can cry for my money, but he's not going to get it.'*

Alcohol is another contributing factor, and again the women blame the men for this weakness. One typical complaint was:

> *'He wants more money to buy alcohol. When he doesn't get it from me, he tries to get it by force. The more he tries, the less likely he is to get it.'*

The women individually and collectively place the blame for wife abuse on the men. They continue to live with their husbands, despite blaming them for the abuse because, according to the women, once the men sober up they are not a problem. In addition, the fish sellers feel quite secure in the village with their work, friends and other support systems. The fact that they see abuse as men's failure liberates them to talk about it freely with other women in the village and seek mutual support. The theory in current literature that the abused women themselves shoulder the blame cannot account for the situation of these fishing village women nor their behaviour when threatened with abuse.

The non-fit of current models of wife abuse

The power issue

Unequal power between men and women is presented in the literature as one explanation for the existence and perpetuation of wife abuse, of men having power over women, and husbands having power over wives (Browning, 1984; Coleman and Weinman, 1980; Rosenbaum, 1986). The fishing village women say their husbands' behaviour has nothing to do with power, but has everything to do with weakness, lack of control and lack of success in their business. One woman voiced a common view when she said:

> *'You think his temper tantrum is power, but I don't let him have power over me. When he is in such a mood, I just go to my friend's place and we have a good time together. I go back only when he has calmed down.'*

The women perceive themselves as equal to men. As one woman put it:

> *'He goes to sea to fish, and I go to the market to sell my fish. Some days he doesn't make any money, while I make quite a bit. Some days it might be the other way round. When the need arises we borrow money from each other.'*

There are definite gender-based roles in these villages. For example, women never go to sea to fish, and men rarely go to sell fish to the suburban housewives. Nevertheless, these gender-based roles have not affected gender equity or the balance of power between men and women in these communities. The women do not let their men control them, either in their activities or in the way they spend the money they earn.

The fishing village men and women often socialise separately. The women spend a lot of time together in the market, and evenings, Sundays and holidays they visit each other and share their joys and sorrows with each other. They see their work as different from the men's, but neither individually or collectively do they see men as superior or having power over them.

Western middle-class men have traditionally held dominant and controlling positions, both in the micro system (family) and in the macro system (society). This dominance has often been legitimised and institutionalised by religious, economic and political subsystems, thus creating a real power difference between women and men. When men feel this traditional expectation of power is eroding, there is an increase in male violence against women. Increased violence is an attempt by men to regain their traditionally sanctioned superiority over women (Hanmer and Maynard, 1987; Dobash and Dobash, 1992). This explanatory model, which may be applicable to the experience of middle-class white women, does not fit the experience of the fish sellers. Although their husbands' perceptions of the situation are not explored in this study, and it is not known whether they see the verbal taunting and physical battering as a means of exerting power over women, the fact that women do not perceive the abuse as an indication of power, but of weakness suggests that power is not the issue in wife abuse in these communities.

The culture of violence theory

The culture of violence theory rests on the assumption that societies accept and endorse the use of violence in sports and entertainment, and even in 'disciplining' the less powerful, such as children, women, slaves and domestic workers. Wolfgang and Ferracuti (1967) state that a society's approval and acceptance of violence co-relates with the presence of violence in that society. Sandy (1981), in her study of 186 societies, demonstrated that males are not genetically programmed to rape and commit violence against women. Male violence against women is a culturally learned behaviour. Her study showed that in societies where roles were gender-based, with little value placed on women's role, power was held by men, and women were mainly seen as men's property. Violence against women was an integral part of such societies. Her study also found that where gender equity was the norm, and a balance of power existed, violence against women was less evident. This theory may be applicable to the cultural and familial values of the middle-class white women. Is it applicable to the fish sellers' situation?

According to the women studied, never in their memory or their mothers' had there been a murder in their close-knit villages. No one is afraid to walk outside at night, they say, and families routinely sleep outside during the hot summer. Do they worry about children wandering about the village untended when both parents are out working? The women say 'no, nothing will happen to them, as the older men and women who are not out working will be watching them.' It is taken for granted that everyone knows everyone else's children, and takes an interest in them. It is almost as though Hilary Clinton's dictum, 'it takes a village to raise a child,' is in action in these fishing villages. Although wife abuse is a part of village life, no kind of extreme violence in sports or other activities is condoned. The men rarely use corporal punishment with their children, and there is little violence between men. The fish sellers do not give in to their men's violence and do not let them control them, either in their activities or the way they spend their income.

Patriarchy and its influence

Patriarchy is the most common familial form of authority. Patriarchy is also the most accepted form at the macro level in wider societal structures, at least traditionally. This unequal power structure is what feminists see as the root cause of the abuse of women (Sugarman and Frankel, 1996; Walby, 1990). The subordination of women is a constant in every patriarchal society, and so is the abuse of women in some form or other (Walby, 1990).

Has patriarchy been a part of the fishing villages' culture historically? The women look forward to having daughters. Their most prized possession, traditionally, has been their suburban fish-selling routes. Interestingly enough these routes are inherited by the daughters, and the daughters also take their mother's name as their surname (for example, Mini, the daughter of Margaret, may be known as Mini Margaret and be registered in that name).

Kerala, the Indian state in which the two fishing villages are situated, is the home of the Nayers who have historically followed the matrilineal (female property ownership) system. The royal family in Kerala has historically, as royals, and currently, as ex-royals, been matrilineal. Furthermore, the communities studied are all Catholic, and so patriarchy in its strongest guise does not define the lifestyle of the women, nor men's and women's attitudes towards each other. In sum, the explanation of wife abuse in terms of patriarchy is not fully applicable in the case of these two fishing villages.

The economic deprivation of women

The current literature on wife abuse holds that women stay in abusive relationships because of their economic dependency on their husbands (Yallo and Bograd, 1988). In many cultures women neither own nor have control of resources and property. The domestic work women do is considered economically valueless. Even wives of the richest men in the community are often penniless, and have to depend upon their husbands to provide them with money for their basic necessities. This dependency model, which is often applicable to white middle-class women in abusive situations, does not describe the situation and lifestyle of the village women studied. As one of them stated:

> *'My husband is the one often asking me for money. I have my own money. Most of the time it is me who buys the food and clothing for the children and myself. In no way do I depend upon him. I can well take care of myself.'*

Although there is a lot of give and take between the husbands and wives, and although they pool their money to cover major expenses, such as putting a new roof on the house, the women have their own income and are not at the mercy of their husbands for everyday family necessities.

Women's low self-esteem model

Women in nuclear families in the patriarchal system are made to believe that if the marriage fails for whatever reason, it is their fault, and that they should by all means try to keep the relationship intact. In many cases, women believe that it is their fault that they have been beaten (Hanmer and Maynard, 1987). They accept the abuse because of their low self-esteem and their belief that they are failures and deserve to be punished (Lempert, 1996).

However, neither individually nor collectively do the fishing village women accept abuse. Although they get hit sometimes, usually they walk out of the situation and seek the company of their female friends. Do these women have low self-esteem? The data show the opposite is true. They do not blame themselves for the men's actions. They put the blame on the men, stating that they are acting 'childish'. Since they don't place the blame on themselves, they have no difficulty talking about their husband's 'antics' to their female friends and neighbours. There is a real camaraderie among the women in the village, such that they can talk and joke about their husbands' behaviour. Neither low self-esteem, nor victim shame, nor victim isolation is a factor in wife abuse in the two fishing villages studied.

The cycle of abuse

The theoretical and explanatory frameworks presented in the literature on wife abuse presume a lifestyle and psychological makeup not at all characteristic of the fishing village women. The cycle of abuse, according to western literature, fluctuates between a sense of 'normality' and physical and emotional battering. The so-called 'honeymoon phase' creates a sense of ambivalence in the women. They minimise the abuse and begin to, or want to, believe that their partners will change. When the 'tension-building phase' starts, they try to do everything in their power to alleviate the tension, but the more they try the worse it becomes as it is the men's control and power that underlie the escalating tension. The women's hope that submissive and adaptive behaviour can prevent violence makes them stay in the marriage (Walker, 1983). Underlying their behaviour are the strong social values, beliefs and expectations of the patriarchal society in which they have been socialised (Walby, 1990). They do not want to break up their family or marriage for fear of being seen as a failure.

Although this explanation of the abused wives' situation does correspond to that of white middle-class women, it does not correspond to the fishing village women's situation. Their response to wife abuse can only be understood within the socio-cultural environment in which their formative and current lives are being played out. To assume their response to wife abuse and their need for help and counselling are the same as what is presented in literature would not only be dangerous but also counterproductive

Discussion and conclusion

Several factors influence the fishing village women's response to wife abuse, and account for the non-fit of their behaviour with what is presented in the literature on wife abuse. First and foremost is the economic independence of the women. Although by any western standards these women are really poor and have little disposable money, the fact that they do not depend upon the men for their basic necessities makes them economically independent. The little money women make selling fish is theirs, and theirs to spend as they want. Not having to give any account of their finances to anyone not only makes them feel free but also creates pride and gives them a positive self-concept.

Her initial impression, when George started her study in the villages, was that the lives of these poor women were full of hardship, exhausting work, and verbal and physical abuse from the men, unmitigated by any enjoyment. She was seeing their lives through her upper-middle-class upbringing, but the data from the women of the village showed that her initial impression was far from the reality of the women's perception of themselves.

Sharing their life stories with other women in the village and market and with their long-standing women customers contributes to the fish sellers' sense of support and comfort. Isolation and loneliness are not factors in these women's lives. There is nothing private or secret about the abuse or any other factor in their lives. They know all about each other and are always helping each other both emotionally and materially. Routinely the women entertain their friends, go to church, do business in the market and get together with other women in the village, all without their husbands. One finds a real bond among the women in the village. In this the women are very different from their western counterparts, whose entire lives revolve around their husbands, leaving them little time or opportunity to have female friends, even when their husbands permit them to do so. Although the fish sellers are poor and without much education, they do enjoy a high self-concept. They do not accept the blame for abuse or marital breakdowns, which they consider the men's fault. They honestly believe it is the men who need to grow up and take responsibility.

The freedom the village women have in controlling their pregnancies and their bodies has also helped them to be really independent. All the women say that they want two children, and that they do not prefer one sex over the other. Once they have two children they go to the hospital and get a tubal ligation, which is free, and for which only the women's consent is necessary. All the women in this study, except two, had had a tubal ligation. The husbands of the other two had had a vasectomy. The women say the men are reluctant to have a vasectomy, and so rather than waiting for their men to make up their minds, they get a tubal ligation because it is they who are really concerned about controlling the size of the family. The small size of the family also gives them a certain sense of power, independence, control and freedom.

References

Alford R (1979) *Health care politics*. University of Chicago Press, Chicago

American Academy of Nursing (1993) *Violence: Nursing debates the issues*. Author, Washington, DC

Bachman R, Saltzman LE (1995) *Violence against women: Estimates from the redesigned survey*. US Department of Justice, Washington, DC

Bohn D (1990) Domestic violence in pregnancy: Implications for practice. *J Nurse Midwif* **35**(2): 86–98

Browning JJ (1984) Violence against women: Toward a profile of the wife assaulter. Unpublished doctoral dissertation, University of British Columbia

Burris CA (1984) Wife battering: A well-kept secret. *Can J Criminol* **26**: 171–7

Campbell JC (ed.) (1995) *Assessing dangerousness*. Sage, Newbury Park, CA

Campbell JC, Harris MJ, Lee RK (1995) Violence research: An overview. *Schol Inq Nurs Pract: Int J* **9**(2): 104–25

Coleman, K.H., Weinman ML, Hsi BP (1980) Factors affecting conjugal violence. *J Psychol* **105**: 97–102

Copeland L (1987) Congressional reauthorization of federal domestic violence program. *Response victim, women, child* **10**: 20–21

Dobash RE, Dobash RP (1992) *Women violence and social change*. Routledge, London

Gopalan V (1984) *Women in Kerala*. Government Press, Trivandrum

Hanmer J, Maynard M (1987) *Women, violence and social control*. Humanities Press International, Atlantic Highlands

Health and Welfare Canada (1993) *Information from the national clearing house on family violence*. Author

Lempert LB (1996) Women's strategies for survival: Developing agency in abusive relationship. *J Fam Violence* **11**(3): 269–89

Nayer PKB (1984) *Kerala women*. University of Kerala, Trivandrum

Pagelow MD (1992) Adult victims of domestic violence. *J Interpers Violence* **7**: 87–120

Pressman B (1984) *Family violence: Origins and treatment*. Educational Practice, Ontario

Reinchert E (1991) International conference on violence against women. *Health Care Wom Int* **12**(4): 451–5

Rosenbaum A (1986) Of men, macho and marital violence. *J Fam Violence* **11**(2): 121–9

Sandy PR (1981) The socio-cultural context of rape: A cross-cultural study. *J Social Iss* **37**(5): 5–27

Staff D (1992) Why so much violence? Centers want to know. *Winnipeg Free Press* Nov 14. Winnipeg: pB2

Stark E, Zuckerman A, Grey D, Robinson J, Frazier W (1981) Wife abuse in the medical setting: An introduction for health personnel. (Monograph #7) Office of Domestic Violence, Washington, DC

Statistics Canada (1993) The violence against women survey. *The Daily* Nov. Ottawa

Sugarman DB and Frankel SL (1996) Patriarchal ideology and wife-assault: A meta-analytic review. *J Fam Violence* **11**(1): 13–23

Walby S (1990) *Theorizing patriarchy*. Basil Blackwood Inc, Cambridge

Walker LE (1983) *The battered women syndrome*. Springer Publishers, New York

Wolfgang MF, Ferracuti F (1967) *The subculture of violence*. Tavistock Publications, London

Yallo KA, Bograd M, eds. (1988) *Feminist perspectives on wife abuse*. Sage Publications, Beverly Hills, CA

4

Self-theory: Metaphysical paradigm (valuing in healthcare practice)

Lourdes Fernandez-Heber

Self-theory is the inner source of energy that guides the healthcare giver in identifying the qualities of care extended to others. Self-care in cross-cultural healthcare practice uses a cultural awareness approach in which the healthcare giver is alert and open to recognising and dealing with values different from her own. In the application of self to healthcare, it has been stated that 'self' is the extension of goodness to others (Watson, 1988; Murdoch, 1992; Rogers, 1961). Self-theory expressed with strong determination guides the nature of the 'valuing process'. Self-theory is the basis of principles and attitudes in the implementation of behaviour or action (Heber, 1986; 1993), and as such encompasses a theology of self. Paul Tillich (1958) describes theology as a response to the totality of man's creative self-interpretation in a particular period. Daily experiences are metaphysical happenings. There is a part of us that has a curiosity to the openness of the experience. Self-reflected experience and virtuous practice in work is an additional knowledge and understanding of truth. Murdoch states that 'The energy of the attentive scholar at work is an artist expressing oneself as spiritual energy' (Murdoch, 1992).

In the healthcare system, extending the inner self in dance/movement for psychiatric clients involves reaching out to others with one's own experience. Dance/movement, especially ethnic dance/movement, relieves stress-related problems and anxiety-related tension (Heber, 1992). The use of 'self' as a resource for dance/movement encourages clients to express their inner feelings. The self approach uncovers the inner feelings of clients participating in group activities and influences their active involvement and self-expression of attitudes and interest for self-recovery.

Action for interaction is the creative approach to self, and the author uses this as the prime mover to self-determination in healthcare practice.

Defining a philosophy is essential in identifying an individual's beliefs and how this affect performance in the teaching/learning process. The study of philosophy involves an examination of essential truths and principles (Fromer, 1981). It is the actual interaction between student and teacher that draws the elements of truth. Defined principles, as acted out in the process of caring, are essential in clarifying a person's philosophical self. According to Burgess (1990), a philosophy seems to clarify and establish an orientation to life. The teacher integrates self into the teaching/learning process so that it provides some guidelines for daily caring. This ongoing process of defining our philosophy is an integral part of our belief system and actualised principles. This action can be identified through students' goals or objectives, indirectly expressed in the principles of nursing or healthcare practice.

Paul Tillich (1958) describes this inner response to the totality of man's creative self-interpretation in which self-reflective experiences are creative and spiritual.

Phenomenological self is a process that unifies the stream of thoughts and experiences a person has about him or herself at a particular point (Denzin and Lincoln, 1994; Sartre, 1977). Phillips (1989) states:

> *'Phenomenological research gets at the lived experience of the whole human field rather than the parts. . . Through this process, the researcher is not removed from the lived experience, but is an active participant in the integral nature of people with their environment. The researcher experiences the wholeness of the situation.'*

A case study is presented to illustrate how self-theory relates to the phenomenon in cultural awareness in healthcare practice. According to Lincoln and Guba (1985), a case study is the best means for summarising all the data that has been previously tested. It is an effective vehicle for demonstrating the interplay be-

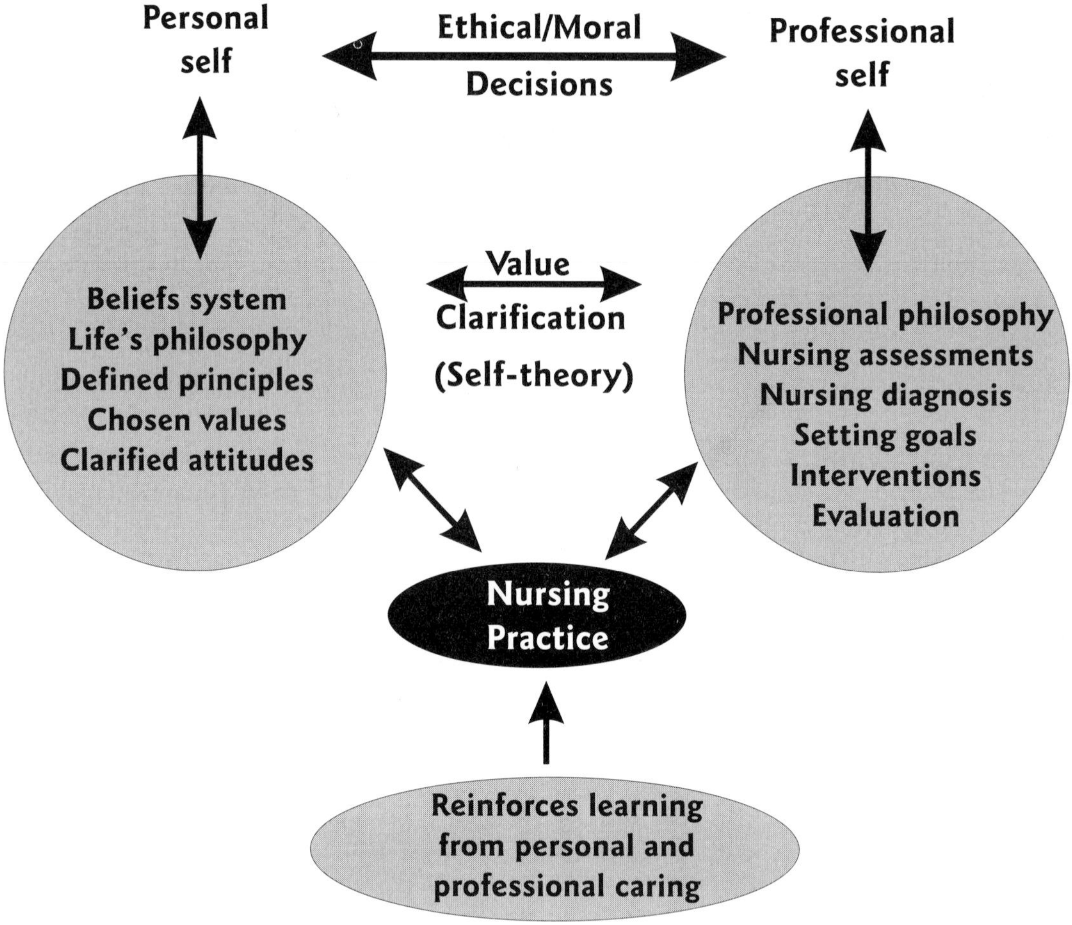

Figure 4.1: Self-theory (value clarification): Linkage to personal and professional self

tween the enquirer and respondents. Case study provides a description necessary for judgements of transferability and represents an unparalleled means for communicating contextual information that is grounded in the particular setting that was studied (Heber, 1992).

The following case study demonstrates the heightened self-awareness and cross-cultural sensitivity of the healthcare giver through the application of 'self':

> A 21-year-old Cree Indian was admitted to the Psychiatric Unit, diagnosed with paranoid schizophrenia. He was uncommunicative for six days and refused to eat. He did not respond to treatment. The nurse suspected that a culturally-based problem might exist and was able to interact positively with the client on that assumption. The client revealed that he was suffering under the spell of bad medicine through a curse from his mother-in-law. Consultation with an Indian Elder and an anthropologist resulted in a recommendation to the staff for traditional medical intervention by a native healer. The client responded to traditional healing and was discharged.

Through this case study, the author was able to apply the principles of self-theory to identify the misdiagnosed illness and promote appropriate nursing intervention. Clark Moustakas (1990) states:

> *'Self-dialogue is the critical beginning, the recognition that if one is going to be able to discover the constituents and qualities that make up an experience, one must begin with*

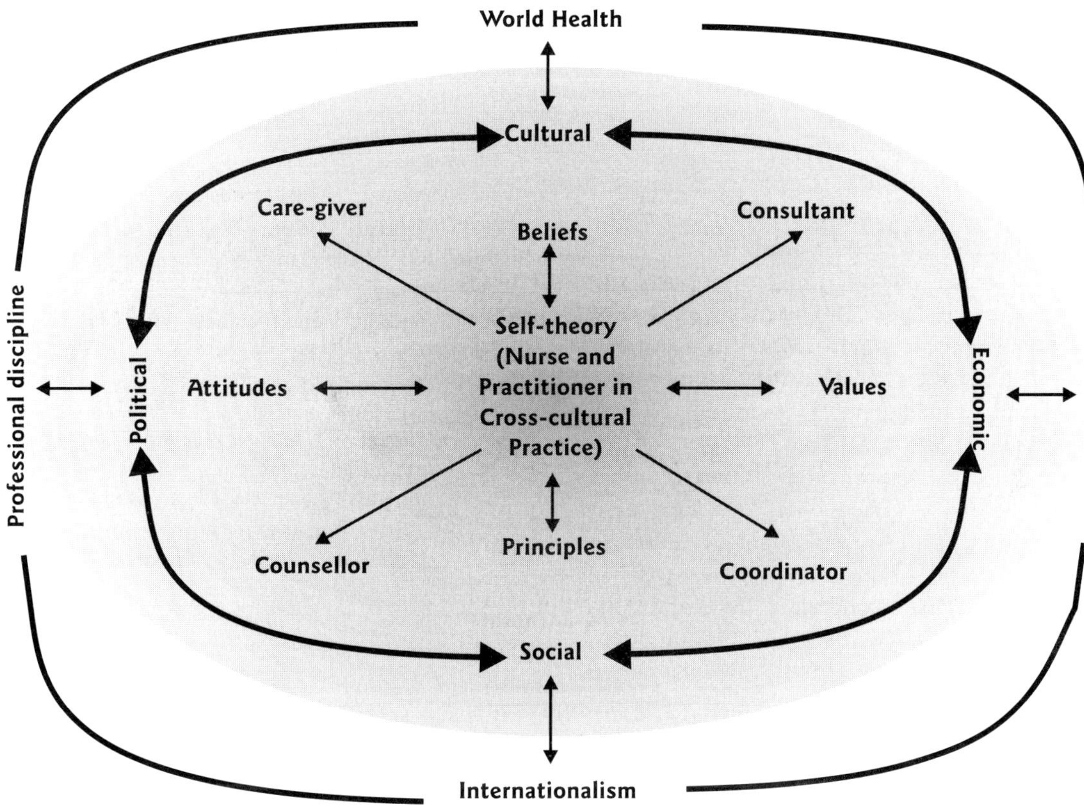

Self-theory: Metaphysical paradigm in healthcare practice

one's self. One's own self-discovery, awareness, and understanding are the initial steps of the process.'

The end product in phenomenological inquiry is a description of an experience as presented through a particular researcher's perspective. The researcher, as the instrument, is identified in other qualitative approaches as well (Salisbury, 1989). As James Coleman (1969) notes, a person's values (see *Figure 4.1*) are chosen by the following criteria: integration of faith; realism and flexibility; and a meaningful and satisfying value system. The valuing process to every healthcare giver has to be flexible and meaningful to each clinical experience in order to provide a consistent yet pragmatic approach to events, issues, people and ideas.

The diversity of the meaning of self, as noted by Peplau (1988), Orem (1991) and Parse (1988), emphasises self-growing, self-caring and self-expanding consciousness through interactive process.

The approach of self is an integration of subjective reality with objective experiences. The application of self is a human triad interaction that involves the educator/therapist or healthcare giver as the prime mover; the client, who is the focus of the human caring and the student, who is the learner/consumer. The triad interaction occurs during cross-cultural counselling sessions for a psychiatric client, and the dance facilitator during the dance/ movement wellness session that provides 'self' as a framework to healthcare practice.

Through self-theory (*Figure 4.2*), healthcare providers can have a better understanding and awareness of cultural diversity in global healthcare, including a better understanding of women and their families.

This chapter examines the triad in clinical teaching and cross-cultural counselling of immigrant clients. Experiences encountered through referrals from psychiatrists and friends gave the opportunity to use the self-theory approach to valuing in the nursing process and applying cross-cultural sensitivity to practice.

Conclusion

An educator isd a role model to every student, and, as such, is committed to an open approach and a trusting rapport in student-teacher relationships.

The nursing educator needs to adopt an open, unbiased approach in a one-to-one teaching style for self-theory to be most effective. The teacher's knowledge of every student is important; that is, reaching out to values and attitudes, and enhancing the cognitive and affective domain of each learner.

Self-theory enhances the perceptions and attitudes of the nurse, practitioner, educator or researcher. This supports individual values, beliefs and principles toward healthcare practice. Through self-discovery, educators and clinicians gain a better understanding and awareness of cultural diversity in primary healthcare practice. Self-theory as a metaphysical paradigm is essential in global health- care practice. It has a holistic approach to human caring, especially among women. According to Murdoch (1992), self is a real innovative and creative human approach, and self-theory is the ultimate guide in the decision-making process. Nursing innovation to practice and alternative policies in health- care, would influence international practice among consultants and project healthcare providers.

A metaphysical paradigm using 'self' moves us to a diversified innovation to caring. As Moustakas (1990) states:

> *'The work of heuristic therapy or research reaches its pinnacle in taking into life active self-awareness, insights, and clarification. The lifting out of the full nature, essence, and meaning of the experiences brings one into touch with creative resources, and enables one to develop a new view of self and life, and makes possible movement toward authenticity, self-efficiency, and well-being.'*

References

Burgess A (1990) *Psychiatric nursing*. Appleton and Lange, Norwalk, CN

Coleman J (1969) *The Quest for Values: Psychology and Effective Behaviour*. Scott, Foresman & Co, Glenview, California: 451–3

Denzin N, Lincoln Y (1994) *Handbook of Qualitative Research*. Sage, Thousand Oaks

Fromer M (1981) *Ethical issues in health care*. C V Mosby, St. Louis

Heber L (1986) Structure of therapeutic self. *Nurse Educ J* **11**(5), 6

Heber L (1992) Ethnic/Movement Dance: Therapeutic Interventions for Psychiatric Clients. *Proceedings of 1st Internationation Nursing Research Conference: Human Caring, Philosophy, Ethics, Politics*. Japanese Academy of Nursing Science, Tokyo, Japan: 42–3

Heber L (1993) Dance/movement: A therapeutic program for psychiatric clients. *Perspect Psychiatr Care* **29**(2): 22–9

Lincoln L, Guba E (1985) *Naturalistic inquiry*. Sage Publications, Newbury Park

Moustakas C (1990) *Heuristic research*. Sage Publications, Newbury Park

Murdoch I (1992) *Metaphysics as a guide to morals*. Chatto and Windus, London

Orem D (1991) *Nursing concepts of practice*. McGraw-Hill, New York

Parse R (1988) Essentials for practice: The art of nursing. *Nurs Sci J* **1**(3): 99–102

Peplau H (1988) The art and science of nursing: Similarities, differences and relations. *Nurs Sci J* **1**(1): 8–15

Phillips J (1989) Qualitative research: A process of discovery. *Nursing Science Quarterly*, Chestnut House Publications, Puttsburgh, PA: 5

Rogers C (1961) *On becoming a person*. Houghton Mifflin, Boston

Salisbury P (1989) Phenomenological research in nursing: Commentary and responses. In: Parse R, ed. *Nursing Science Quarterly*, Chestnut House Publications, Puttsburgh, PA: 11–18)

Sartre J (1977) *Being and nothingness*. Simon and Schuster, New York: 155–8

Tillich P (1958) *Dynamics of faith*. Oxford University Press, New York

Watson J (1988) New dimensions of human caring theory. *Nurs Sci J* **11**(4): 175–181

5

Women in community health

Maria Elena Colomé and Marilyn Maturell

Introduction

A high percentage of Cuba's healthcare workers are women, including nurses, specialists, paramedics and social workers. A high percentage of the present enrolment in medical schools and health technician schools is also female. Women represent a substantial proportion of medical scientists and internationalist workers.

When the revolution triumphed, Cuba lost the majority of its doctors. The revolutionary government had to take up the task of training doctors who would be capable of meeting the needs of the population. With the establishment of the rural medical service for newly graduated doctors, and the willingness of the few experienced doctors who remained in the country to work in the most remote places in Cuba, public healthcare began to function in every corner of the island. Health services were expanded and given priority. They were made available, free-of-charge, to all the population. Medicaments used in hospital were also given free-of-charge. The principles of preventive medicine started to be applied, and the population began to take an organised and conscientious part in healthcare delivery. More medical care facilities were built, and a massive vaccination campaign was undertaken against the most frequent infectiousness diseases. The infra- structure of a nation-wide health system was created and priority programs were launched, such as integral care for women and children.

To guarantee healthy babies, Cuba's public health system provides specialised counselling to pregnant women and couples with a high risk of having children with genetic diseases; the doctors are both scientific and human in their approach. They use intrauterine diagnostic methods at an early stage in foetal development to avoid the birth of a deformed or seriously genetically ill child. The opening of maternity homes in rural areas has also helped to reduce the maternal and infant mortality rate. These institutions serve women who, due to the remoteness of where they live, might have trouble reaching the hospital in time. They spend the last weeks of their pregnancy there, under the watchful eye of the specialists, who prepare them physically and psychologically for giving birth without fear and who teach them useful tips on caring for the newborn.

The Maternity Law guarantees preferential treatment for the woman and child. It gives a working woman the right to medical care throughout her pregnancy, the birth and after- wards. Working women have paid maternity leave at 34 weeks of pregnancy if the pregnancy is simple, and 32 weeks if it is multiple. After delivery, the woman has the right to six months' leave. Pay is distributed in three payments, the first prenatal and the other two postnatal. After this six months period, she is paid at 60% of her salary until the baby is a year old. All women with children under 16 years of age have the right to take unpaid leave without affecting their labour bond.

In Cuba the general life span is 73 years; for women it is 75. As a result, the number of elderly persons has progressively increased. It has, therefore, been necessary to seek solutions to the present situation with respect to caring for the elderly, trying whenever possible to let them maintain their family ties. Care for the elderly in Cuba means care for those 65 years and over. Its goal is to give them all the medical attention they need plus the indispensable social concern to provide for their well-being at this stage of their lives. Medical care for the elderly is guaranteed by the national health system, which covers the whole country and is completely free of cost. The day-care centres for the elderly, known in Cuba as 'grandparent homes', help those who have arrived at the third age to pass their time in a family atmosphere, where the staff provides the warmth and support necessities.

The national sex education program draws up the work guidelines, co-ordinates activities and advises on the work related to sex therapy, orientation and education, including family planning and family education. In the area of family planning, the couples decide exactly how many children they want and when will be the best time to have them. The conditions were laid down for women to choose an abortion if they became pregnant by accident and did not have the ability to raise a child at that time.

Concurrently, systematic work was undertaken to inform the population about the availability of contraceptives and to instill in them an awareness of using them so they could be used in a responsible and consciously chosen manner. All of this contributes to ensuring that children are loved and desired by their parents and have a healthy development.

The family doctor holds seminars that concerned with helping to solve a problem that Cuba still faces today: pregnancy among very young girls. The doctor helps to form a responsible awareness, especially among young people, of what the basic conditions are for establishing intimate relationships, including the protection provided by contraceptives to avoid unwanted pregnancy. The goal is to educate the new generations to form relationships based on mutual love, respect and affection; to be able to create happy and stable marriages and families that incorporate sex as one element of their lives, which, correctly viewed, contributes to the positive development of a person's personality, and to his/her physical, psychological and social well-being.

In Cuba, another important program for women is the early diagnosis of cancer of the neck of the uterus. This cancer is one of the most frequent causes of death in women. The mortality has diminished significantly, due in great measure to the programme of early diagnosis. The objective of Cuba's national programme of early diagnosis of cervico-uterine cancer is to diminish the mortality by detecting the disease at the earliest possible stage, to permit early and effective therapy and adequate treatment at each of the clinical stages of the cancer. The programme is applied across the country for all women aged 20 years and over who have been sexually active. The test is repeated every two years from ages 20 to 59 years. For a woman over 60 years who has the test for the first time, if the result is negative it will be repeated in a year and five years later; if the results continue to be negative, the test is no longer necessary.

Development

For this work, samples from the Dr Carlos J Finlay Policlinic in Santiago, Cuba were chosen. The centre had 271 workers, 231 women (88.9%) and 30 men. It had specialists in paediatrics, gynecobstetrics, otorhinology, dermatology, internal medicine and integrated general medicine. The centre serves a general population of 28,670, of whom 15,351 (53.6%) are women.

The fecundity of women in the fertile age was 41%. Fecundity in the age range 20 to 24 years was 76%; from 25 to 29 years it was 75.6%. It diminished according to age because fecundity was controlled.

There were 41 medical offices with 48 doctors, 29 of whom were women (60.4%) and 19 men. All families in the health district were distributed among these doctors; everybody received doctors' services free-of-charge, with service targeted to the woman, the adolescent, the adult, the child and the elderly.

Women in our society receive special attention. Family doctors work in different areas; for example, they give talks to adolescents on various topics, especially sex, to prevent adolescent pregnancy until the girls are really ready to be mothers. Education focuses on preventive measures, covering smoking habits, alcoholism, prostitution, etc.

Another important group is women in the fertile age group. Doctors explain to them about family planning. If the woman has risk factors, such as hypertension, diabetes, a history of birth defects, obesity, smoking or poor diet, the doctor works with her before she becomes pregnant so that she can have a healthy baby.

The family doctor also works with women over 60 years of age. These women carry out different activities guided by their doctor, such as exercises, theatre debates, talking about sex, traditional and natural medicine, and the family. These women are invited to give chats to the youngest or pregnant women to share their experiences as mother, maternal nurses and other roles. This group of women receives periodic check-ups from their doctors, who take their vital signs, etc. There is also a compound gerontological cabinet for each doctor, nurse, therapist and social worker who work with this group of women; it is controlled by the geriatrician of the Policlinic.

People surveyed in this health area included 72 women: 6 were single adolescents, five were students and one was a housewife. Twenty were between the ages of 20 and 29 years; 18 were 30 to 39 years; 8 were 40 to 49 years; and 20 were over 50 years.

The majority of women in their twenties had a junior high school education and were married. Eight were workers, eight were housewives, four were students. Six were pregnant. Three suffered from asthma and one from hypertension. In the group aged 30 to 39 years, most had a junior high school education, were workers and were married. Many of the women in the 40s' age group had university qualifications, were workers and were married. Most of those over 50 years had minor qualifications, junior school, and were widows or housewives. Seven were retired. The pathology of this group was hypertension.

All these women were satisfied with the service they received from the family doctor because:

- they received good treatment
- they received adequate orientation
- they received careful attention in spite of economic difficulties
- they had been visited when they had been hospitalized
- the doctor was concerned about the health and personal problems that affected members of the community they attended
- they were visited periodically at home by their family doctor, even though they were not sick.

Pregnant women are examined in the first weeks. If the pregnancy is high risk, the woman is checked by the family doctor and a specialist twice a month until the 28th week. If it is low risk, she is visited once a month in her house and once in the doctor's office. After 37 weeks, the doctor begins to see her weekly. Pregnant women take special tests during pregnancy to check for malformations in the fetus and to achieve healthy children; or to interrupt the pregnancy if this is considered necessary. All childbirths in a hospital are without cost. After childbirth, women are assisted for 42 days by the family doctor for their area, and the newborn are vaccinated with BCG and antihepatitis B without cost to the mother.

In this community, a social worker works with the family's doctor and contributes to prevention, cure and rehabilitation by working with the team and compiling an evaluation of social factors. They attend women of fertile age who have a history of mental deficiency, severe psychiatric pathology or incompatible genetic pathology, and adolescents in unstable sexual relationships. They also attend women of fertile age who are at risk due to antisocial conduct, such as a marked affectation of the family dynamic, children of several unions and/or inadequate attention, sexual promiscuity or severe socio-economic problems.

The social worker evaluates a situation, and provides for free medication and economic aid in cases where this is required. She has a programme for attending to women. She attends pregnant women with social and economic problems, family conflicts, low weight and chronic pathologies associated with pregnancy, and adolescent women at social risk. She promotes issues, such as how to prevent early pregnancy, maintain education and avoid prostitution. She also attends single mothers with social problems, helps to achieve family planning, deals with situations, such as children supporting their parents, secures labour bonds or social aid (either in money or in kind, ie. clothes and shoes), and provides for medication when a pathology exists.

The social workers carries out a social study of women over 60 years old who lack family attention, administering internal or semi-internal admission to a grandparents' home according to the social diagnosis of each case. She also determines other needs, such as free medication or social aid. She is involved in different activities, such as:

- collective birthdays
- celebration of weddings
- visiting museums
- visiting historical places
- theatre debates
- literary club
- camping
- educational chats
- exchanges of experiences
- forming mutual aid by means of the interrelation of the group.

Conclusions

From the sample taken, it could be noted that the percentage of women working in public health has increased through the years.

In the survey carried out in the health district, of the 72 women checked, the majority had passed high school, and the ones who had not were over 50 years old. This demonstrates the attention that has been given to women in education during the last years.

We should also note that most of the women were workers and married, demonstrating the women's stability. Of the surveyed women, eight were pregnant, six of whom were in their twenties and two in their thirties. This shows the attention women have received in terms of family planning. The major illness was hypertension, especially in women over 50 years of age. Other illnesses included: arthritis, diabetes, asthma, migraine and peptic ulcer.

The family doctor has provided new levels of health and satisfaction for the population. Activities are programmed around the family, but without forgetting the importance of the individual. The doctor's objective is to promote health through positive change in knowledge, lifestyle and sanitary customs to prevent illness, and to guarantee early diagnosis of disease and integrated medical attention. The doctors educate the population on the importance of and their responsibility for immunisation.

In the community, the family doctor is assisted by a social worker who helps with prevention, cure and rehabilitation. The social worker carries out educational activities to promote hygiene and especially works with populations with difficulties.

It is very important to point out that women working in community health have a special role in social development. Nowadays, women as health workers have contributed to keeping the community free of health disorders and other problems related to a person's well-being.

The work of the family doctor is based on preventive medicine directed towards the individual, the family and the community. The objective for the year 2000 is to improve the state of health of the population through the Maternal Infant Attention Program and to focus attention on adolescents, the elderly, and chronic transmissible and non-transmissible diseases.

Section II:

The trauma of sexual abuse and violence across the life span

Sexual abuse of girl children and violence against women is a complex and serious health issue. Theories and research on sexual and physical abuse have mushroomed over the past two decades. Statistics shed light on the shocking prevalence of such abuse on women and girl children across the globe. Shelters for victims of domestic violence and state intervention for removing children from abusive environments are only superficial responses to the vast problem of women's victimisation across their life spans. Often inadequate or inappropriate, intervention and treatment are meted out to these victims by the existing social systems, including the healthcare system. Little progress is made in preventing this deep-rooted problem in society, and often the system fails to identify and prescribe the best combination of treatment for survivors of childhood sexual abuse and victims of domestic violence. This chapter attempts to shed some light on the life-long impact of abuse on its victims and the complex intervention and documentation needed in caring for the abused women and girls.

Janna Lesser's chapter discusses the various difficulties adolescent mothers must face when raising their children. Pregnant adolescents and young mothers have a high reported incidence of childhood mistreatment. Research indicates that childhood abuse is associated with many emotional and behavioural problems, such as depression and parenting difficulties. Lesser's ethnographic interviews with 15 adolescent mothers, with reported histories of physical and/or sexual abuse, demonstrate the strength these mothers present, in spite of their difficult situations. The desire of these young mothers to give their children a better life and to better themselves by part-time schooling and work, and their resilience, have not been given much attention by society at large. Emphasising these strengths would be a major part of the intervention programmes for these adolescent mothers and a break in the vicious cycle of abuse.

Mary Hampton and Inger Frombach present the results of their investigation into gender differences in the prevalence of post-traumatic stress disorders (PTSDs) in a sample of 87 adult patients at a cancer clinic. Cancer diagnosis and treatment are not only stressful, but potentially traumatic, leading to development of PTSD symptoms. Their study showed a higher percentage of women than men qualified for a diagnosis of PTSD; surprisingly, it was not the life-threatening diagnosis of cancer, but the treatment women received that emerged as most predictive of PTSD for women. The well-documented findings that women are treated differently by the medical establishment and the androcentric approach to treatment may have created more stress, leading to PTSD in women. Based on their study results, the researchers present some recommendations for cancer care for female patients.

Carol Jackson's chapter discussed the life-long trauma of childhood sexual abuse and some of the ways the survivors deal with life events. The successful birth of a child is perceived as a joyful event by society, and it is for most women. However, to women who have survived sexual abuse, this is often not the case, and Jackson discusses the difficult experiences of pregnancy and childbirth for women survivors and how, by having recourse to dissociative conditions, including dissociative identity disorder, these women deal with such experiences in their lives. Her chapter sheds some light on the impact of childhood sexual abuse and trauma on survivors, and offers some suggestions for sensitive support by health professionals who work with women survivors during their pregnancy and child-bearing.

Gloria Geller's chapter also deals with issue of childhood sexual abuse and its effect on survivors. Using questionnaires and focus groups with women survivors and service providers, her research identified the existing healthcare system's shortcomings for sexual abuse survivors, especially those who are experiencing dissociative problems. It also discusses the cost to society for untreated and unsupported survivors of sexual abuse, how the system should modify its approach to treating survivors and the legacy of their trauma.

Joan Wagner, Shirley Yakimishyn *et al* describe the work of the Victorian Order of Nurses for abused women and their children in women's shelters in a Canadian city. Women who have been abused experience feelings of anxiety, panic, depression or stress-related illness that are directly related to the abuse. These women are also often worried about the effect of abuse on their children. In providing services to people in crisis, such as women in shelters or teenagers who are the product of violent home environments, and who may have been victims of physical or sexual abuse, the VON has identified the need for care on the basis of 'client-identified need'. The chapter discusses the special needs of abused women and children, both in their care and in documentation.

6

Depression in abused adolescent mothers: a qualitative study

Janna Lesser

The high incidence of a history of childhood maltreatment has been identified in a number of samples of pregnant teenagers and adolescent mothers. Research findings indicate that a childhood history of abuse is associated with many of the emotional and behaviourial problems that teenage mothers may experience; for example, depression and parenting difficulties. Negative parental child-rearing practices, including abuse, are thought to lead to depression (Gotlib and Hammen, 1992). Additionally, recurring and chronic stressful life events can lead to the onset of depressive episodes in already vulnerable individuals (Hammen, 1991). Because adolescent mothers with a history of abuse frequently present a mixture of problematic personal characteristics (ie. low self esteem, impaired coping skills) and problematic contextual factors (ie. poverty, poor education, sexual exploitation, inequality and exposure to community violence), this population is particularly vulnerable to high levels of stressful life events and subsequent depressive symptomatology. Finally, many mothers suffering from depression have been found to show negative styles of communication with their children (Hamilton *et al*, 1993), and research suggests that there exists a cyclical intergenerational patterning of depressed mood involving parental rejection of children (Whitbeck *et al*, 1992).

Despite reported negative outcomes, some teenage mothers have described having children as a positive force that helps them to alter their course from a previously self-destructive path to a more productive and hopeful one (Arenson, 1994). In an ethnographic study of the responses of a sample of 36 pregnant adolescents attending preparation for motherhood classes, we found that these teenagers had the desire and expectation to give their children the 'ideal' mothering that they themselves never received (Lesser *et al*, in press). The hope underpinning this theme was that by bestowing these 'ideal' mothering qualities upon their babies, they would somehow heal their own traumatic childhood wounds. We titled this term 'reparation' to express the adolescents' desire to repair and heal the wounds they had suffered, often at the hands of their own parents. The findings of this qualitative study indicate that, for these adolescents, pregnancy implied a desire, and thereby an opportunity, to heal childhood wounds.

In an effort to obtain a description of adolescent mothers' perceptions of their psychological status throughout the postpartum period, a series of home-based ethnographic interviews with young mothers was conducted. Some of these mothers were the same young women who attended the prenatal classes mentioned above. Maternal role attainment theory (Mercer, 1981; 1985) and a cognitive-interpersonal model of depression (Gotlib and Hammen, 1992) provided the conceptual framework for this study.

Literature background

While there is a growing body of research in the areas of adolescent pregnancy and parenting, little is known about the more personal experience of these teens. Recent qualitative descriptive studies of pregnant and parenting adolescents have identified surprising strengths in these youths (Anderson, 1990; Arenson, 1994). One of the major purposes of Arenson's (1994) qualitative descriptive study was to 'uncover new and more optimistic information about adolescent parenting as an impetus for evaluating our long-held negative views of this group'. Six out of the seven adolescent mothers in Arenson's sample described having a baby as an event that greatly improved their chaotic and self-destructive lives. Improved family relation- ships, a new identity and meaning for life, and motivation to pursue education and get a better job were some of the positive changes described by Arenson's subjects (1994).

Anderson (1990) described the pregnancy- related decision-making processes of a group of detained pregnant adolescents and expectant teenage fathers in her qualitative research paper, 'Pregnancy Resolution Decisions in Juvenile Detention'. She found, as did Arenson, that, though 'troubled and troublesome', these teenagers presented some surprising strengths and resolutions for the future that were engendered by their new expectant parenting roles. The purpose of this chapter is to describe the affective component of depressed adolescents' maternal role obtained by eliciting adolescent mothers' perceptions of their maternal role and their experiences of depression.

Methods

Participants were recruited from the UCLA Early Intervention Program (EIP) being conducted in collaboration with the San Bernardino County Department of Public Health, after they had completed the 24-month postpartum evaluation. San Bernardino County has a population of pregnant adolescents and young mothers that is larger than the state average. Many of these young women are ethnic minorities and living in poverty in both urban and rural communities.

The sample included 15 adolescent mothers who reported symptoms of depression, either during pregnancy or postpartum (as measured by the CES-D), or reported a history of suicide attempts. Ten of the 15 had reported a history of physical and/or sexual abuse. Of these ten, five had received an intensive early intervention programme (EIP), while five had received only traditional public health nursing intervention. The remaining five participants had also received the EIP intervention, but did not have a history of abuse.

Ethnographic interviewing is a methodological approach to gathering data that is a form of ethnographic fieldwork. The ethnographic interview is designed to discover what people think, what they believe and the meaning of their behaviour through a series of questions about their everyday experiences (Spradley, 1980). During the interview, the researcher uses answers from general questions to structure specific questions and thereby obtain pertinent details (Anderson, 1989).

Domains explored during the ethnographic interviews, included the kinds of feelings experienced by teenage mothers who are depressed; the types of events that trigger depressive feelings in teenage mothers (such as relationship conflict and/or loss and family problems); the kinds of chronic stressors that teenage mothers must face (adverse early or current family environments, poverty, exposure to violence); and the kinds of feelings that teenage mothers have about their baby and about their child-care responsibilities.

Examples of interview questions include the following:

1. What would a typical day be like for a teenage mother? What kinds of things do the teenage mothers that you know do during the day?
2. What are the kinds of things that pregnant teenagers do to prepare to become parents? What kinds of things do they do to stay healthy and to have a healthy baby?
3. How do teenage mothers describe a 'good' mother? How do teenage mothers describe a 'bad' mother?
4. What are the kinds of things teenage mothers do to become good mothers?
5. What are the kinds of problems teenage mothers have that make it hard to be a good mother?
6. What kinds of problems do the teenage mothers that you know talk about?
7. What kinds of things make teenage mothers sad, depressed, stressed out, angry, happy or proud?
8. What types of things do teenage mothers do if they feel unhappy?

Data collection procedures

After completing informed consent procedures, as directed by UCLA Human Subject's Protection Committee, and completing their home-based ethnographic interview, each young women received a payment of 10 US Dollars. Each interview lasted between one and two hours.

Analysis

The first five ethnographic interviews were transcribed from tape recordings into computer files and analysed using content analysis for a preliminary coding of categories and the identification of themes. These data segments were then sorted into clusters according to the emerging patterns or categories, noting commonality and differences. Key words and phrases from each of the themes were listed separately on index cards. After the next 10 mothers had completed their interviews, the index cards were given to these young women for consensual validation. Each young woman was asked to identify which words and phrases (if any) accurately reflected her own postpartum experiences, thereby validating or invalidating initial interpretations. Newly emerging information was added and presented to the next interviewees.

Transcripts from the 15 ethnographic interviews and any additional observational field notes the researcher recorded were transcribed into computer files and analysed further using content analysis.

Findings

At the time of their interviews, eight of the participants had one child, four were pregnant with their second child and three had two children. Six young women were married or living with their boyfriend, four were living alone or with a friend, and five were living with their mother. Ten participants were Latina, three African-American and one Caucasian. Two of the babies' fathers were in prison. One father had been killed in a gang-related incident and one was seriously wounded by a gunshot to his head. Three of the participants described their pregnancy as the impetus to get out of their gang. These young women reported that they had no difficulty dropping out of the gang, generally a dangerous undertaking, noting that their gang respected motherhood.

Two overall categories identified in the study are described in this chapter: maternal protectiveness and transformation. The first category, maternal protectiveness, reflects the adolescent's concern about the health, welfare and future of her children. Within the category of maternal protectiveness, two primary themes emerged: responsible maternal role behaviours and child mental health promotion practices.

Recurring examples of the theme of responsible maternal role behaviours identified in the interview data include planning for a better future, working towards financial independence, being a good role model, controlling one's temper, and protecting one's child or children from exposure to parental fighting.

One participant expressed how maternal responsibility motivated her to return to school so that she could achieve a better future as a medical technician:

> *'Just having her made me more responsible. You know, once you have a baby you've got to stay with them . . . and another one [a second child] made me even more responsible, and I wanted to go to school even more, so I was just waiting for my pregnancy to be over, and to start school, and once it was, I started school the next year.'*

Additionally, despite her married status, financial independence became a goal:

> *'I depend on my husband a lot. I just thought about it, and I thought what about if we ever would not be together, then what would I do? Then it would be even harder, because I'll feel like I have nothing, and I'll probably get really depressed and down. And I have to know that if we separate, I know that I'd still go on because I'll have something for me, that I can do, that I've been doing for a while.'*

Another young woman, working and attending college classes, expressed the following similar thoughts:

> *'[Becoming a mom,] I had to mature a lot faster. . . It changed me in a good way, because I feel now I have even something more to live for . . . something to work hard at (an educa tion) . . . I really have to set my goal and really strive for it, because I have a kid to support. . . I know now that I have to go to work and I have to bring home money, because if I don't eat, that's fine, you know, but my kid has to eat, my kid has to have diapers, my kid has to have clothes, my kid has to have a place to sleep.'*

The importance of trying to be a good role model for her children as well as the challenges of controlling her temper was vividly expressed by one young woman:

> *'I see my mom's character, she screams a lot and she gets angry really fast, it's hard for my mom to control her temper, and I see myself going the same way, before I had them. I said to myself, "I remember my mom used to yell a lot, I hated Mom yelling so" . . . I'm the same way, I seen myself just being my mom all over again, so I just remember that I don't want to be like that, because I hated my mom screaming at us all the time for nothing . . . especially for the*

> *whole neighbourhood to hear it, and so I remember that I don't want them [her children] to go through the same thing.'*

The theme of child mental health promotion exemplified in the above statement is reflected as well in the following exemplar, a statement made by a young mother attending high school and pregnant with her second child. In describing what she believes is one of the essential qualities of good mothering, she advises:

> *'Sit back and think about what you are doing. Think what fighting does to him, what's it going to do to him, what's he going to think? Is it going to mess him up in the long run? That's what I'm afraid of, of messing him up, doing something bad to him now and then later on in his life, he would be bad or something. So just always think about stuff that you say to them, or how you treat them.'*

Transformation, the second category identified from the interview data, emerged as an extension of maternal protectiveness, in particular as an extension of responsible maternal role behaviours. Examples of transformation were evident in such reported behaviour changes as dissociation from gang affiliations, cessation of heavy drug and alcohol use, returning to and finishing high school, and enrolling in college or vocational training programs. All these behaviourial changes required that the adolescent develop her inner strength. For these young women, the maternal role was transforming in that it provided new possibilities of experiencing herself as she gained access to previously untapped strengths within. Emerging as a crucial step in the process of transformation is reparation, the theme identified previously in pregnant adolescents; that is, the teenager's desire to repair and heal her childhood wounds through bestowing the mothering qualities upon her children that she felt she had missed. One young mother described the positive changes that had occurred in her mental health since becoming a mother:

> *'All my life I had problems with depression, maybe back to age 11, and I would get really depressed, so when I had kids it was something good, because I found more — not more love, but having something that was more mine, kind of brought me up on my feet a little bit.*

Another young woman described her own difficult transformation from a frightened, pregnant child to an independent mother, working and going to college:

> *'At first when I found out I was pregnant, I thought everything had just collapsed on me and closed down, and I thought I'm not going to be able to graduate, I'm going to be on welfare, I just thought the worst of everything. But really it's all on yourself. If you really want to do it, a kid's not going to stop you from your goals. It's just going to be a little difficult, it's maybe going to be a trip or something, but it's not going to be a total fall, I mean you'll fall, but you have to learn how to get up and climb those steps again...'*
>
> *You have to be really strong and be able to stand up on your own and say, "No. This is what I want. This is what I have to do" to get where I want to get. And you have to be physically, morally also, strong. And you have to stop thinking actually you're 18, 17, 16, whatever, and start thinking, not so much as an age but as a parent.'*

One young mother, a college student, remarked:

> *'A teenage mom is probably the smartest teen in the whole world. It takes a lot of smarts to be able to figure out how am I going to get the money to do this? How am I going to be able to take care of this child?... Like for me, it's hard for me to go to school and everything. I'm not the same as someone who doesn't have a child, I have to work harder than they do ... a lot harder. So I guess instead of saying teen moms are smarter, I should say they are stronger... It's like you are in a race with someone who's not pregnant or doesn't have kids, in the same race with them, running the same amount of time, but theirs is maybe five miles, and mine is maybe ten ... that's the way I see it. I'm running a lot more, but we're still in the same spot.'*

Clinical applications

In this chapter, the postpartum experience of teenage mothers is presented from the vantage point of young women living the experience. From a scientific perspective, this information provides a kind of theoretical understanding that is necessary for clinicians working with this population of women. In order to be successful, psychological interventions for adolescent mothers must be grounded in these young women's psychology and in their hopes and dreams.

Acknowledgements

The author's dissertation committee: Deborah Koniak-Griffin, RND, EdD, FAAN (chair); Nancy L R Anderson, RNC, PhD; Adeline M Nyamathi, RN, PhD, FAAN and Constance Hammen, PhD.

References

Anderson NLR (1989) The manipulator reputation in juvenile detention: Collective labelling in a total institution. *J Child Adolesc Psychiatr Nurs* **2**: 28–33?? is this the correct title for the journal??

Anderson NLR (1990) Pregnancy resolution decisions in juvenile detention. *Arch Psychiatr Nurs* **4**: 325–31

Arenson JD (1994) Strengths and self-perceptions of parenting in adolescent mothers. *J Pediatr Nurs* **9**: 251–7

Gotlib IH, Hammen CL (1992). *Psychological Aspects of Depression: Toward a Cognitive-interpersonal Integration*. John Wiley and Sons, New York

Hamilton EB, Jones M, Hammen C (1993) Maternal interaction style in affective disordered, physically ill and normal women. *Fam Process* **32**: 329–40

Hammen C (1991) Generation of stress in the course of unipolar depression. *J Abnorm Psychol* **100**: 555–61

Lesser J, Koniak-Griffin D, Anderson NL (in press) Sometimes you don't feel ready to be an adult or a mom: The experience of adolescent pregnancy. *J Child Adolesc Psychiatr Nurs*.

Mercer RT (1981) A theoretical framework for studying factors that impact on the maternal role. *Nurs Res* **30**: 73–7

Mercer RT (1985) The process of maternal role attainment over the first year. *Nurs Res* **34**: 198–204

Spradley JP (1980) *Participant observation*. Holt, Rinehard & Winston, New York

Whitbeck LB, Hoyt DR, Simons RL *et al* (1992) International continuity of parental rejection and depressed affect. *J Personal Soc Psychol* **63**: 1036–45

7

Gender differences in post-traumatic stress disorder in a sample of cancer patients

Inger Frombach and Mary Ruckles Hampton

Introduction

Since there continues to be an androcentric bias in research appearing in dominant medical journals, there is a need for more data reporting gender-specific responses to treatment (Charney and Morgan, 1996; Meyerowitz and Hart, 1995; Muecke, 1996). One study that looked at responses by gender to the initial diagnosis of cancer found no differences, but also suggested that future research investigate long-term responses to cancer by gender (Sneed *et al*, 1992). The authors were interested in the long-term, severe trauma reaction described by many cancer patients and whether there were gender-specific responses in this reaction (Lorde, 1980). Post-traumatic stress disorder (PTSD) is a psychiatric category used to describe a severe and chronic psychological response to a traumatic event that elicits intense fear, helplessness or horror because of threats of death or serious injury (American Psychiatric Association, 1994). PTSD symptomatology includes chronic symptoms of intrusion (flashbacks and nightmares), avoidance (psychological numbing) and increased physiological arousal such as hypervigilance, irritability and difficult sleeping. Chronic PTSD was specified as PTSD where symptoms lasted one month or longer.

Until 1994, illness was specifically excluded as a stressor in the diagnostic criteria for PTSD (APA, 1994). Recent research has found intrusive and avoidant symptomatology as well as persistent anxiety or increased arousal characteristic of PTSD to be elevated in cancer populations (Alter *et al*, 1996; Cordova *et al*, 1995; Kelly *et al*, 1995; Stuber *et al*, 1994). Investigations into the relationship between stress and health have shown that high levels of stress can result in reduced immunological functioning, increased cardiovascular reactivity, and, ultimately, higher morbidity rates (Uchino *et al*, 1996). Therefore, the negative effect of this increased level of PTSD among cancer patients is a significant health hazard and needs to be understood more fully. Recent research on patients with cancer of various types has provided valuable insight into the physiological and psychological benefits of reducing stress levels in cancer patients through increasing support in the form of support groups and behavioural interventions (Fawzy *et al*, 1993; Gruber *et al*, 1993; Levy *et al*, 1990; Spiegel, 1992). However, a comparison of factors by gender that might predict development of PTSD could further enhance our understanding.

This study investigated gender differences in the prevalence of PTSD among a heterogenous sample of cancer patients. We were interested in whether women and men experienced differential levels of chronic, traumatic stress in response to cancer and, if so, whether specific aspects of the cancer experience would predict development of this reaction. A biopsychosocial model guided our inquiry, meaning that measurements from several domains of participants' experiences with cancer were included for investigation (Anderson *et al*, 1994; Faragher, 1996; White *et al*, 1992). We also used prevailing theoretical models of PTSD that use a combination of variables, including environmental stressors, available social supports, individual coping resources and the nature of the stressor to predict development of this disorder (Breslau *et al*, 1995; McFarlane and Girolama, 1996; Peterson *et al*, 1991).

Method

Procedure and participants

Over a four-month period, 225 consecutive patients attending a local cancer clinic were given a package of questionnaires by the receptionist, together with a stamped return envelope. Potential participants were excluded from the study if they were less than 18 years old or had a central nervous system disorder. In addition, since the focus of our study was a chronic condition, participants must have been diagnosed with cancer at least 12 months previously. Participants who did not fully fill out the questionnaire package were excluded. Some 87 (39%) patients met the criteria and were included as participants in this study: 59 women (mean age 58 years; range 28 to 78) and 28 men (mean age 64 years; range 38 to 89). About twice as many women as men received research packages and twice as many women as men returned questionnaires. Thirty-two women reported breast cancer as their primary diagnosis; nine reported lymphoma, three colon cancer, three ovarian cancer and 12 other forms of cancer. Twelve men reported prostate cancer as their primary diagnosis; five had colon cancer, three lymphoma and eight other forms of cancer.

Instruments

A background questionnaire asked for basic demographic information as well as disease and treatment-related information. With the consent of participants, medical parameters with respect to the stage of illness, currently and at time of diagnosis, were confirmed from medical records. Seven questionnaires using Likert-type rating scales were included in the research package. The Impact of Events Scale (IES), found to be highly predictive of a diagnosis of post-traumatic stress disorder, was used to assess the frequency of the common symptoms of avoidance and intrusion associated with PTSD (Horowitz *et al*, 1979). This scale has been used to assess acute and chronic emotional response to traumatic life events in many settings and has been validated for use in the cancer population (Kelly *et al*, 1995). Scores of 20 or higher on the IES were used as criteria for diagnosis of PTSD. To establish a control for potential traumatic occurrences in participants' lives unrelated to or in addition to the cancer diagnosis, three open-ended questions were added to the IES. Participants were asked to:

1. Identify the stressful life event they were considering while filling out the Impact of Events Scale;
2. Identify any events prior to the cancer diagnosis that the average person would consider traumatic; and
3. Identify any events they had experienced since their cancer diagnosis that the average person would experience as traumatic.

Research and theoretical literature often distinguishes between the stress related to the life-threatening nature of cancer and the stress of cancer treatments, with life threat being a fundamental criteria for PTSD (Anderson *et al*, 1994; Stuber *et al*, 1994). We included the Appraisal of Life Threat and Treatment Intensity Questionnaire, which distinguished between these two aspects of the cancer experience (Stuber, 1995). Questions relating to appraisal of life threat were: 'I thought I would die when I was diagnosed with cancer' and 'I could still die from cancer'. Questions relating to treatment intensity included: 'Cancer treatment was emotionally upsetting for me' and 'Cancer treatment was/is hard for me'. Participants rated responses on a five-point Likert-type scale ranging from disagree to agree. Treatment intensity was quantified by asking participants to check-mark on the background sheet the kinds of treatment they had received (ie. chemotherapy, radiation, hormone, surgery, other) as well as numbers of treatments (1 to 5, 5 to 10, more than one cycle of treatment, etc).

The Ways of Coping—Cancer Version (WOC-CA) was used to assess five different individual coping strategies commonly used by cancer patients: seeking or using social support; focussing on the positive; distancing; cognitive escape-avoidance; and behavioural escape-avoidance (Dunkel-Schetter *et al*, 1992). The scale also asks participants to identify the most stressful aspect of their illness from a list of commonly experienced stressors. We added a space under 'Other' for participants to write in an aspect not covered in the list. The Constructed Meaning Scale (labelled 'Meaning of Illness' for this study) was included, since the ability to construct meaning in a cancer diagnosis seems to be helpful in adapting to the stress of this life-threatening illness (Fife, 1995).

Based on the literature review, the presence or absence of social support is useful in predicting development of PTSD symptomatology, and serves as a moderating variable in stress levels (Blanchard and Harper, 1996; Uchino *et al*, 1996; Quick *et al*, 1996; Shannon, 1996). Three measures of social support, previously used in medical settings, were included in order to distinguish between the different sources of support (Blanchard *et al*, 1995). One scale measured perceived social support from family, another measured perceived social support from friends and a third from healthcare professionals involved in participants' care (Procidano and Heller, 1983; Fife, 1995).

Results

T-test analysis of IES scores revealed that a significantly greater proportion of women than men participants qualified for a diagnosis of post-traumatic stress disorder ($p< 0.01$). Sixteen (27%) of the female participants had scores of 20 or higher on the IES, with twelve (20%) indicating specifically cancer-related PTSD and four (7%) with symptomatology not related to cancer. Three male participants (10%) scored 20 or higher on the IES, all specifying cancer- related PTSD. These figures compare to the prevalence in community-based populations of 5% to 14% (American Psychiatric Association, 1994). Time since diagnosis (ranging from 12 months to 10 years) did not serve as a moderating variable.

Other gender differences significant through t-test analysis included total number of treatments ($p >0.0001$), with women reporting a much greater number of treatments than men. Women reported more kinds of treatment, including surgery, radiation, chemotherapy and hormone treatments. Men reported receiving primarily surgery and radiation treatments. Women also reported significantly more problems with healthcare professionals on the Ways of Coping Questionnaire ($p < 0.05$).

Correlation coefficients were computed between scores on the Impact of Events Scale and other measures to determine which variables were associated with PTSD symptomatology. Analysis of these correlations reveal gender differences (see *Table 7.1*). For female participants, environmental and relationship stressors such as treatment intensity and problems with health care professionals are strongly related to high IES scores. Two individual variables (cognitive avoidance and low meaning of illness) were related to high IES scores. For male participants, more measures of individual coping strategies (behavioural avoidance, cognitive avoidance and psychological distancing) were correlated with high IES scores. One environmental stressor (surprise at diagnosis) correlated with higher IES scores. For both women and men, cognitive avoidant coping was related to high IES scores.

Table 7.1: Correlates of high post-traumatic stress disorder scores

Women (PTSD = 27%)	Men (PTSD = 10%)
Treatment intensity	Behavioural avoidance
Problems with healthcare professionals	Cognitive avoidance
Cognitive avoidance	Distancing
Low meaning of illness	Surprise at diagnosis

Table 7.2: Predictors of post-traumatic stress disorder

Women ($n=59$; $R^2=.51$)	Men ($n=28$; $R^2=.36$)
Treatment intensity	Behavioural avoidance
Problems with health-care professionals	
Cognitive avoidance	

Predictors of post-traumatic stress disorder identified by stepwise multiple regression analysis also revealed gender differences (see *Table 7.2*). Among the women participants, three variables predicted over half the variance in development of this disorder: treatment intensity ($R^2=0.23$); problems with healthcare professionals as identified on the WOC-CA questionnaire ($R^2=0.17$). Examples of cognitive avoidant coping from the Ways of Coping questionnaire are: 'Went over in my mind what I would say or do'; 'Depended mostly on others to handle things'; and 'Prayed'. Surprisingly, it was the treatment rather than the degree of life threat from cancer that emerged as most predictive of PTSD for women. T-test analysis of gender differences on items from the Treatment Intensity Questionnaire revealed that women subjectively experienced the treatment as significantly more intense than did men ($p<0.05$). For male participants, only behavioural avoidant coping was predictive of PTSD symptomatology ($R^2=0.36$). Examples of behavioural avoidant coping are: 'Did something just to do something'; 'Took it out on other people'; and 'Avoided being with other people'.

Since treatment intensity was revealed to be so strongly predictive of PTSD symptomatology for women, correlation analysis was conducted between this measure and other variables. Several statistically significant ($p<0.01$) relationships were revealed. *Table 7.3* lists the variables highly correlated with high scores on the Treatment Intensity Questionnaire. Young women reported more subjective distress at treatment intensity. Low levels of perceived social support from health care professionals as measured by the Social Support from Health Care Professionals Questionnaire were also highly associated with experience of intense treatment. Diagnosis at a late stage and high levels of pain associated with treatment were correlated with high treatment intensity scores. Interestingly, low meaning of illness was significantly correlated with both treatment intensity and higher IES scores, but only for female participants.

Women responded in written form on the questionnaires at much greater length than did men, and listed a wider range of stressors (Morse and Field, 1995). There were clear gender differences in thematic analysis of stressors identified on the Impact of Events Scale and the WOC-CA (see *Table 7.4*). Men's responses centred around concerns of business and loss of money as a result of their having cancer. Women also cited many concerns about job loss and strain as a result of cancer, but listed a greater variety of stressors. Examples of these stressors included such things as loss of other family members to cancer, difficulty continuing care-giving responsibilities, helplessness in depending on others for rides to treatment, as well as anger at the way they were treated as patients. Themes of loss of significant relationships, such as death of a spouse, child or family member emerged as stressors in the non-PTSD-related events identified by female participants.

Table 7.3: Correlates of treatment intensity for women

Age (negatively correlated)
Low levels of perceived social support from healthcare professionals
Pain
Low meaning of illness scores
Stage of disease at time of diagnosis

Table 7.4: Examples of the most traumatic aspects of the cancer experience

Women	Men
'Fear of my infant children growing up and never knowing me'	'My cancer and my company, which I closed due to my illness'
'My family and grand-kids. I'd like to be around for them'	'The merger of the company I work for and my cancer'
'Just dealing with having cancer and trying to figure out family and friends' feelings'	'My business has since closed with severe financial repercussions due to my ongoing medical problems. I could not emotionally or physically carry on'

Women's problems with healthcare professionals showed up in four places: (1) low scores on the Social Support from Health Care Professionals Scale; (2) unsolicited written comments on the Social Support from Health Care Professionals questionnaire; (3) written responses identifying problems with healthcare professionals on the Impact of Events Scale; and (4) written responses to the 'Other' category on the Ways of Coping Questionnaire. In fact, it was particularly through women's written responses in the 'Other' category on the WOC-CA questionnaire that we were alerted to the degree to which women experienced interpersonal difficulties with healthcare professionals. Not one male participant listed problems with healthcare professionals as stressors. Women also wrote, in some instances, narratives of their experiences in healthcare settings in which they were subjected to misdiagnosis, abusive treatment and sexist comments. *Table 7.5* lists examples. Themes of disrespectful treatment, lack of helpful information, communication difficulties and not being listened to emerged as common stressors for the women participants. Comments written on the Social Support from Health Care Professionals questionnaire revealed that the difficulties they experienced went beyond lack of support to actual abusive treatment.

Table 7.5: Examples of women's comments about problems with healthcare professionals

'They are so busy, one feels guilty taking their time'
'I found my oncologist to be difficult, unapproachable, and not very communicative'
'My surgeon/gynaecologist is very supportive, helpful, explains in detail and I feel truly cares. My oncologist is often abrupt and impatient with my questions. I have also been extremely upset by callous comments made regarding my physical appearance; of flippant answers to questions I felt required a more tactful approach'

Discussions

Of the women participating in this study, 27% qualified for a diagnosis of PTSD compared to 10% of the men. This suggests that there are gender-specific responses to the cancer experience. Surprisingly, it was the treatment rather than the threat to life that emerged as most predictive of development of PTSD for women. Insight into predictors can show us where to focus preventive efforts. For women, the environmental stressors of treatment intensity and problems with healthcare professionals were strongly predictive of PTSD. For male participants, an individual measure, the use of behavioural avoidant coping was the only variable that emerged as predictive of PTSD. Correlation analysis also confirmed gender differences with women experiencing more problems with the treatment setting and men experiencing more problems with individual coping.

This research suggests that treatment for cancer and problems with healthcare professionals chronically traumatises a large percentage of women, and creates an iatrogenic response in the form of a PTSD reaction (Illich, 1982). Male participants did not identify problems with treatment or healthcare providers. Narratives written on questionnaires by women participants reflect the isolation and horror of the treatment experience and give clear examples of androcentric behaviour by healthcare professionals. The results clearly indicate that androcentric bias in the delivery of cancer treatment has very negative effects on women's health (Muecke, 1996). While many women want aggressive cancer treatment, other women are questioning the need for such harsh treatments, and still others wish to complement medical treatment with other gentler therapies. However, the problem for these women overall is that they are treated, and expected to behave, as passive recipients of care rather than active agents in the treatment process (Findlay and Miller, 1994). Lessening treatment intensity for women has to do with changing ways in which our settings respond to the voices and experiences of women.

The finding that, for women, lack of support from healthcare professionals rather than lack of support from either family or friends was strongly predictive of PTSD and highly correlated with PTSD, suggests that strengthening support in the healthcare setting is a high priority. Participants clearly identified a major source of difficulty to be communication problems with healthcare professionals. Previous research has demonstrated that communication difficulties in physician-patient dialogues contributes to difficulties women encounter in medical settings (Grace, 1995; Lerman *et al*, 1993). Our research confirms other research that demonstrates patients' need for treatment from physicians that includes information, interpersonal respect and an interest in patient ideas (Brody *et al*, 1989). It also indicates the iatrogenic effect on women of more intense treatment, lack of social support from healthcare professionals and problems with healthcare professionals.

A related finding in our research is that low meaning of illness scores were significantly correlated with both treatment intensity and higher PTSD scores for women participants. This result is consistent with Fife's (1995) findings that the ability to find meaning in an illness contributes to a sense of control and mastery. Enhancing personal control also mediates the impact of trauma in development of PTSD symptoms (Meichenbaum, 1996). Support groups may be one way to strengthen support in treatment settings. They have been shown to help women with breast cancer develop strategies for negotiating with the medical establishment as well as provide opportunities for patients to come to an understanding of their experience (Cooper and Faragher, 1993; Spiegel, 1992). Expanding our goal for treatment beyond mortality and morbidity rates to include enhancement of quality of life would contribute to lessening the intensity of treatment for women patients (Anderson, 1992). Access to complementary therapies can also be a way to lessen the subjective appraisal of treatment intensity (Stalker *et al*, 1989).

Gender differences in response to the cancer experience were also clearly demonstrated in responses to open-ended questions asking participants to identify major stressors. Male participants listed problems with work, due to cancer, to be the greatest stressor. Women's concerns included work-related stressors, but also were more varied in content. A major theme that emerged was relational concerns for family and friends. Other major stressors included difficulty continuing care-giving responsibilities, helplessness in having to depend on others and disrespectful treatment from healthcare providers. Women wrote narratives about losses of other family members to cancer and grief over deaths of significant others since they had been diagnosed with cancer. This reinforces other researchers' observations that the importance of the social context of women's lives tends to be overlooked in medical encounters (Borges and Waitzkin, 1995; Thorne *et al*, 1997; West, 1993). The women participants in this research took the opportunity on questionnaires to share their stories — they wanted, and perhaps needed, to talk about what had happened to them. Telling our stories to others who understand the unique aspects of fear and loss that affect us is a form of prevention of PTSD and has been helpful to survivors of other forms of trauma (Herman, 1994; Pennebaker *et al*, 1988). Sharing information and experiences with other women can lead to women's empowered ability to make choices and decisions based on good information that includes the whole of a woman's life (Pellisier and Venta, 1996).

In conclusion, our results reinforce Batt's (1994) observations that women diagnosed with cancer suffer the shock and personal trauma of cancer; yet, just as traumatic for women is the institutionalisation they encounter when they become 'patients' in a system that is controlled by androcentric values. Feminist revisioning of cancer institutions would make treatment, education and research more meaningful to our lived reality and lower the incidence of iatrogenic disorders.

Implications

Based on results of this research, we make two recommendations for cancer treatment settings: (1) reduce treatment intensity for women through systemic changes of treatment delivery; and (2) prepare women to deal with the system and with treatments. Models exist in the literature for implementing these suggestions. Gray *et al* (1991) suggest changes in our healthcare settings geared toward empowerment of patients and expanding treatment parameters beyond the biomedical boundaries. This model includes access to psychological and family support services, consumer representation of all committees and integration of complementary therapies. Malterud (1993) suggests concrete ways that healthcare providers can adapt communication patterns to hear and respond to concerns of women as well as to communicate effective information and treatment choices. And finally, various types of groups for cancer patients and families who wish to use them can enhance quality of life and serve as forums for sharing information (Fawzy *et al*, 1995; Wellisch, 1993).

References

Alter CL, Pelcovitz D, Axelrod A *et al* (1996) Identification of PTSD in cancer survivors. *Psychosom* **37**: 137–43

American Psychiatric Association (1994) *Diagnostic and Statistical Manual of Mental Disorders*, 4 edn. APA, Washington, DC

Anderson BL (1992) Psychological interventions for cancer patients to enhance the quality of life. *J Consult Clin Psychol* **60**: 552–68

Anderson BL, Kiecolt-Glaser JK, Glaser R (1994) A biobehavioural model of cancer stress and disease course. *Am Psychologist* **49**: 389–404

Batt S (1994) *Patient No More: The Politics of Breast Cancer*. Gynergy Books, Charlottetown, PEI

Blanchard CG, Albrecht TL, Ruckdeschel JC, Grant CH, Hemmick RM (1995) The role of social support in adaptation to cancer and to survival. *J Psychosoc Oncol* **13**(1/2): 75–95

Blanchard CG, Harper GR (1996) Coping with the stress of cancer. In Cooper CL (ed.), *Handbook of Stress, Medicine and Health*. CRC Press, New York: 357–74

Borges S, Waitzkin H (1995) Women's narratives in primary care medical encounters. *Women Health* **23**(1): 29–56

Breslau N, Davis GC, Andreski P (1995) Risk factors for PTSD-related traumatic events: A prospective analysis. *Am J Psychiatry* **152**: 529–35

Brody DS, Miller SM, Lerman, CE, Smith DG, Lazaro CG, Blum MJ (1989) The relationship between patients' satisfaction with their physicians and perceptions about interventions they desire and received. *Med Care* **17**(11): 1027–35

Charney P, Morgan C (1996) Do treatment recommendations reported in the research literature consider differences between women and men? *J Wom Health* **5**(6): 579–84

Cooper CL, Faragher EG (1993) Psychosocial stress and breast cancer: The inter-relationship between stress events, coping strategies and personality. *Psycholog Med* **2**: 653–62

Cordova MJ, Andrykowski MA, Kenady DE, McGrath PC, Sloan DA (1995) Frequency and correlates of posttraumatic stress disorder like symptoms after treatment for breast cancer. *J Consult Clinic Psychol* **63** 981–6

Dunkel-Schetter C, Feinstein LG, Taylor SE, Falke RL (1992). Patterns of coping with cancer. *Health Psychol* 11: 79–87

Faragher EB (1996). Life events, coping, and cancer. In: Cooper CL, ed. *Handbook of Stress, Medicine and Health*. CRC Press, New York: 159–76

Fawzy FI, Fawzy NW, Hyun CS *et al* (1993) Malignant melanoma: Effects of an early structured psychiatric intervention, coping, and affective state on recurrence and survival 6 years later. *Arch Gen Psychiatry* **50**: 681–9

Fawzy FI, Fawzy NW, Arndt LA, Pasnau RO (1995) Critical review of psychosocial interventions in cancer care. *Arch Gen Psychiatry* **52**: 100–13

Fife B (1995) The measurement of meaning in illness. *Soc Sci Med* **40**(8): 1021–8.

Findlay DA & Miller LJ (1994) Medical power and womenÆs bodies. In Bolaria BS & Bolaria R (eds.), *Women, Medicine and Health*. Fernwood Publishing, Nova Scotia: 115–39

Grace VM (1995) Problems of communication, diagnosis, and treatment experienced by women using the New Zealand health services for chronic pelvic pain: A quantitative analysis. *Health Care Wom Int* **16**: 521–35

Gray RE, Doan BD, Church K (1991) Empowerment issues in cancer. *Health Val* **15**(4): 22–8

Gruber BL, Hersh SP, Hall NRS *et al* (1993) Immunological responses of breast cancer patients to behavioral interventions. *Biofeedback Self-Reg* **18**(1): 1–22

Herman J (1994) *Trauma and Recovery: From Domestic Abuse to Political Terror*. Pandora, London

Horowitz M, Wilner N, Alvarez (1979) Impact of events scale: A measure of subjective distress. *Psychosom Med* **41**: 208–18

Illich I (1982) *Medical Nemesis: The Expropriation of Health*. Pantheon, New York

Kelly B, Raphael B, Smithers M *et al* (1995) Psychological responses to malignant melanoma: An investigation of traumatic stress reactions to life threatening illness. *Gen Hos Psychiatry* **17**: 126–34

Lerman C, Daly M, Walsh WP *et al* (1993) Communication between patients with breast cancer and health care providers: Determinants and implications. *Cancer* **72**: 2612–20

Levy SM, Herberman RB, Whiteside T, Sanzo K, Lee J, Kirkwood J (1990) Perceived social support and tumour estrogen/progesterone receptor status as predictors of natural killer cell activity in breast cancer patients. *Psychosom Med* **52**: 73–85

Lorde A (1980) *The Cancer Journals*. Spinsters/Aunt Lute, San Francisco

Malterud K (1993) Strategies for empowering women's voices in the medical culture. *Health Care Wom Int* **14**: 365–73

McFarlane CA, de Girolama B. (1996) The nature of post-traumatic stressors and the epidemiology of post-traumatic reactions. In: van der Volk BA, McFarlane AC, Weisaeth L, eds. *Traumatic Stress: The Effects of Overwhelming Experience on Mind, Body and Society*. The Guilford Press, New York: 129–54

Meichenbaum D (1996) *Treatment of Clients with Post-Traumatic Stress Disorder (PTSD): A Cognitive-Behavioral Approach*. University of Waterloo, Waterloo, Ontario

Meyerowitz BE, Hart S (1995) Women and cancer: Have assumptions about women limited our research agenda? In: Stanton AL, Gallant SJ, eds. *The Psychology of Women's Health: Progress and Challenges in Research and Application*. American Psychological Association, Washington, DC: 51–84

Morse JM, Field PA (1995) *Qualitative Research Methods for Health Professionals*, 2 edn. Sage Publications, Thousand Oaks, CA

Muecke M (1996) The gender analysis imperative: Introduction to the special issue. *Health Care Wom Int* **17**: 385–92

Pellisier JM, Venta ER (1996) Introducing patient values into the decision making process for breast cancer screening. *Women Health* **24**(4): 47–67

Pennebaker JW, Kiecolt-Glaser JK, Glaser R (1988) Disclosure of traumas and immune function: Health implications for psychotherapy. *J Consult Clin Psychol* **56**: 239–45

Peterson KC, Prout MF, Schwartz RA (1991) *Post-traumatic Stress Disorder: A Clinician's Guide*. Plenum Press, New York

Procidano ME, Heller K (1983) Measures of perceived social support from friends and family. *Am J Comm Psychol* 11: 1–24

Quick JD, Nelson DL, Matuszek AAC, Whittington JL, Quick JC (1996) Social support secure attachments, and health. In: Cooper CL, ed. *Handbook of Stress, Medicine and health*. CRC Press, New York: 269–87

Shannon C (1996) Dealing with stress: Families and chronic illness. In: Cooper CL, ed. *Handbook of Stress, Medicine and Health*. CRC Press, New York: 357–74

Sneed NV, Edlund B, Dias JK (1992) Adjustment of gynaecological and breast cancer patients to the cancer diagnosis: Comparisons with males and females having other cancer sites. *Health Care Wom Int* **13**:11–22

Spiegel D (1992) Effects of psychosocial support on patients with metastatic breast cancer. *J Psychosoc Oncol* **10**(2): 113–20

Stalker MZ, Johnson PS, Cimma C (1989) Supportive activities requested by survivors of cancer. *J Psychosoc Oncol* **7**(4): 21–31

Stuber ML (1995) Stress responses to pediatric cancer: A family approach. *Fam Sys Med* **13**: 163–72

Stuber ML, Gonzalez S, Meeske K *et al* (1994) Post traumatic stress after childhood cancer II: A family model. *Psycho-oncol* **3**: 313–9

Thorne S, McCormick J, Carty E (1997) Deconstructing the gender neutrality of chronic illness and disability. *Health Care Wom Int* **18**: 1–16

Uchino BN, Cacioppo JT, Kiecolt-Glaser JK (1996) The relationship between social support and physiological processes: A review with emphasis on underlying mechanisms and implications for health. *Psychol Bull* **19**(3): 488–531

Wellisch DK (1993). Beyond the year 2000: The future of groups for patients with cancer. *Cancer Pract* **1**(3): 198–201

West C (1993) Reconceptualizing gender in physician-patient relationships. *Soc Sci Med* **36**(1): 57–66

White NE, Richter JM, Fry C (1992) Coping, social support and adaptation to chronic illness. *W J Nurs Res* **14**(2): 211–24

8

Carrying more than a baby: women survivors of child abuse and childbearing

Carol Jackson

Missing voices: The secrecy of abuse

Australian and international studies indicate one in four or five girls and one in nine boys have experienced sexual assault during childhood (Critchley, 1996; Finkelhor *et al*, 1990; Fleming, 1997; Goldman and Goldman, 1986; Kilpatrick *et al*, 1992; Tomison, 1996). In Australia, during 1994/95, there were 30,615 substantiated cases of child abuse (Angus and Hall, 1996). Of these proven cases, 16% (4,890) were of child sexual assault. Some 3,716 (76%) of these assaults were on girls. The total population of Australia is over 18 million; there are about 2 million girls under 16 years of age. Using this figure, the total percentage of sexually abused girls under the age of 16 would be 0.19%. However, we know from many studies, including those cited above, that 20 to 25% of girls are sexually abused. This means that, of the total population of 2 million girls, 450,000 have been assaulted — a very different figure from 3,716. What has happened to them? The reality is that many children have consciously hidden, or unknowingly dissociated, their abuse (Williams, 1994).

For various reasons, the majority of children who experience sexual assault never report the abuse to their parents or the authorities (Fleming, 1997; Williams, 1994). Participants in Fleming's study did not tell because of shame. In her study, Rivera (1991) found that even if the children disclosed, their words were disregarded, or not understood. A large proportion of her participants were blamed and punished for 'telling lies'. They did not 'tell' again. Commonly, disclosure occurs only after the person is in a situation of physical and psychological safety, removed from contact with the abuser. Hence, the reports of adult women survivors of childhood assault who have always remembered their abuse, but were in no position to report it. Another major reason for not disclosing, and the focus of the rest of this paper, is that the abusive episodes have been dissociated and are not available to conscious recall (Briere, 1996; van der Kolk, 1996; Whitfield, 1995; Williams, 1994). This is called traumatic dissociation and it is a survival mechanism.

When in a situation of terror and the resulting autonomic nervous system (ANS) arousal, inactivation of Broca's area in the left cortex occurs, resulting in alexithymia (Everly, 1995). There are no corresponding words laid down for what is happening, just snapshot pictures (Rolls and O'Mara, 1993), smells, sounds, touch and so on (Jackson, 1995). Traumatic dissociation of memories is common in very young children who believe their physical or psychological existence is in danger.

Dissociation in children

How difficult would it be for a child to keep in her conscious mind that the people who were supposed to provide nurture, love and protection — the parents — were instead the source of physical and emotional terror? Quite apart from the need to respond positively to the parents at times other than the abuse, it is vital that children maintain the facade that their parents actually care; it is a matter of survival. From the testimony of many adult survivors, it has become apparent that children, trapped in abusive, unsupportive families, frequently make use of their innate abilities of dissociation (Kluft, 1985). They deny what is happening and this results in an absence of memories of the abuse. When children have no means of escape from ongoing abuse — and what four-year-old does? — it is common for them to develop 'abnormal states of consciousness in which the ordinary relations of body and mind, reality and imagination, knowledge and memory, no longer hold' (Herman, 1992). For example, Heather, an adult with

Dissociate Identity Disorder (DID), said she had experienced:

> *'. . . severe sexual abuse and neglect within my family on a daily basis from infancy and had already learned to "dissociate." Of course, I did not know the term then, but young children are quite adept at it. To me it meant "waiting for the other girl to come" while I floated on the ceiling, watching what happened to the other girl, but not feeling it.'*
>
> (Jackson, 1996).

I do not believe that the initial occurrence of DID can happen in children older than five to six years old. All 24 people with DID that I have worked with had experienced the initial traumatic event before the age of four years. Each believed she was going to die. (An adult body on a tiny chest crushes it, and causes difficulty with breathing. An erect adult penis forced into a two-year-old's mouth effectively blocks the child's airway.) When one takes into account the smallness and fragility of the pre-schooler's body, and the immaturity of the child's personality, the age limit makes sense. Observations of infants show a rapid flow and change in behavioural states, ie. from crying to laughing almost concurrently. The fluidity of their behaviour indicates a general lack of specialisation, even though different states are discernible (Putnam, 1989; Sparshott, 1997; Wolff, 1987). Myelination is still occurring and permanent states are still being determined. In addition, the ability to dissociate is higher in children, peaking before adolescence (Ross, 1989). If uncontrollable arousal of the ANS occurs in these early years, and the infant/child successfully uses dissociation to 'escape', future life-threatening events will elicit the same survival mechanism — if it works, why change it? But after myelination of the hippocampus is complete, the response to extreme ANS stimulation is more likely to be Post Traumatic Stress Disorder (PTSD) or a dissociate disorder other than DID, or Dissociative Disorder Not Otherwise Specified (DDNOS) (APA, 1994).

These survival mechanisms are especially prevalent in, but not exclusive to, young children in incestuous families. The other group of children affected are those who witness their parents or care-givers being physically attacked, tortured or murdered. Apart from domestic violence, the obvious situation that springs to mind is children caught up in wars. The extra needs for these children are frequently unrecognised, but there are ongoing implications for both the children and, if they are lucky enough to gain refuge, the countries that accept them.

Dissociation: Retrieval of memories — flashbacks

Just as traumatic memory is encoded and stored differently, so too is retrieval. People describe flashbacks as fleeting visual glimpses of physical sensations of past experiences that, over time, become crystal clear, then disappear. All or some of the senses may be involved. Typically, the flashbacks come with increasing clarity and frequency, and may cause great distress. Flashbacks are often the first sign of dissociated memories resurfacing. Not everyone who has flashbacks has multiplicity — far from it. Flashbacks are a common phenomenon in people with PTSD. They are also common in those who have been traumatised to the level of having to dissociate a physical or psychological life- threatening event, such as rape victims or prisoners of war. Flashbacks seem to occur in a similar way for people with or without multiplicity, but the outcome differs. The fleeting snapshot pictures, sounds or smells, and so on, signify flashbacks are the same for both groups. Human beings are 'geared' to survival, so normally flashbacks will only begin to surface when the person is ready to manage the memories.

Sometimes flashbacks occur prematurely. They can be caused by an assault on the person's usual means of control and containment. (and on their internal systems). Situations when this happens may:

- be anniversaries
- involve high levels of pain (for example, during labour or with an acute back injury)
- happen when there is a perception that the person or loved one, ie. your child is, or is likely to be, in danger (Jackson, 1994).

The author has found that the following may initially trigger flashbacks:

- the client loses a close support person
- during labour and birth (especially of a girl)
- the client's situation is now either very safe or is becoming increasingly dangerous. Factors, such as an angry confrontation with the teacher of a survivor's child, chronic painful illnesses, or

life-threatening car accidents have been stated as causal factors in triggering flashbacks

- the survivor's child is reaching the age when the survivor was initially abused
- the death of the non-offending parent
- the death of the abuser (Jackson, 1991).

This is a time of crisis for the person. Singletons may experience increased nightmares, intrusive thoughts and disruption of daily living. For people with multiplicity (DID), the unexpected flashbacks may initiate devastating situations — psychotic-type responses, days or months of dissociation where another personality or personalities takes over, or self-harm episodes, ie. burning, cutting and suicide attempts. The symptoms may be the impetus for the singleton to seek counselling. For many people with multiplicity, the symptoms are taken as a psychiatric crisis and can result in incarceration.

Because the control of who is 'on the circle' (usually the host personality) has evaporated, the panic-stricken personalities of the internal system of people with DID, rapidly cycle through to the external world, staying only long enough to say a couple of words, or grunt, or appear violent or paralysed. To onlookers, this behaviour appears fractured and senseless, and has been labelled psychotic (Steingard and Frankel, 1985). A fictional example of this process is described in the novel *The Prince of Tides*. Savannah, Tom's sister, has been hospitalised because of a psychotic episode occurring after a suicide attempt. Her psychiatrist has taped what Savannah said during the psychosis, and asks Tom, 'Is there anything in this that you recognize as significant?' Tom replies, 'I recognise a lot of it. Everything seems significant.' Further on, he adds, 'She's screaming out her autobiography to you . . . to anyone who's listening . . . to herself' (Conroy, 1992).

Maintaining control over the pace of the surfacing of memories is certainly important to the safety of the people abused in childhood, whether or not they have DID. The physiological and emotional pain has been contained until the person has reached a stage in life where there is enough stability and support to cope with processing the effect, sensation and knowledge of the childhood trauma. While the feelings and knowledge arising from the controlled filtering of memories are very difficult and painful, they are manageable. When that control is taken away — by triggers or unintended discovery of the internal system in people with DID — the flashbacks can escalate into uncontrolled abreactions, resulting in chaotic crises that may destroy the person physically or psychologically.

Maintaining control is, therefore, important. Women survivors who have no conscious memory of abuse will consistently display a dislike or fear of gynaecological examinations, to the point where they refuse to even think about having routine smears or breast examinations. Think about the women who delay receiving antenatal care, or who become rigid and distraught on examination (Seng and Petersen, 1995). Any gynaecological or obstetrical procedures can initiate a flashback for these women.

Dissociation and gynaecology

Invasive procedures resulting in flashbacks

Jenny Kitzinger's article, 'Recalling the Pain' (1990), should be mandatory reading for anyone who orders or carries out invasive procedures in the urogenital region of women. The paper begins with a description of four nurses catheterising a very old woman. Three nurses restrain the woman while one attempts to pass the catheter. Throughout she pleads for her father to leave her alone. This was the first time the old woman had given any inkling that she had been sexually abused as a child. The nurses were so overwhelmed that they neither talked with the woman, nor between themselves, about the incident.

Intended sexual assault by a doctor resulting in flashbacks

NB: The women mentioned in the passages that follow, who are identified by letters of the alphabet, have been or are currently clients of the author. They have willingly given permission for their stories to be told in the belief that health workers will gain some understanding.

> **A** 30-year-old woman, was referred [to the Centre Against Sexual Assault where I was working as a counsellor/advocate] because of Rape Trauma Syndrome (Burgess and Holstrom, 1975), a reaction she sustained after a particularly invasive gynaecological examination, which was eventually reported to the authorities. (The doctor has since

been charged and found guilty of similar offences perpetrated on other women patients.) During sessions, she disclosed about time gaps, hearing voices, inability to see certain parts of the body and numbness. Since the doctor's examination, very frightening flashbacks and chaotic dissociation had begun. During one of these episodes, different personalities would appear in rapid succession — almost too hard to keep up with. **A** was diagnosed as having Dissociative Identity Disorder — DID (previously known as multiple Personality Disorder), with 14 female and two male personalities. She had first been sexually abused by her grandfather at the age of two. Abusive (not all sexual) episodes that she had never dissociated, occurred from other family members and school friends throughout her adolescence. She tried to tell many times but each time she was punished.

A was living a more or less peaceful life within several years of her first flashbacks. She had no suicidal ideation, or parasuicide episodes that had been a fairly frequent part of her life since early teenager years. The twice yearly depressive episodes (present since the age of fifteen years) disappeared. Her older child commenced pre-school and fitted in well. About two years later, after I had left the Centre Against Sexual Assault, she contacted me explaining that she badly wanted to have another child. I will continue the story of this pregnancy and labour in a later section.

Metrorrhagia

B had a long history of intermittent metrorrhagia for which no cause could be established. During the counselling process she remembered two extremely violent incidents of abuse at the age of 12 years — she was the victim of a gang rape and required hospitalisation for one week, and a month later, witnessed a rape. Approximately two months later, she began menstruating. She was 30 years old when she finally remembered these events as well as multiple abuse from her father and brother from the age of 5 years. In addition, her five year old son was the outcome of a rape. Her menstruation returned to normal with no surgical or medical intervention.

Like the women in William's (1994) study, she had dissociated the memories of her rape and her hospitalisation. She did not have Dissociative Identity Disorder.

C is in her early fifties. After the birth of her first two children (both boys), she was hospitalised for severe post-natal depression. Two children (both girls) later, her menorrhagia was so severe that a hysterectomy was performed — she was 28 years old. Since the first birth, she had many years of psychiatric care, and several diagnoses including bipolar depression, manic depression, and BPD. She was diagnosed with DID approximately 7 years ago, but no treatment was commenced. She successfully completed 3 years of DID work in 1993, graduated in the top 1% in her university course, and is now working full time. During our work together, a 13 year old part disclosed that she and another part used to menstruate after **C** resulting in 3 weeks in a row of bleeding. This continued until the hysterectomy was performed.

I had not seen this situation reported anywhere else until I recently saw the film *Dialogues with Madwomen* (Light-Saraf, 1993), during which one of the women interviewed expressed the same phenomenon.

Antenatal

Pseudocyesis has been reported (Hennessy and Polk-Warner, 1990). **Hyperemesis**, to a level requiring intravenous rehydration and weeks of hospitalisation, has occurred in three of my clients with DID.

Negative reaction to pregnancy

There may be dismay when the pregnancy is confirmed. Frequently, the women's concerns are about the ability to 'cope', or their mothering capacity. Keep in mind that very young pregnant women may be current victims of sexual abuse or incest, and that the baby may be an outcome of the abuse. The following is an abstract from one of my student's reflective journals:

> As the class goes on, I remember other people I have met along the way. The 13-year-old girl who I nursed during my midwifery training. She came in antenatally, and until her admission, her parents had been unaware that she was pregnant. Mum was distraught, shocked and disbelieving as her daughter rarely, if ever, left home. There was no knowledge of an interest in boys. Dad, on the other hand, was jovial, teasing her about 'no bikinis this year', etc. His reaction always baffled me.

Looking back, maybe it was Dad's baby. I never suspected: I wonder if anyone else did? Some months later, after an horrific labour she delivered a live baby girl and placed the child for adoption. I hope someone was looking out for that young girl (13 years ago — maybe not).

Denial of pregnancy

(See also Miller, 1990; Nicholson *et al*, 1996; Spielvogel and Hohener, 1995.)

D, a 40-year-old woman was in an abusive and intermittent relationship. She had been sexually abused from the age of 8 years by her paternal uncle and grandfather. At the time of her daughter's birth she was in full-time employment as a bank teller. On the day of the birth, **D** attended the doctor because of abdominal pain that had woken her during the night. At 1pm that afternoon she gave birth to a 7 lb full-term girl. She had no idea she was pregnant. For at least six months after the birth she steadfastly denied having intercourse with anyone.

Unawareness of pregnancy and labour in women with DID

Van der Hart *et al* (1991) also reported several cases where women were unaware of their pregnancies. Other personalities had conceived, carried and in some cases given birth to the infants.

A, a survivor with multiple personalities whose story appears above, stated that she had not conceived, and was not present for the birth of either of her children. She had great difficulty developing an attachment, because she did not know that they were hers. She rang me two years after finishing therapy saying that she wanted another baby so that she could go through the normal process of birth and attachment as a whole person. After much family discussion, she and her husband decided that they would go ahead.

It was a totally new experience for her, and her healing was dramatically tested. The two older children had been full-term vaginal births of approximately 4 hours labour, and for which, she stated she was not present. For this pregnancy, she had an emergency Caesarean at 32 weeks and the baby remained in hospital for 7 weeks post delivery. He was readmitted for bilateral herniorrhaphy a week after discharge. Although this whole experience was very difficult, especially the period of separation, and readmission, **A** remained integrated, and was delighted with her accomplishment. At our last contact in 1995, the baby had just had his fourth birthday, and the family were managing well.

Perinatal

Van der Leden and Raskin (1993) reported that women who were survivors had statistically significant shorter labours than those who were not abused, and suggested that the survival strategy of dissociating from painful experiences may be the reason. The experience of **A** supports these findings in that she dissociated and another alter was present for the delivery. However, for other women this has not been the case. Labour has been the initiating factor for the surfacing of previously dissociated memories of childhood sexual assault (initial flashbacks). Parratt (1993) found three of her six participants first remembered their abusive childhood experiences during childbirth. In an Australian survey of people with MPD/DID, six women identified themselves as mothers and each one identified the birth as the catalyst for flashbacks. For them, the level of pain interfered with the control of the dissociated memories generally maintained by the internal system. Trying to control the pain, the dissociation and/or the memories simultaneously were too difficult. In addition, just as the old woman in Kitzinger's article thought she was being abused, the experience of labour placed these women in a situation of powerlessness and feeling that they were being sexually abused. Five of the six were hospitalised for severe PND or puerperal psychosis (Jackson, 1994). With my DID clients who are mothers (not many of them are), 70% were also hospitalised for severe PND/psychosis. All had been diagnosed with varying degrees of postnatal depression.

Sex of the baby

Girls: Some women have been delighted that the baby was a girl: 'I will teach her how to look after herself'; 'I will protect her'. If the reaction is negative, the reason I have commonly been given is, 'Girls will become victims — that's their lifescript'.

If the woman holds a belief such as this, there is a real danger of distancing herself from her newborn daughter. Together with her belief that she is 'damaged goods' because of her own sexual abuse (Sgroi, cited in Long, 1986), and the underlying fear that she feels powerless to protect her baby daughter from harm, it is likely she will distance herself from the source of her vulnerability — her infant. This type of reaction is common in parents of premature infants who attempt to delay forming attachments because of a fear that their baby may die (Controle, 1981; Goldberg and Taylor, 1988; MacArthur and Dezoete, 1992). The implications are poor attachment and a seeming disinterest by the mother in her baby.

Boys: Some women express pleasure that the baby is a boy, wrongly believing that boys are not likely to be sexually abused. Conversely, the woman may believe that he will grow up to become an abuser. If the woman is currently in a situation of domestic violence, this fear may be strong.

No matter how irrational these types of beliefs seem, to the woman they are valid. If we are really in the business of supporting people, then we must listen and not dismiss such statements. This becomes even more important when a woman talks about issues such as being contaminated, or harming the baby because of her touch.

Breast-feeding

Because of the WHO 'Baby Friendly Hospital' scheme, in Victoria at present, there is a concerted effort to have every woman breast-feed. Although totally supportive of breast-feeding, I believe this current trend may be problematic for many women who were sexually abused as children.

Most survivors, men and women, find touching difficult and even frightening. Most survivors also have a strong dislike of their own bodies. In addition, many hold cognitively immature, but strong beliefs about their skin and body fluids, including blood and breast milk, being contaminated. The idea of feeding the baby with the inherently intimate, tactile contact between mother and baby, together with a belief that her breast milk is contaminated, is terrifying. Another factor that I have not seen written about, but which has been disclosed to me is the bodily response of the woman when the baby suckles. The feelings are quite sexual and out of her control — replicating the situation when they were being abused as children.

And we ask them, sometimes threateningly, to put their babies to the breast and wonder why some women refuse, become angry or burst into tears!

Contamination

> **E** was abused sexually and emotionally by her father and four brothers from infancy and emotionally and physically abused by her mother. Apart from several admissions for hyperemesis during the first two trimesters, the pregnancy was uneventful, resulting in the full term birth of **Z**. **E** was initially frightened to touch him but soon overcame that feeling and then could not 'put him down'. Unfortunately, **Z** developed pyrexia and jaundice and was placed in an humidicrib. **E** was devastated and confided many months later that she believed that her touching was responsible for her baby becoming ill. She resolved not to make him sick again. After that period of separation (24 hours) **E** would only touch **Z** when she absolutely had to. She could not play with him; she could not look at him. She tried to breast-feed but ceased this after one week because both she and **Z** were unsettled. At 2 weeks of age she tried to drown him during his bath. By the time he was 6 weeks of age, she was regularly hitting him. During his twelfth week of life **E** fractured **Z**'s skull.

Her perceived inadequacy as a mother ('making' her baby sick because of her contaminated touch, failing to breast-feed, her inability to touch him or play with him, and failure to quieten her baby's crying) escalated her into uncontrolled panic and terror.

Abuse continuing into adulthood

> **F** presented to the centre because of a rape two weeks earlier, and brought with her her three month old baby girl. **F** had always remembered her sexual abuse, and had left home at 16 years of age to escape. Apart from keeping contact with her younger sister, **F** had severed all connection with her family. She was 24 years of age and this was a planned, deliberately fatherless baby. Soon after sessions started, she disclosed that her father found out where she was living, and had threatened to assault the infant if she did not re-establish a sexual liaison with him. To protect her infant, she agreed. The rape was done by him.

The resolution of this situation was not without difficulty; however, it was resolved. **F** now runs a self-help group for women survivors of incest, and she and her school age daughter are fine. I have included her story because this young woman was strong and assertive, had put herself through university, yet agreed to her father's demands in order to protect her child. **Abuse can continue into adulthood for some women.**

Child sexual assault and contaminated body fluid as the cause of abnormality

> **G** gave birth to **Y**, a planned first baby. **Y** was breech and there was great difficulty during her birth. She took 45 minutes to breathe and by day two was having continual convulsions. I worked with the parents over a period of 3 years, supporting the family through their grieving process and through a very difficult time with their marital relationship. Formal contact ended when **Y** received a permanent placement in an institution, but the family kept in contact through the birth of the next two children and **Y**'s death. About two months after **Y**'s death, and six years after **Y**'s birth, **G** rang, very anxious and upset. She disclosed (for the first time to anyone) that she had been sexually abused by her brother at age 12 years. She had believed that this had caused **Y** to be disabled because of the 'bad genes'.

I was stunned that she had held onto that belief during all those years — we had a very close working relationship and I believed that she and her husband trusted me. **It was with this revelation that I began to realise just how difficult it is for *anyone*, child or adult, to disclose that they have been abused.**

Implications for all nurses — The seven As

The extent of childhood sexual abuse, and the feelings that arise when one becomes aware of the ramifications of the abuse, often seem overwhelming — too big to tackle. Reading about or hearing survivors' stories may be too difficult. It may be easier to dismiss their testimonies or ignore them and change the subject because you, as a worker, feel unable to effectively help. The list below could be used as a guide to assist you in supporting adult survivors of childhood sexual abuse.

- **Be aware of the effects of CSA.** Making yourself familiar with the short- and long-term effects of childhood sexual abuse will help you recognise the actions and/or behaviours of survivors. An excellent resource for nurses is the January 1994 issue of *The Journal of Nurse-Midwifery*, which contains many articles about adult survivors of childhood sexual assault. For example, Holz's contribution from that journal lists the following behavioural clues as 'red flags' of incidences of child sexual assault (Holz, 1994):

  1. addictions
  2. self-destructive tendencies
  3. multiple somatic complaints without physical cause
  4. poor self-esteem
  5. phobias
  6. sexual dysfunction
  7. inappropriate affect.

  See appendix for other recommended literature.
- **be alert to non-verbal signs and behaviours** as discussed in this paper
- **'actions speak louder than words' — treat *all* clients/patients with respect.** People who have survived childhood abuse learn to be very aware of dangers in their environment. Hypervigilance is one mechanism that is used. Most adult survivors appear to have an acute ability to 'read' the verbal and, more important, the non-verbal behaviours of other people. They will carefully check out how you relate to them and to other patients/clients before they feel safe enough to disclose. If they do not feel safe, it is unlikely they will speak out
- **allow the opportunity for the woman to disclose if she wishes.** The best support for survivors who disclose their abuse is just listening and believing. Affirming statements include, 'I believe you', 'You are not to blame for what has happened', 'You have done nothing wrong' and 'I will do my best to help you'. If you suspect the client/patient is a survivor, you can gently ask questions such as, 'I knew another person who (felt, acted, spoke like you — she was a survivor of child sexual abuse. I'm wondering if you could also be a survivor and if you would like to talk to someone about it?' This is fairly innocuous and gives a

choice of answer. You really do not have to do or say more than this. If the woman thinks you are safe, and perceives that you might treat her and her story with respect, she may want to discuss the situation further. If she does not think it is safe, or the events are still dissociated (and therefore not available to conscious memory), at least when she is ready to disclose, she will have had an example of someone in a helping profession who could listen and was willing to hear her. And the freedom to talk about long 'hidden' secrets in the knowledge that, when you are ready, you might be heard and treated with respect, is a great gift to give anyone.

- **appropriate referral but only if requested**. The dynamics that enable abuse of children are those of power and control. As adults, survivors of child abuse strive to gain and maintain control over their lives. It is important that we, as nurses, do not usurp their control by making decisions for them, coercing or manipulating them because we think "it would be good for you." This is often the sort of statement told to them during childhood. We need to explore whether suggestions or advice are for the person's benefit, or for ours. Indeed, most of us would feel more comfortable if we knew the survivor was to receive counselling. But this must be the survivor's decision. In situations of mandated reporting, it is vital that the person be told of your professional responsibilities.

  Having appropriate posters displayed, or pamphlets easily but privately available (for example, in a holder behind the toilet door) may encourage a survivor to know that help is available when she is ready.
- **advocacy**. You can advocate, educate and intervene when other hospital or agency staff dismiss the survivor as being difficult, infantile or manipulative, and you can suggest appropriate intervention and referral. Depending on your work situation, you may be able to facilitate a support group, or upgrade your skills and provide individual counselling. Lobbying for longer term, affordable and appropriate services is another way to support adult survivors of child abuse.
- **awareness of your own attitudes, or one's own unresolved history and of vicarious traumatisation**. *Self-awareness*. There is little point raising awareness of abuse if you have a belief that you will never see, or have to work with families or children in these situations. It is, therefore, important to awaken one's self-awareness and to challenge ingrained attitudes about abuse.

  Unresolved history. There is also a risk to patients/clients when workers have their own unresolved legacy of abuse. Findings from a pre-module survey that my students complete two sessions before 'tackling' the violence and abuse modules indicate about 30% have been victims or witnessed some form of childhood or current abuse. This figure rises to approximately 60% after the modules. Once safety networks are in place, and the students begin to explore the theoretical models, such as adult survivors of child abuse, domestic violence, etc, and to address and work on the individual feelings that arise, the issues surrounding abuse and violence do not seem as formidable, threatening or insurmountable.

  Vicarious traumatisation (McCann and Pearlman, 1993). This occurs through being overwhelmed by the stories of survivors. You may hear about cruel, terrifying and sadistic actions that some adults inflict on some children. You may experience reactions, such as anger, sickness, disgust and sadness. It is important for you to work through personal issues that may colour your ability to support the woman, prior to offering such support. Develop both a support system where you can talk through the rougher times, and methods to combat stress. These need to be implemented because it is vital that your feelings are kept in control. This does not imply that you should not be empathetic. However, please remember that survivors have spent a lifetime being responsible for other peoples' feelings and actions. If, for example, your anger at the offender is too great, you will effectively make the client 'clam up' and cease talking. You are taking away the client's anger by using your own — and you do not have that right. If you take in too much information that is distressing, and you demonstrate your distress either verbally or non-verbally, there is a strong tendency for one of the following to occur: (a) for you to stop listening, or (b) for the person to control her responses to a level she perceives you can manage.

Survivors are very protective of everyone but themselves.

Summary

The legacy of child sexual assault may surface in many ways, some of which are mentioned above. As nurses we are in an ideal position to become advocates for women survivors of child abuse, especially during the ante-, peri- and post-natal periods. Some women may disclose the abuse, but many will not. Some women do not have conscious memory of the abuse until the time of labour or after the birth. The women may or may not remember the abuse, but may be reacting in ways that indicate that childhood abuse has occurred. Please take into consideration that the 'difficult' patient, or a woman with an aversion to breastfeeding, or the one who does not play with her baby, may be a survivor.

Most of the information and experiences in this chapter have been given, first with hesitation and fear, and then with hope, by the women who lived through them. The hesitation and fear were mostly because the author was the first person to be told about their experiences — or rather, the first person who listened. The few who had spoken out on previous occasions had been ignored or dismissed. Those who had no words, only actions that they themselves did not understand at the time, were routinely given strong non-verbal and verbal messages that they were 'no good', or were in some way 'letting their babies down'. The hope the women hold is that researchers, policy makers and health workers will hear their stories and explore more closely the effects of childhood abuse and neglect in relation to childbearing and childrearing. It is the hope of the author, too.

Further reading: about healing

Adults

Bass E, Davis L (1988) *The courage to heal*. Harper and Row, New York

Briere J (1996) *Therapy for adults molested as children: Beyond survival*, 2 edn. Springer, New York

Cameron M (1995) *Broken child*. Kensington Books, New York

Cohen B, Giller E, Lynn W (1991) *Multiple personality disorder from the inside out*. Sidran Press, Lutherville, MA

Davis L (1990) *The courage to heal workbook*. Harper and Row, New York

Daugherty L (1984) *Why me?* Mother Courage Press, Racine, WI

Feldmeth J, Finley M (1990) *We weep for ourselves and our children: A Christian guide for survivors of childhood sexual assault*. Harper, San Francisco

Gil E (1988) *Treatment of adult survivors of childhood abuse*. Launch Press, Walnut Creek, CA

Gil E (1990) *United we stand: A book for people with multiple personalities*. Launch Press, Walnut Creek, CA

Herman J (1992) *Trauma and recovery*. Basic Books, New York

Hocking S *et al* (1992) *Living with your selves: A survival manual for people with multiple personalities*. Launch Press, Rockville, MD

Kluft R, Fine G, eds. (1993) *Clinical perspectives on multiple personality disorder*. American Psychiatric Press, Washington, DC

Lew M (1990) *Victims no longer: Men recovering from incest and other sexual child abuse*. Harper Collins, New York

Loring M (1994) *Emotional abuse*. New York: Lexington Books

Lynn S, Rhue J, eds. (1994) *Dissociation: Clinical and theoretical perspectives*. The Guilford Press, New York

Maltz W (1992) *The sexual healing journey: A guide for survivors of sexual abuse*. Harper Perennial, New York

Putnam F (1989) *Diagnosis and treatment of multiple personality disorder*. The Guildford Press, New York

Ross C (1989) *Multiple personality disorder: Diagnosis, clinical features and treatment*. John Wiley & Sons, New York

Sanford L (1990) *Strong at the broken places: Overcoming the trauma of childhood abuse*. Avon Books, New York

Salter A (1995) *Transforming trauma: A guide to understanding and treating adult survivors of child sexual abuse*. CA:Sage, Thousand Oaks

Starck P, McGovern J, eds. (1992) *The hidden dimension of illness: Human suffering*. National League for Nursing Press, New York

Waites E (1993) *Trauma and survival: Posttraumatic and dissociative disorders in women*. W W Norton, New York

Whitfield C (1995) *Memory and abuse: Remembering and healing the effects of trauma*. Health Communications Inc, Deerfield Beach, FL

For partners and parents

Crowley P (1990) *Not my child: A mother confronts her child's sexual abuse*. Avon Books, New York

Davis L (1991) *Allies in healing: When the person you love was sexually abused as a child*. Harper Perennial, New York

Dympna House Collective (1990) *Facing the unthinkable*. Dympna House Inc, Haberfield, New South Wales

Gil E (1992) *Our growing the pain together: A book for spouses and partners of adults abused as children*. Dell Trade Paperback, New York

Hooper C (1992) *Mothers surviving child sexual assault*. Tavistock/Routledge, London

For children

Adams C, Fay J (1981) *No more secrets*. Impact, San Luis Obispo, CA

Blank J, Quackenbush M (1986). *A kid's first book about sex*. Five Mile Press, Hawthorn, Victoria

Freeman L (1987) *It's my body*. Parenting Press, Seattle

Hessell J (1987) *What's wrong with bottoms?* Century Hutchinson, Auckland

Johnsen K (1986) *The trouble with secrets*. Parenting Press, Seattle

Kehoe P (1987) *Something happened to me and I'm scared to tell*. Parenting Press, Seattle

Marsh J (1988) *Incest info. for girls*, 2 edn. J S McMillan, Sydney

Otto M (1987) *Tom doesn't visit us anymore*. Women's Educational Press, Toronto

Seuss Dr (1993) *Oh! The places you'll go*. Random House, New York

Sweet P(1986). *Something happened to me*. Boobook Publications, Balgowlah, NSW

References

American Psychiatric Association (1994) *Diagnostic and statistical manual of mental disorders*, 4 edn. American Psychiatric Press, Washington

Angus G, Hall G (1996) *Child abuse and neglect in Australia, 1994–5*. Child Welfare Series No. 16. Australian Institute of Health and Welfare, Canberra

Briere J (1996) *Therapy for adults molested as children: Beyond survival*, 2 edn. Springer Publishing Company, New York

Burgess A, Holstrom L (1975) Assessing trauma in the rape victim. *Am J Nurs* **75**(8): 1288–90

Conroy P (1992) *The Prince of Tides*. Bantam Books, New York

Contole J (1981) Coming home. *Knox Prem Support Group Newsletter*, no. 3

Critchley C (1996) Girls suffer more abuse. *The Melbourne Herald-Sun*, July 27

Everly G (1995) citing a paper by Henry J (1993) Alexithymia and PTSD. In: Everly G, Lating J, eds. *Psychotraumatology: Key papers and core concepts in post-traumatic stress*. Plenum Press, New York

Finkelhor D, Hotaling G, Lewis I, Smith C (1990) Sexual abuse in a national survey of adult men and women: Prevalence, characteristics and risk factors. *Child Abuse Neg* **14**: 19–28

Fleming J (1997) Prevalence of child sexual abuse in a community sample of Australian women. *Med J Aus* **166**: 65–8

Goldberg J, Taylor P (1988) *Premature infants: Their continuing care at home*. Longman Cheshire, Melbourne

Goldman R, Goldman J (1986) *Children's sexual thinking*. Routledge and Kegan Paul, London

Hennessy M, Polk-Warner G (1990) Case study of pseudocyesis: Consideration of the diagnosis of sexual abuse. *Nurs Prac* **2**: 31–2

Herman J (1992) *Trauma and recovery: The aftermath of violence — from domestic abuse to political terror*. Basic Books, New York

Holz K (1994) A practical approach to clients who are survivors of childhood sexual abuse. *J Nurse Midwif* **39**(1): 13–18

Jackson C (1991) *Multiple personality disorder*. Paper presented at the Australian & New Zealand Association of Psychiatry, Psychology and Law Conference, Melboure University, November

Jackson C (1994) *We do have that problem here — MPD in Australia*. Paper presented at Western Clinical Conference of the Orange County Association for Multiple Personality and Dissociation 7th Annual Conference, Costa Mesa, CA, April 14–17

Jackson C (1995) *Dissociation and traumatic memory*. Paper presented at the Australian Association of Trauma and Dissociation 4th Annual Conference, Melbourne, Sept. 15

Jackson C (1996) Dangerous secrets: What it means to be labelled MPD. Unpublished master's thesis, RMIT Faculty of Nursing

Kilptrick D, Edmunds C, Seymour A (1992) *Rape in America: A report to the nation*. National Victim Center, Arlington, VA

Kitzinger J (1990) Recalling the pain. *Nurs Times* **86**(3): 38–40

Kluft R, ed (1985) *Childhood Antecedents of Multiple Personality*. American Psychiatric Press, Washington, DC

Light-Saraf (Producer), Light A (Director). (1993). *Dialogues with madwomen*. (Film)

Long S (1986) Guidelines for treating young children. In: MacFarlane K, Waterman J, Conerly S, Damon L, Durfee M, Long S, eds. *Sexual abuse of young children*. Cassell, London: 225–30

MacArthur B, Dezoete A (1992) *Early Beginnings: Development in Children Born Preterm*. OUP, Auckland

McCann L, Peralman L (1993) Vicarious traumatizations: The emotional cost of working with survivors. *Treat Abuse Today* **3**(5): 28–31

Miller L (1990) Psychotic denial of pregnancy: Phenomenology and clinical management. *Hos Comm Psychiatry* **41**(11): 1233–7

Nicholson J, Geller J, Fisher W (1996) "Sylvia Frumkin" has a baby: A case study for policymakers. *Psychiatr Serv* **47**(5): 497–501

Parratt J (1993) *Survivors of Incest, Their Experiences and Feelings During Childbirth*. Paper presented at the National Midwives Conference, Adelaide

Putnam F (1989) *Diagnosis and treatment of multiple personality disorder*. Guilford, New York

Rivera M (1991) Multiple personality disorder and the social systems: 185 cases. *Dissociation* **4**(2): 79–82

Rolls E, O'Mara J (1993) Neurophysiological and theoretical analysis of how the primate hippocampus functions in memory. In: Ono T, Fuhada M, Squire L, Raichie J, Perrett D, eds. *Brain Mechanisms in Perception and Memory*. OUP, Oxford: 276–300

Seng J, Petersen B (1995) Incorporating routine screening for history of childhood sexual abuse into well-woman and maternity care. *J Nurse Midwif* **40**(1), 26–9

Sparshott M (1997) *Pain, Distress and the Newborn Baby*. Blackwell Science, London

Spielvogel A, Hohener H (1995) Denial of pregnancy: A review and case reports. *Birth* **22**(4): 220–6

Steingard S, Frankel F (1985) Dissociation and psychotic symptoms. *Am J Psychiatry* **142**: 953–5

Tomison A (1996) Protecting children: Updating the national picture. *Nat Child Protect Clear House Newslett* **4**(2): 4–6

van der Hart O, Faure H, van Gerven M, Goodwin J (1991) Unawareness and denial of pregnancy in patients with MPD. *Dissociation* **4**(2): 60–73

van der Kolk B (1996) Trauma and memory. In: van der Kolk B, McFarlane A, Weisaeth L, eds. *Traumatic Stress: The effects of Overwhelming Experience on Mind, Body and Society*. Guildford, New York: 279–302

van der Leden M, Raskin V (1993) Psychological sequelae of childhood sexual abuse: Relevant in subsequent pregnancy. *Am J Obstetr Gynecol* **168**(4): 1336–7

Whitfield C (1995) *Memory and Abuse: Remembering and Healing the Effects of Trauma*. Health Communications Inc, Deerfield Beach, FL

Williams L (1994) Recall of childhood trauma: A prospective study of women's memories of childhood sexual abuse. *J Consult Clin Psychol* **62**(6): 1167–76

Wolff P (1987) *The development of behavioral states and the expression of emotions in early infancy*. Unversity of Chicago Press, Chicago

9

Participatory action research project on the needs of women survivors of sexual abuse

Gloria Geller

Introduction

A variety of studies conducted in the recent past have found the prevalence of child sexual abuse to be more common than was previously thought to be the case (Report of the Committee on Sexual Offences Against Children and Youths, 1984). The devastating effects of child sexual abuse in the immediate and long-term periods have been coming to light in recent years (Finkelhor *et al*, 1986; Geller, 1991; Bagley and King, 1991). The Report of the Committee on Sexual Offences Against Children and Youths found that approximately one in two females and one in three males have been victims of unwanted sexual acts and about four in five of the incidents occurred when they were children or youths. Finkelhor *et al* (1986) note that sexual abuse had a 'noxious' impact on the victim, in the immediate and long-term periods.

In a study conducted by the author, primarily in Saskatchewan, women who had been sexually abused as children and youths identified a wide range of reactions to the abuse. Such reactions to their abuse included feeling fear, suicidal, angry, unsafe, isolated and distrustful. The women said they had withdrawn from other people, blamed themselves for the abuse and that they suffered from low self-esteem (Geller, 1991). The long- term effects of the abuse included: abuse of drugs and/or alcohol; eating disorders; a history of psychiatric hospitalisations; depressions; suicide attempts; insomnia; anxiety/panic attacks; dissociation; nightmares and flashbacks to the abuse experiences. Respondents also said they had relationship difficulties due to their lack of trust.

A history of exposure to severe trauma in childhood, both sexual and physical forms, often results in post-traumatic stress disorder (PTSD). Symptoms of PTSD include insomnia, sexual dysfunction, dissociation, anger, suicidality, self-harm, drug addiction/alcoholism (Matsakis, 1992; Gil, 1988). Dissociation is one of the means by which victims and survivors of child sexual abuse have learned to deal with sexual abuse (Gil, 1988). Dissociation is a disturbance of alteration in the functions of identity, memory or consciousness. Three types of dissociative disorders include multiple personality disorder, depersonalisation and psychogenic amnesia and psychogenic fugue. Dissociative disorders include phenomena, such as feelings of reality replaced by feelings of unreality; memory of important events or specific time periods that cannot be recalled (Gil, 1988); and/or the development of two or more distinct personalities or personality states within an individual, which at some time take full control of the individual's behaviour (Herman, 1992; Gil, 1988).

With the increasing evidence of the prevalence and detrimental effects of child sexual abuse throughout the life of the survivor, it is also evident that the cost of responding to the needs of survivors to the healthcare system is significant. The Canadian Panel on Violence Against Women (1993) reported that there is a significant cost to the healthcare system resulting from the misdiagnosis of thousands of women in Canada who receive inappropriate medical care. Another study (Rivera, 1991) noted that individuals dealing with dissociative disorders who had been sexually abused in childhood had been treated on the average for 6.8 years before an accurate diagnosis was made. An example in this study was given of a woman who spent more than 227 months in the healthcare system at the cost of $870,000 (£350,000). Once correctly diagnosed, the 18 months of treatment cost $21,903 (£8600). The high cost of untreated dissociative individuals is compounded by the cost of drug and alcohol abuse treatment, social assistance payments to individuals not able to work consistently prior to appropriate treatment, child welfare and legal costs.

Evidence of the long-term effects of child sexual abuse and concerns that many survivors of sexual abuse who are using social, health and justice systems are often misdiagnosed and/or do not receive help to deal with their abuse, influenced the author's decision to undertake a needs assessment on women survivors of sexual abuse. This chapter addresses the process of undertaking this participatory action research project, presents key findings of the needs assessment and discusses the efforts the working group have taken to seek changes in the nature and type of services available to women survivors of sexual abuse in Regina.

Participatory action research 'Partners'

The dissociative disorders working group (DDWG) was formed in 1994 after a week-long workshop held in Regina on dissociation and multiple personality. A number of people working with survivors felt isolated with no one to call on to discuss issues. Professionals had limited opportunities in the local community to debrief and consult. They experienced considerable difficulty obtaining diagnosis and/or treatment options in the community. Furthermore, group members felt that survivors with dissociative behaviours were not receiving appropriate or adequate service and at times were revictimised by the medical model of treatment. The working group's initial goal was to provide a coordinated interagency approach to services for women survivors of sexual abuse.

Meanwhile, the Social Administration Research Unit (SARU) submitted a proposal to the Health Services Utilization Research Commission in the Spring of 1994 to undertake a needs assessment on women's mental health services needs. The needs assessment would be focused on the Regina Health District and would endeavour to expand upon the 1993 report to the Regina Health Board by the Mental Health Working Committee which did not address women's mental health services needs. The report did, however, state that there was a need for appropriate service delivery models to address physical, emotional and sexual abuse and that services were inadequate and fragmented (Mental Health Working Committee, 1993). The report also noted the need for research and evaluation of mental health services. When seed funding was made available to pursue research on the mental health services needs of women, it was decided to use these funds to undertake a needs assessment on women survivors of sexual abuse.

In the winter of 1995, the Dissociative Disorders Working Group called a meeting to discuss a needs assessment. The author advised the members at the meeting of her intention to do such a needs assessment. At that meeting a decision was made to work together on a needs assessment.

Methodology

Survey and focus groups with service providers

A list of 82 community service providers was drawn from among individuals known to be working with survivors, in public health and community based organisations. All the service providers received a questionnaire and consent form in the mail together with an invitation to attend a day-long focus group needs assessment to be held May 26, 1995, at the University of Regina (Geller and MacNeil, 1996).

The DDWG supplied the names of service providers, helped to design the focus group format, reviewed and helped adapt a similar survey undertaken in Saskatoon by the Saskatoon Inter- agency Council (Watkinson, 1994). The DDWG group members facilitated the small group focus group discussions. Once a first draft of the findings had been completed, the DDWG supplied feedback on the document and the recommendations to be made, based on the research.

The questionnaire (completed by 38 of the 82 people it was distributed to) was designed to:

1. describe the level of service offered to survivors based on the role of each agency;
2. determine the main approaches used by agencies providing direct and indirect survivor services;
3. identify the difficulties service providers encounter working with survivors; and
4. examine service areas in need of development, or existing services in need of improvement.

The focus groups for service providers was structured to collect data about the needs of women survivors and the services available to them. Thirty-five people of the 82 service providers, who were invited to the all-day event, participated in the focus groups. Of this number, 18 service providers had also completed the questionnaire. In all, 50 service providers were involved in the needs assessment. The goals of the focus group meeting were to:

1. identify problems service providers encounter in addressing the needs of women survivors of childhood sexual abuse;
2. do a needs assessment and identify gaps in the service delivery system;
3. discuss service delivery models.

Four groups worked together throughout the day in order to respond to questions concerning the needs of women survivors of sexual abuse. Along with the facilitator, each group also had a researcher who took notes and tape-recorded the discussions. A volunteer from each group recorded the key issues from each group on a flip chart. The following were the items discussed by each group:

1. discuss and identify problems service providers and others experience when dealing with women survivors of childhood sexual abuse. The goal of this question was to establish the context in which each participant works and to identify the problems they encounter;
2. discuss what dissociation is with the group and identify the problems service providers encounter when working with women survivors who experience dissociation;
3. discuss and identify the needs and gaps in services provided to survivors and those with dissociative disorders;
4. discuss service delivery models used by the participants and identify the approaches they find most useful in dealing with survivors' needs. The goal was to come up with a list of what does and does not work for survivors.

Focus group with survivors of sexual abuse

In order to obtain some input from survivors of child sexual abuse, the facilitator of a self-help group for women survivors of child sexual abuse was contacted. An arrangement was made for the author to meet with the group and talk to them about the needs assessment. A meeting was held in March 1995, as part of their regular group meeting time. An arrangement was made to conduct the needs assessment in May 1995. The group would start earlier than usual and pizza and drinks would be supplied.

The eleven women who attended the survivor meeting were asked to voluntarily participate in the focus group meeting and to sign a consent form. Before responding to any questions, the purpose of the focus group meeting was explained. It was made clear that the information they provided during the meeting was confidential and that they could refuse to answer any questions. Ethics approval had been obtained from the University of Regina Ethics Committee prior to conducting this research.

Women were also asked to fill in a survivor questionnaire, similar to one created by the Saskatoon Interagency Council (1994), and return it to their group facilitator within the following two weeks. Seven of the 11 questionnaires were returned.

Two open-ended, unstructured questions were asked of the women attending the focus group meeting. Each woman was asked to tell the story of her abuse experiences, describing the help she sought at the time of the abuse, or at some later time, from whom she sought help, what was helpful and what was not helpful. The second question concerned what kind of help survivors need, what would have helped them at the time of their abuse and what services they currently required.

The context for this focus group was a supportive one since the group had been meeting for some time and most of the women knew one another. An effort was made to focus on the help the women had sought and obtained rather than on the abuse experience(s). Nevertheless, the sharing of this information raised strong emotions for all those in attendance, including the researchers. It is crucial that when such information is gathered support is available to participants.

Limitations of the needs assessment

The information gathered for this needs assessment came from a cross-section of the Regina community of service providers working with survivors of sexual abuse. Our sample was a stratified one and did not represent the whole range of individuals, groups and organisations working in this area, in particular the medical and psychiatric community. However, it is believed that the results of the needs assessment is useful for the identification of needs of women survivors of sexual abuse in the Regina Health District and it is likely to be relevant to other communities in the province.

A relatively small group of survivors is included in this report. While a more detailed evaluation of services available to survivors, based on their experiences, would more accurately reflect their needs, the facts are that the author has previously conducted detailed interviews with survivors. The Saskatoon Interagency Needs Assessment includes the views of survivors, and there is a growing body of information about survivors and their needs. Therefore, this needs assessment builds on existing knowledge.

Research findings

For the purposes of this chapter, some of the significant findings of this project are presented, including:

1. the gaps in service that were identified by survey respondents;
2. problems identified by focus groups;
3. needs of survivors who experience dissociation;
4. issues with respect to service delivery models; and
5. some information obtained from the focus group with survivors of abuse.

Gaps in services identified by survey respondents

Those who completed the questionnaires identified a wide range of gaps in services in the Regina Health District in the following areas.

1. *Counselling services*

- immediate, long-term and follow-up counselling
- easy access to affordable services and counsellors, elimination of waiting lists
- supportive counselling
- financial support to women to attend counselling and support groups
- trained and experienced therapists and cooperative psychiatrists able to deal with survivors.

2. *Services to a variety of populations*

- culturally appropriate services, including native-focussed counsellors
- services for survivors who experience dissociation and multiple personalities
- services for male survivors of sexual abuse
- specialised practitioners in the area of multiple personalities
- services for survivors' families

3. *Assessment, diagnosis and integrated services*

- correct diagnoses of sexually abused women who have been misdiagnosed with long-term, chronic mental illness such as schizophrenia
- good, knowledgeable psychiatrists to assist with dual diagnosis in women
- unified treatment approach from initial crisis management stage to long-term support and counselling services
- analysis and diagnosis of abuse issues early in treatment of all women seeking services, especially in dissociation treatment
- more social work/psychological staffing in psychiatric units to provide adequate case management.

4. *Specific approaches*

- more understanding and awareness by physicians, psychiatrists and counsellors and better education of service providers — courses do not provide a practical clinical focus that could assist individuals through the healing process
- a safe place for women to receive counselling outside the medical system
- a non-medical approach to severe trauma caused by abuse
- a more holistic approach to healing — many survivors have had too much concentrated cognitive work while their affect remains primarily unhealed
- self-help models to move through crisis when ready
- more counsellors with a feminist perspective who have knowledge of dissociative disorders
- coordinated and unified service approach with communication between agencies providing services using a client-centred model

5. *Residential services*

- long-term residential care where women have the opportunity to build a healthy life-style
- a safe house for women experiencing dissociation/MPD
- stabilisation/crisis hostel rather than hospitals
- YWCA provides accommodations for women discharged from hospital, but does not receive funding for supportive services.

Focus groups with service providers

Those who participated in focus groups identified a number of problems in their efforts to respond to survivors of sexual abuse. These are discussed below. The needs of survivors who experience dissociation are also presented and the most and least effective approaches to responding to the needs of survivors are indicated.

1. *Problems identified by focus groups*

a) Inability of existing services to respond adequately to women survivors of abuse.

Many agencies and organisations that offer services in the community do not have the mandate, resources and capability of adequately serving women survivors of abuse. Shelters for battered women find that many of the women and children they serve have been sexually abused. Generally speaking, the shelters do not specialise in treating survivors of sexual abuse, nor do they provide follow-up services for women who have left the shelters. Survivors with multiple personalities are viewed as being inappropriate clients in shelters.

It was noted that there are numerous barriers to accessing services by survivors and that service providers frequently must advocate on behalf of survivors in order to obtain services. Fragmentation of services are barriers for survivors seeking to obtain services. Isolation, divide-and-conquer and trust issues were viewed as being the causes of this fragmentation, making it difficult for service providers to work together.

b) Inappropriate and inadequate models/ approaches in current usage in dealing with women survivors of abuse

Many concerns were expressed by respondents about the use of the medical model as an approach to helping women survivors of sexual abuse. An assumption of the medical model is that people do not know what they need and come to the doctor to be diagnosed and treated. The feminist approach tends to assume that the client does know what her needs are. This approach seeks to empower the client to take control over her own life.

It was felt that psychiatric diagnosis and labels can be harmful, since those so labelled often take on the label as their identity. It was felt that psychiatrists, in general, do not have the understanding, knowledge and time to deal with survivors. It was also felt that the work done by counsellors in community agencies is not given the proper recognition by medical and psychiatric professionals.

Another issue raised in this area concerns the fact that sexual abuse is viewed as a secondary issue to other presenting problems, such as depression and addictions. The tendency is to deal with these symptoms of depression, addiction, etc, rather than the underlying problem, the abuse.

A further issue concerns the fact that the current emphasis on brief or short-term counselling within the mental health system and through employee assistance programmes, does not recognise the needs of survivors of abuse for access to long-term counselling. Many survivors experience periods of ongoing crisis and require a range of services over a long period of time. It was felt that the pressure to change within a few sessions revictimises people who want to heal.

c) Inadequate and insufficient understanding and knowledge of the effects of trauma and inadequate training and educating in dealing with women survivors of sexual abuse

Several respondents indicated that workers in their agencies were not trained to deal with sexual abuse, even though they had to work with survivors in their jobs. The primary problems identified in this area are the lack of knowledge of the long-term effects of trauma by mental health professionals and the lack of training of service providers to deal with abuse.

d) Issues concerning dissociative disorders

Within the mental health system in Regina there has been disbelief, particularly among psychiatrists, in multiple personality disorder as a phenomenon. Respondents said there is a lack of support from the mental health system for service providers who work with survivors who exhibit dissociation. There is a lack of training, information and understanding about dissociative disorders.

e) Problems of specific populations of women

Different populations present different types of problems when the issue of sexual abuse is considered. Street women who have been sexually abused may give greater priority to such things as life skills, education and family issues rather than focus specifically on sexual abuse. Sexually abused adolescents whose abuse is reported to the Department of Social Services are forced to disclose to a number of people, which makes them shut down. It also takes a long time for the Department to respond to reports of sexual abuse.

Another issue concerns that of addictions, a common problem among women who have been abused. These women require services responsive to both the abuse and the addiction. Rural women lack resources and services. Often, they have special needs that include transportation and childcare if they are to access services.

Native women have special needs as well. The models and approaches used in the mainstream, including the medical model, often do not incorporate the values of native culture and philosophy. Native people will go to a sweat lodge and to elders for healing rather than to a non-native male. It was stated that doctors and psychologists do not understand cultural healing approaches such as sweat lodges, Sundance ceremonies and spiritual healing circles.

f) Parenting issues

The generational effects of abuse become apparent as women survivors endeavour to raise their own children. Young mothers who have been abused often do not know how to care for their children. Native people may have lost some of their ability to parent when they were taken from their families and communities and placed in residential schools. Large numbers of mothers of children who have been sexually abused have themselves been abused. Finding out about their children's sexual abuse may bring a flood of memories about their own sexual abuse. In crisis, some mothers are not able to care for their children and children are taken into foster care. There is no safe place for the whole family to go when mothers are in crisis.

2. Needs of survivors who experience dissociation

As is evident from the name of the group, the Dissociative Disorders Working Group, the needs of both the women who experience dissociation and the service providers who work with them are of particular concern. Questions were addressed to the needs of this group as part of the focus group discussions. A one-page handout gave a definition and indicators of multiple personality. People who are dissociative may or may not have full-blown multiple personality in which there are at least two personalities that take full control of the person's behaviour at times. A variety of symptoms related to dissociation and multiple personality were indicated in the handout, including various kinds of behaviour symptoms, amnesia symptoms, process symptoms, previous experiences with the psychiatric system, affective symptoms, post-traumatic stress symptoms and somatoform symptoms.

In our data-gathering process, it was important to identify needs and gaps in services for survivors who are dissociative. These include:

a) Information, knowledge and training

A general framework is needed to educate people with dissociative disorders about themselves as well as to educate service providers, and the broader community. It was noted that local psychiatrists were reluctant to confirm a dissociative disorder diagnosis, preferring to diagnose a mental illness such as schizophrenia instead.

b) Resource and services

Extensive services were identified including:

- assessment of people with dissociation and multiple personality
- crisis services, especially for those on long waiting lists who may have suicidal impulses
- a safe place to receive help, be nurtured, express their emotions and heal
- referral services
- psychiatric service
- funds to finance therapy
- support groups
- support for service providers who work with dissociative survivors.

3. *Service delivery models*

A discussion of service delivery models ended the day's discussion. If the needs of survivors of abuse are to be met, it is important to ensure that the services to be provided are effective. Many of the respondents were critical of an approach that is based upon the medical model, one in which a 'patient' comes in with 'symptoms', which are then 'diagnosed', and a 'treatment plan' is developed in order to 'cure' the patient. It is important to recognise that survivors of abuse are not mentally ill, but are survivors of a violation of their very beings. For some years now, more effective approaches to working with survivors of abuse and people exhibiting symptoms of post-traumatic stress have been developed. We present below a summary of what the respondents identified as effective methods as compared to least effective ones.

Effective service delivery approaches

- a safe house or shelter that is community based and has a multidisciplinary team and a flexible approach
- a client-centred approach that involves survivors in determining what their needs are
- feminist models are effective. Aboriginal approaches are effective, as are approaches that are holistic and empowering of the individual
- approaches that are culturally sensitive
- creative approaches that include music, movement, body work, art and play therapy, guiding imagery, and bio-psychosocial approaches are effective
- a wide range of therapeutic choices that are accessible. Different approaches addressing a wide range of issues at different times are effective.

Least effective service delivery approaches

- the medical model is considered to be the least effective model for working with women survivors of abuse
- short-term intervention is not effective
- cognitive approaches may not be helpful. Long-term trauma is embedded at the cellular level and belief systems are fairly entrenched
- traditional addiction treatment
- power imbalance in therapeutic relationship.

Focus groups with survivors of abuse

Data gathered from the survey completed by survivors of abuse include: demographic information about the women, information about the abuser, help sought, effects of the abuse, services accessed and legal advice required. In the focus group process women's help-seeking experiences were offered by each woman. Each woman's story is included in the needs assessment report. The women were given an opportunity to read this part of the report and to suggest any changes to their particular stories. A summary of their help-seeking efforts is included here.

The women had sought help from immediate family members and friends, from health care professionals and from counsellors. It was very rare for the police and the criminal justice system to be involved. In most cases, unfortunately, the people who they approached did not offer the kind of help that was needed at the time the abuse was occurring or had occurred, so, for the most part, the suffering continued for a long time before help and healing became possible.

For a number of the women the process has been a long and torturous one and the effects of abuse have been far-reaching. Some of the women became pregnant and had children from the abuse. Many had, or continue to have, problems with substance abuse. Some have had extensive involvement with the mental health system. Some have had the unhappy experience of watching yet another generation of their own daughters undergo similar experiences. Help, when it has come, has more often than not come from others who have had similar experiences who offer support and encouragement for healing. Others, after a long period of searching, have finally found a counsellor who has been able to help them. Not all of the women who spoke had, at the time of the focus group, found the help they were seeking.

The women identified a variety of needs they had as children and as adults. Their experiences illustrate the difficulties children have with being heard when they disclose abuse. Family members, the medical profession, members of the public and the general community must be able to respond to the victim when she seeks help.

The women had problems accessing resources and services in Regina. There are long waiting lists and inappropriate and inadequate treatment. Each woman had an opportunity to speak about what she believed victims and survivors need. Overall, the women identified the needs of survivors of abuse to include: counselling services, a holistic treatment model, competent well-trained therapists, residential and crisis services, community-based services, safe places for children, education for the public, survivors, victims and professionals.

Recommendations

There are 21 recommendations made in the needs assessment report (Geller and MacNeil, 1996). These were grouped according to the six key problem areas indicated above, which emphasized the inadequacy of existing services to respond to survivors of abuse, including women who were dissociative. Two specific recommendations were made to the Regina District Health Board with respect to actions to be taken. These recommendations are:

> *That the Regina District Health Board participate and assist in the development of a women's wellness centre. The Centre would incorporate: assessment; individual and group counselling; 24-hour crisis service; a safe, short-term residential setting; parent programs; support, individual and group counselling for children; support, education and counselling for partners and family members; use of a multi-disciplinary, holistic approach supported by appropriately trained personnel.*
>
> *That the Regina District Health Board appoint the Dissociative Disorders Working Group to head a task force to implement a cost-benefit analysis and develop a women's wellness centre in Regina.*

Actions following from the needs assessment

Copies of a draft of the needs assessment were sent to members of inpatient psychiatric services in Regina. A meeting was called between the Dissociative Disorders Working Group, the author and members of in-patient psychiatric services, including the chief psychiatrist for Regina, the head nurse of the Regina General Hospital and social workers from the General Hospital and the Pasqua Hospital. At the meeting on October 1, 1996, it was agreed by those representing in-patient psychiatric services that many women survivors of sexual abuse who entered the hospital could be better served in a community facility and that there was a need for such a facility and services in Regina. The representatives from psychiatric services were not prepared to endorse the needs assessment, especially since there remains considerable disagreement concerning the diagnosis of dissociation and multiple personalities. It was decided that a two-page brief should be written and distributed among those who had attended the meeting.

A copy of the needs assessment, together with the brief, was submitted to all the board members of the Regina District Health Board and a presentation was made to the board on February 27, 1997. In June 1997, the Regina District Health Board appointed a task force to review the services available and the gaps in the services for women and men survivors of sexual abuse in the health district. A number of those who were appointed to the task force had participated in the needs assessment. One representative of the DDWG was asked to sit on this committee. An initial report was to be presented in October 1997.

In addition, at a meeting in May of the Dissociative Disorders Working Group, after some discussion about establishing a safe place in an existing residential service for abused women, the group members agreed to develop a proposal to establish a residential crisis service for women survivors of abuse. At the time of writing, work has commenced on this proposal.

Conclusion

The need for a residential centre, outside the hospital, for women survivors of abuse who are in crisis, has been recognised as a need across the country. Several attempts have been made by women's groups and coalitions to establish such residences, but up to this point it has been very difficult to obtain the necessary funds. In one situation, in Prince Edward Island, a building was obtained, but the group has not been able to locate operating funds to maintain the residence and so the building is being used for other purposes. In Saskatoon, Tamara's House, has been seeking funds to establish a residence for several years. Tamara's House has office space in which a variety of programs are offered to survivors of sexual abuse, but a building is not yet in the offing.

An important issue for those involved with this project has been the implicit desire to establish alternative services for women survivors of sexual abuse that offer feminist services. At a time when women's services have become somewhat more mainstream and when funding for mental health and social services have been greatly downsized, feminist approaches to working with women, long proven to be very effective for many women, are under considerable stress from the backlash that exists in various sectors of the community. One of the challenges faced by groups, such as the DDWG, is that efforts are made to reach out to the traditional mental health and social services sectors, and that services offered should empower women toward healing from a history of childhood sexual abuse. The fact that the group has decided to work towards establishing a pilot project for women in crisis is an important step in ensuring some level of autonomy in determining what are the needs of women. At the same time, the fact that the District Health Board has responded to the recommendation for a task force to look into the needs of survivors of abuse in the Regina Health District indicates that this participatory action research project has been effective in influencing this decision. This process has been an empowering one to those of us seeking to improve the ways in which women's mental health needs are responded to in our community.

References

Bagley C, King K (1991) *Child sexual abuse: The search for healing*. Tavistock/Routledge, London and New York

Canadian Panel on Violence Against Women (1993) *Changing the Landscape: Ending Violence — Achieving Equality*. Ottawa

Committee on Sexual Offences Against Children and Youth (1984) Sexual offences against children and youth, vol 1. *The Badgely Report*. Canadian Government Publishing Centre, Ottawa

Finkelhor D *et al* (1986) *A Sourcebook on Child Sexual Abuse*. Sage Publications, Beverly Hills

Geller G (1991) *Justice for women victims and survivors of abuse*. Occasional Paper No. 4. Social Administration Research Unit, Regina

Geller G, MacNeil D (1996) *Needs assessment: Mental health services needs of women survivors of sexual abuse*. Social Administration Research Unit, Regina

Gil E (1988) *Treatment of Adult Survivors of Childhood Abuse*. Launch Press, Walnut Creek, CA

Herman JL (1992) *Trauma and Recovery: The Aftermath of Violence from Domestic Abuse to Political Terror*. Basic Books, USA

Matsakis A (1992) *I can't get over it: A Handbook for Trauma Survivors*. New Harbinger Publications Inc, Oakland, CA

Mental Health Working Committee (1993) *Report to the Health Board*. Regina, Saskatchewan

Rivera M (1991) *Multiple Personality: An Outcome of Abuse*. Education/Dissociation, Toronto

Watkinson AM (1994) *A Report on the Needs of Adult Survivors of Child Sexual Abuse in the Saskatoon District*. Saskatoon Interagency on Survivor Services, Saskatoon, Saskatchewan

10

VON People in crisis program: Highlights of a working manual

Joan Wagner, Shirley Yakimishyn, Tessa Merry, Sharlene Wolbeck and Donna Zachariah

Introduction

The Victorian Order of Nurses (VON) (Edmonton Branch) People in Crisis (PIC) Program provides client-driven nursing services to various shelters and agencies in the Edmonton community. This health facilitation occurs at the level of the individual, the family, the agency serving them (ie. the shelter that VON contracts with) or the community. PIC staff participate in various community coalitions that serve to bring involved agencies together with a common voice to respond to pertinent issues related to violence and abuse. Active involvement with community coalitions, such as the Edmonton Council Against Family Violence, Edmonton Council against Child Abuse and Neglect and the Interagency Committee on Spousal Abuse, further illustrate the various levels at which client-driven interventions happen under the mandate of the PIC Program.

History of Edmonton People in Crisis

The PIC program originated due to the vision and foresight of a volunteer board member. At the time that the first Women in Need (WIN) shelter for abused women opened in Edmonton, Daisy Wilson served on both the VON board of directors and the board of the Edmonton Women's Shelter. She recognised the shelter residents' need for nursing service. As a result, in 1979, the VON began providing nursing service to WIN House for one hour per week. Service was increased to one afternoon per week with the opening of the second WIN House.

WIN House was established by concerned community members and operated with the assistance of a volunteer board of directors. Funding was obtained through fundraising projects, charitable donations and other non-governmental sources. Small amounts of government funding have become available to the shelters over the years.

In 1984, the Safe Place women's shelter opened and requested and received similar nursing services from the VON. Over the next 10 years, other community agencies with volunteer boards of directors requested the specialised VON service:

- the Youth Emergency Shelter
- WINGS, a second-stage housing for battered women
- Lurana Family Center, an overflow shelter for battered women; now a well-used shelter called Lurana Shelter
- Atonement Home, for abused and neglected children apprehended by Child Welfare (transferred to Boyle Street Co-op in 1996 and now known as Stepping Stones)
- group programming to women and their children leaving WINGS for independent living (developed at the request of the women)
- a VON primary health clinic in the Boyle Street Co-op (initially intended to serve youth but eventually opened to all)

Two innovative publications on family violence were also completed during this time period: *Trust Is the Key* (November 1992) and *From Victim to Advocate* (May 1995).

Funding

VON donated the nurse's time to the WIN Houses from 1979 to 1984, since there was no additional shelter funding available. With the opening of the second WIN House and the request for a similar nursing service for Safe Place, VON applied to the United Way for funding. The Edmonton United Way has been funding the PIC Program since 1985. In 1991, with a small grant from VON Alberta, and later from NOVA Corporation, a primary health clinic was opened in the Boyle Street Co-op.

Services provided to clients through the PIC Program

Meeting the health needs of abused women

To survive on a day-to-day basis in an abusive relationship, women may be forced to neglect both their own and their children's health. In addition, nurses working in the shelters find that many women who have been abused experience feelings of anxiety, panic or depression, or have stress-related illnesses that are directly related to the abuse they experienced. They frequently complain of headaches, insomnia and chronic fatigue. An example of a severe case of forced neglect is a battered woman whose husband abandoned her in the country with her sick children without any means of communication or transportation. Some women experience complications in pregnancy as a result of abuse; others have contracted sexually transmitted diseases (STDs) from an abusive partner. They may find out that he was unfaithful when they discover they have an STD. Many women have sought medical help for distress in the past and have been discouraged by attitudes, previous negative experiences with medication or a feeling that they have not been listened to by professionals. VON nurses have found that women want to become informed health care consumers.

Effects of abuse on children

Abuse can affect children in many different ways. A child may be diagnosed as having an attention deficit disorder or hyperactivity as a direct result of the abusive environment. Some- times a young child may imitate his father and hit and call his mother abusive names or be abusive to his siblings. Many children come to the shelter sick with colds, influenza, running noses, asthma, rashes, diarrhoea and middle-ear infections. Abused children do not have the opportunity to learn decision-making skills, or to feel a sense of autonomy or self-efficacy.

The VON nurse recognises the child as client, and thus the child's self-knowledge is encouraged, believed and respected. The children are encouraged by the nurse to make decisions about their own health and self. The nurse works to promote achievement of these and other developmental milestones in every interaction with children. Mothers and children may seek specific help, a referral from the nurse or may need to review what has happened, what has worked in the past and what has not, and make an informed decision after exploring all available options.

The VON nurse works with parents and centre staff as part of the team at Stepping Stones to identify risky health situations, to prevent illness and injury, and to promote health and well-being of families and individuals. With the help of talented VON volunteers, VON nurses facilitate weekly health support (research-based play therapy) groups for the children. These groups serve a number of functions, encouraging emotional expression, providing opportunities for building self-esteem and managing stress, as well as giving all the children an opportunity to receive attention and nurturing from the nurse without having to be 'sick'.

Meeting the needs of youth

VON nurses work as part of the team with Youth Emergency Shelter staff to provide service to and advocate for youth aged 16 to 18 years. Many of these teenagers are products of violent home environments and may have been victims of physical or sexual abuse at home. Some are suicidal. Many have numerous health concerns. Some require assistance with their medication.

The VON nurses work with staff to provide medication monitoring and guidance on medication use to youths. Ongoing health counselling on pertinent issues, such as diet, hygiene, sexuality and birth control, are important components of nursing time spent in the shelter. The nurse also provides basic physical assessments as required and refers teenagers with concerns to the appropriate health professional. This nursing service has become an invaluable part of the shelter support to youth.

Meeting the needs of men and women in the inner city

Primary healthcare is provided to the individuals who attend the Boyle Street Co-op drop-in centre on a regular basis. These individuals either live in the inner city or use the drop-in centre as an important part of their socialisation. They are frequently living in poverty and have experienced physical, sexual, psychological, emotional or financial abuse. Many are abusing drugs and/or alcohol.

The primary nurse at Boyle Street Co-op describes the focus of care as the client's autonomy: 'their body, their health, their decision, their choice'. Part of the healthcare service provided is regular, free foot care, which has become very important to these people. Years of neglect and poor care have resulted in serious foot problems for many individuals attending the programmes

VON also provides free foot care to clients of Operation Friendship, a centre that provides accommodations for 'hard-to-house' seniors aged 55 years and over who have developed behaviour patterns (alcoholism, violence) that are incompatible with most rental situations.

Provision of health information to shelter clients and staff

Health counselling on issues that are identified as problematic by shelter clients and staff are part of the nurse's daily routine. Some mothers know little about normal child development and others are worried that the child may be delayed because of coming from an abusive environment. An in-depth study of the children 0–18 years of age began in November 1984 at WIN House to identify children's problems and determine the most appropriate interventions to meet their needs. VON was asked to help with the project by providing Denver Development Screening Tests (DDSTs) for the children aged six years and under. An increase to almost a full-time nurse was a direct result of this testing process and the identification of their health needs. DDST screening is still done at the mother's request and the testing has been proven useful to introduce discussion. The mothers and children enjoy the DDST, which offers opportunities for mothers to ask for further information about toilet training, feeding problems, immunisations and behavioural management.

In addition to the health counselling offered to women and children at WINGS, the VON nurse facilitates a weekly health group that offers a wide range of topics ranging from women's health issues, nutrition, AIDS, to self-esteem and stress management. Since many women and children have difficulty sleeping, relaxation training is offered for those who are interested.

VON nurses provide in-services to shelter staff and volunteers and help staff set up health-related programming and policy. Examples are communicable disease programmes and medication workshops, which are all accompanied by staff in-services. In-services are given on mental health issues, including stress management, depression, suicide and any other health topic requested by shelter staff. Values clarification workshops have also been provided.

Family violence education to the community

VON Edmonton also works with other agencies within the community, upon invitation, to provide family violence education. This education occurs through oral presentations, written articles and provision of educational opportunities. The Office of the Prevention of Family Violence has supported two VON health education initiatives: partial funding for developing the *Trust Is the Key* manual and funding for developing a workshop, both for nurses and other health professionals dealing with family violence. VON Alberta supported development of a health promotion package for abused women's groups called *From Victim to Advocate.*

The VON PIC program provides clinical placements for nursing students in their final year of the master's degree program at the University of Alberta. Opportunities to learn group facilitation have also been provided to nursing and counselling students in master's programs. An important component of the community education program has been the provision of guest lectures on family violence at the University of Alberta to degree nursing students in their final year.

Conclusion

The Victorian Order of Nurses (Edmonton) People in Crisis Program has used a 'client-driven' methodology to develop a unique approach to primary nursing within the shelter and agency environment. The nurses have responded to the expressed needs within the community and developed innovative techniques of health facilitation and documentation as demonstrated through the philosophy and standards documented in Appendix A and Appendix B. VON People in Crisis nurses have become recognised expert nurse care providers in the area of domestic violence within the Edmonton community.

Appendix A: Philosophy and standards of PIC Program

Philosophy

A philosophy of continuous improvement is vital to this program. The VON PIC Program is dedicated to the collaboration with others in developing and delivering client-driven nursing services that provide supportive environments where healthy lifestyle changes can occur. Essential philosophical components of these standards include principles of health facilitation, flexibility, trustworthy interactions and recognition of clients as the experts in their lives

Standard 1: Client-driven service

Criteria:

- shared continuous needs assessment, evaluation and adaptation demonstrated in all provider-client relationships (partnership with client, which is an egalitarian relationship — consensus)
- work within the values and beliefs of the client agency
- establish relationships with clients based on mutual respect and dignity.
- flexibility demonstrated throughout all elements of service provision
- confidentiality demonstrated in accordance to client needs and client protection.

Standard 2: Health facilitation

Criteria:

- healthcare services provided based on principles of primary healthcare
- participation in the provision of supportive environments to enable people to change their lifestyle to improve their health
- provision of a supportive environment that includes physical, psychological, emotional and spiritual elements
- a skilled health service that is characterised by excellent communication skill, good information, client decision-making using problem-solving techniques and realistic goal-setting
- there will be evidence of advocacy for responsible caring for others and for health facilitation within the community, for example, working on the advisory committee for the Edmonton Council Against Family Violence advocating the principle 'Edmonton strives to be a violence-free zone'.

Standard 3: Personnel

Criteria:

- personnel must be flexible, dedicated, non- judgmental, highly skilled (with professional preparation at a minimum of baccalaureate degree in nursing and in-service training), and with a willingness to undertake continuous learning both formally, informally and most importantly from clients
- the individual must demonstrate the ability to work within the philosophy of a client-driven service.

Standard 4: Collaboration

Criteria:

- collaboration with others in the development of health and social policy will be demonstrated by:
  - accessibility
  - development of joint proposals
  - collaboration with other agencies to advocate for clients
  - collaboration with other agencies to provide needed community services
  - community interagency involvement
  - development and delivery of a model of a caring, client-driven service.

Standard 5: Volunteers

Criteria:

- dedicated, caring, creative volunteers are an important component of PIC work with groups of children
- volunteers serve as important role models, participate in creative play and appreciate the special charm and talent of each child
- positive male role models who can demonstrate non-violent problem-solving, respect and caring

are desperately needed by children who have experienced and witnessed male violence

- volunteers assist children in gaining success, confidence and well-being in play
- volunteers are screened to protect the children
- volunteers are given orientation and ongoing support
- volunteers participate in ongoing programme development, problem-solving and continuous programme evaluation.

Appendix B: Documentation standards for PIC services

Need for development of documentation standards

The PIC nurses provided the services to the shelters on a 'client need' basis. Experiences with this special group of clients who came from traumatic environments and were in a state of physical and psychological crisis revealed special needs, not only for service, but also for documentation. The PIC nurses responded to the needs voiced by their clients and tailored their documentation accordingly.

Shelter staff watched the evolution of the VON 'client-driven' documentation with great interest. Discontent with their own documentation procedures culminated in several requests to the VON for assistance with documentation. The VON Edmonton PIC staff developed the following document to be used as a resource for all interested community agencies.

Principles of VON People in Crisis Program Documentation

1. **Client-driven** clients are enabled to assume ownership of their records, whenever possible and appropriate through:

(a) being kept informed of what is recorded in their personal health record;

(b) actively assisting the nurse in deciding what will be recorded;

(c) constant access to personal files;

(d) release of health records to the client for storage whenever possible.

2. **The client**: the client may be individual, parent or child, family/community or agency.

3. **Safety**: **All documentation is completed following a principle of the most good for the most vulnerable combined with the least harm to the most vulnerable. The client's safety needs are paramount. The decision about what and how to document must be based on the provision of physical safety for the client and respect for client confidentiality.

VON nurses do not take client files out of a crisis shelter. VON PIC staff work as a team with clients and shelter staff and maintain confidentiality. Confidentiality often extends to physical location of clients and shelter sites due to their vulnerability.

** "Who needs to know what?" is the guideline used to provide direction and balance in documentation. The health records are legal documents. Accurate VON PIC documentation has been used in court to assist our clients.

4. **Maximum time spent on service delivery**: paperwork must be kept to an absolute minium to maximize the time available to spend with the client. Continuous review and improvement of documentation to update and streamline is a significant part of this process.

Goals/purpose of documentation

- to advocate
- to empower and support the client
- to obtain needed services/community connections
- to communicate as a team member
- to set an example of appropriate documentation that fits a client-driven model
- to provide a beginning model for clients to record and retain their own health records (encouraging clients to take responsibility for their own health action).

Note

Supplementary reading

Cearns F and Edmonton Area Interagency Committee on Wife Assault Services (1993) *Wife Assault Hurts All of Us*. City of Edmonton Community and Family Services

Hutchinson P, Lord J (1993) The process of empowerment: Implications for theory and practice. *Can J Comm Ment Health* **12**(1): 5–22

VON, Edmonton Branch Newsletter. Von (Edmonton) *Happenings — VON Canada 1897–1997*. VON Edmonton Branch, Edmonton, Alberta, Canada

Section III

Reproduction, motherhood and the social control of women

Every society imposes control on women's reproductive capacities and motherhood experiences — of how and when they should have children and how they should care for them. These social norms are imposed on women overtly and covertly, and when women deviate from the social norms, they often experience stress, anxiety and guilt. How and when to breast-feed the baby and how many children she should have (or not have) are some of the issues over which a woman seems to have little control.

The concept of breast-feeding the infants waxes and wanes, based on the social attitude at a particular point in time. The very powerful baby formula industry created the myth that commercially made formulas, not breast milk, is good for babies, and mothers felt guilty not feeding formula to their children. The pendulum had swung to the other extreme in the second half of this decade, when women were made to feel guilty if they did not breast-feed their babies.

Mariza Almeida and Elizete Passos collected data in Brazil on the feelings and experience of women who for some reason weaned their babies earlier that what was believed to be the appropriate time. Some of the women's feelings about breast-feeding were indifference, sacrifice, a feeling of being exploited, pleasure and a feeling of duty. However, a feeling of guilt was more often expressed by women who had to stop breast-feeding before the time they thought it was right to do so.

Women in many countries across the globe find themselves having no say in the decision about how many children they are having, or the right to use family planning measures to limit family size. Women's low status, lack of education, lack of control over economic resources and total dependency on husbands and family for their basic needs, and the patriarchal culture under which they live, are all factors that affect their lack of reproductive control. Valeri Ehlers's chapter addresses the population problem in Africa, especially South Africa, and women's lack of control over reproduction. She also presents factors that could enhance the status of women in Africa and the relationship between education, socio-economic development and their impact on curbing population growth in South Africa.

The patriarchal culture, through social norms, dictates women's use of contraceptives and controls child-bearing. Deviating from this social norm is often unacceptable. However, the patriarchal hold on women and the control over their reproductive behaviour is slowly changing in many countries. In the last decade, Ireland has seen some changes in this regard. Abby Hyde's chapter discusses the contraceptive practices of 51 unmarried pregnant women prior to conception. Although non-marital pregnancies are still considered a problem in Ireland, there is a degree of acceptability of non-marital child-bearing in selected situations and Hyde elaborates on this from her qualitative data.

Women's experience of childbirth and women's experiential knowledge about pregnancy and childbirth have been muted with the rise of obstetrics and gynaecology, and the control of these areas by medical men. The medical men became the pregnancy and childbirth experts and the pregnant women who were the real experts became the 'patients'. With the publication of *Our Bodies, Ourselves* by the Boston Health Book Collective, a group of non-professional women made it clear that women sharing their knowledge of the so-called 'expert medical knowledge' in everyday language empowers women, creating an arsenal for women seeking help from the healthcare system. Maureen Laryea's chapter discusses the importance of predecessorship for women during pregnancy and childbirth. She defines predecessor as a non-healthcare professional who has been through the experience of childbirth and is willing and capable of sharing her experience with pregnant women preparing for childbirth.

Health professionals tend to see breast-feeding purely from its biological perspective, and promote it for the health of infants and as a maternal obligation to the child and to society. However, breast-feeding is a much more complex issue for the women concerned. In Brazil, even though 97% of women start breast-feeding, 43% stop before the child is three months old. Ana Nakano and Marlie Mamede interviewed 22 nursing mothers and collected observational data about the mothers' breast-feeding behaviour. Their chapter discusses the complex nature of breast-feeding and society's and the mother's expectations on the rights of mother and infant, and the interplay of those rights.

11

Women's feelings about breast-feeding and early weaning

Mariza Silva Almeida and Elizete Passos

Introduction

Despite government programmes to encourage breast-feeding, studies show that premature weaning continues, either because of mothers' own desires or other factors.

The practice of breast-feeding has grown considerably in the last few decades. Science has stressed the physiological and economic benefits rather than women's feelings, thoughts or expressed views. The ideological pressures and social factors that have led to this conflict between the role of the mother and the role of the professional have not been analysed.

The objective of this study is to explore the significance of early weaning, specifically in terms of the feelings of the women who wean their children early. Particular attention is paid to studying the female condition, to the values passed on to women during formative years, to the support that society gives to breast-feeding, and to the motivations and ideological pressures on women to cease breast-feeding.

Reich (1989), using a psychological and sociological perspective, sees sentiments as measured social constructs that are influenced by economic, social and cultural relationships forming a dialectic process. Breast-feeding and weaning vary according to place and time, and are directly associated with the values of a mother's society. For this reason, the practice of breast-feeding and weaning in the period 1950 to 1995 is investigated.

Method of study

The choice of the dialectic of historical materialism

Historical materialism teaches that our understanding of feminine sentiments is part of the historical process, and that this understanding is not unchanging; it goes through transformations. A qualitative method seems most pertinent to the theme because it allows the same analysis or object to be examined from multiple social and economic perspectives.

The first element of the dialectic method involves analysing the collected historical facts, historical development and historical transformation. Another essential element in this methodology is to categorise the totality and the internal contradictions of the ideologies, beliefs and values surrounding discussions about breast-feeding and weaning.

Besides explaining the behaviour of individuals within their context and material conditions or overall economics, the dialectic theory tries to understand the reality in order to transform it. For Lowy (1985), the more we understand reality, the more we will have conditions to transform it. The more we are involved in transformation, the more we can contradict the ideologies, utopian beliefs and values. This is inevitable because it is through the process of knowing that we transform reality.

Methodology

The study is based on a survey of teaching staff at the Centre of Hydration and Rehabilitation, Assistencial Sanitary District of Barra-Rio Vermelho, and at other places (homes and work) where we could find women of different socio-economic conditions who weaned children in the last 45 years and were not currently breast-feeding children. Semi-structured interviews of 36 women were conducted between January and April, 1995.

The data were analysed and articulated within the socio-historical context of the referential theory about the human species, breast-feeding and weaning. Official documents encouraging breast-feeding were also used, as were magazines and newspapers that provided stimuli for either breast-feeding or weaning. Categories to order the data collected emerged from the words of the women interviewed. These constructed categories were based on a minimum of formal theory. Onto this structure, we progressively elaborated an explanation based on selected anterior referential theory. The empirical reality we found was correlated to fundamental philosophical theory. In the end, the analysis was completed not in one moment, but through a process of correlating facts — by a dialectic process that considered the question in totality, and its internal contradictions within the interplay of multiple relationships.

This methodology led to four categories: from femininity to maternity; from breast-feeding to weaning; from education to conviction; and from conviction to feeling.

From femininity to maternity

The study attempted to identify the construction of feminine identity, a woman's path to motherhood, the changes in the concept of motherhood and cultural influences on nursing. Societal influences are important during a female's formative years in each generation in changing and forming women physically, in terms of their concepts and how they define the value of motherhood, and implicitly in terms of the process of nursing and weaning. This also involves cultural influences that are the basis of a woman's formation.

From breast-feeding to weaning

The study tried to identify current views of nursing and associated historical-sociological conditions; the public politics that encouraged nursing, as well as the ideologies of these politics; and the factors that discouraged maternal nursing, which had a large influence on the weaning process and the formation of women's feelings on the subject.

From education to conviction

It is important to consider women's experiences from childhood onwards, and the contribution of social processes on their lives, their ways of being and their self-guidance. The facts presented gave an opportunity to know them better, bringing us to believe that the major economic and social changes in our country during the last 45 years were not enough to change values and beliefs formed over a long period of time.

From conviction to feeling

We studied the meaning of premature weaning for women on the social rather than the psychoanalytic level, trying to capture through the women's words their convictions. We focussed on motherhood and the process of nursing to explore feminine feelings when women wean their children before the time considered to be adequate.

The meaning of weaning

In developing the work, we observed in the women's words a confirmation of the power of public opinion, which condemned mothers who did not nurse their children. This can still be felt, even in the twentieth century, thanks to the spread of negative communication that left a deep mark on the female unconscious. In this way, it was easy for them to accept responsibility for everything that happened to their children, especially anything bad.

Thus, the expression of feelings may or may not be valued, since women represent emotion and attitudes. The way women verbalise their feelings and the interrelationships of their emotions shows that they value these feelings and relate them to their day-to-day difficulties and resources. From this point on, the women in this study show feelings of indifference, sacrifice, relief and pleasure, among others, during the process of nursing and weaning.

Final considerations

This study showed that roles were not formed according to the biological nature of men and women but through false conceptions and prejudices that define women by their biological capacity to procreate and their lesser physical strength.

From this research we concluded that women's behaviour has been manifested in different ways through the years, depending on the type of society and the social class to which they belong. Society and class lead to the construction of their values, desires and different needs.

Difficulties in various areas, mainly politics and economics, have prevented government programs from achieving expected success. In this process, breast-feeding continues to be undervalued.

Since no educational practice is neutral and unbiased, the education received by the women interviewed reinforced the values, prejudices and ideologies related to breast-feeding, to whether natural breast-feeding was encouraged or discouraged.

The established social rules of conduct direct women into conflict with existing ideologies, newly acquired knowledge and daily reality. Many feelings are involved in this conflict, depending on the time period and situation, as well as bio-sociological or even social factors specific to an individual's life history.

The interviewees were aware of the obligations imposed upon them, their duties and the knowledge that showed the importance of their actions. However, these coexisted with difficulties, lack of social support for motherhood and breast- feeding, and with a lack of understanding that breast-feeding is a fundamentally socio-anthropologic issue.

The historical weaning of life and the transitory socialisation process to which they were subjected clearly shows the dialectic of feminine feelings about early weaning. Throughout the period studied, we observed different social values and positions about breast-feeding. Segments of society used various strategies in their own economic interests, and mothers found themselves in the middle of this dispute trying to reconcile antagonistic interests. As we have seen, women from the 1950s to the early 1970s, who were not subjected to the mechanisms or discussions that made them to blame, did not express this feeling. By contrast, in later years women carried a feeling of guilt.

The results of this study made us believe that we should not make the mother the only one responsible for breast-feeding or for the consequences of weaning; the process should be shared by everyone — the family, the husband and the society. We must not ignore the relationship between the individual and the collective, nor incite feelings of guilt, anxiety and sacrifice within women.

References

Lowy M (1985) *Ideologia e a Ciêcia Social Elemento par Análise Marxista*. Cortez, Sao Paulo

Reich W (1989). *Análise de Caráter* (trans. Branco ML, Pecegueiro MM). Martins Fentes, Sao Paulo

Supplementary readings

Badinter E (1985) *Um Amor Conquistado: O Mito do Amor Materno* (trans. Dutra W). Nova Fronteira, Rio de Janeiro

Demo P (1991) *Avaliaçao Qualitativa*, 3 edn. Cortez, Sao Paulo

Heller A (1993) *Teoria de Los Sentimentos*, 3 edn. trans. Cuso F. Fontamara, Mexico

Minayo MC (1992) O Desafio do Conhecimento. Pesquisa Qualitativa em Saúde, 3 edn. HUCITEC/ABRASCO, Sao Paulo

12

Women and population control in African countries

Valerie Ehlers

Introduction

The rate of population growth on the African continent exceeds 2%, but the total fertility rate is reported to be 4.2 for the Republic of South Africa and 7.6 for Malawi (Cornwell, 1996). The high population growth rate exacerbates problems, such as deforestation, desertification, erosion, pollution and access to scarce water resources.

The growing gap between job opportunities and the size of the labour force is fundamental to African development. It is expected that by the year 2000 the labour force for the 42 sub-Saharan African countries (see *Figure 12.1*) will have grown from 154 million in 1980 to 265 million — an increase of 111 million workers in merely 20 years — and as these people are already born, it is too late for birth control.

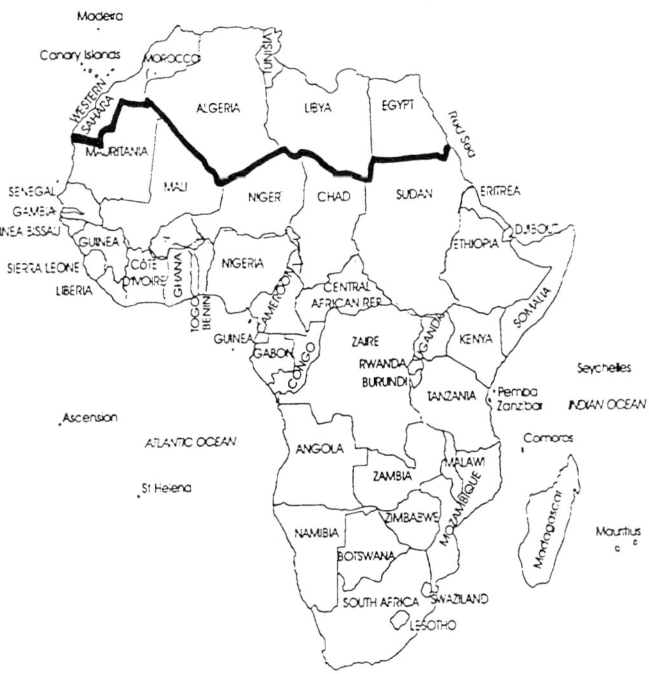

Figure 12.1: Sub-Saharan Africa

> *Africa is a continent of exceptionally high fertility and very low contraceptive use. In 1992 the total fertility rate . . . was approximately 6.5, compared to 3.6 for all developing countries. Contraceptive use rates were only 11 percent on average, compared with approximately 51 percent for all developing countries and 71 percent for the industrial countries.*
>
> (World Bank, 1994)

Africa's high fertility rates need to be viewed within the total societal context with special reference to the women of Africa.

Factors contributing to the high population growth rate in African countries

Numerous factors influence the birth rate of many countries. This chapter addresses medical issues, women's position in society, socio-economic factors and the abortion debate as factors influencing the number of children born to African women.

Medical issues

According to Zopf (1984), the population explosion in Africa is due mainly to improved nutrition and sanitation, and the medical revolution.

Improved environmental health and medical care

In first world countries, medical technology developed over a period of 150 years. This gradual medical development coupled with the industrial revolution made it possible for birth rates to decline simultaneously with death rates in these countries. In African countries, mortality rates declined drastically when the colonial powers provided improved healthcare to the populations of their African colonies. However, in Africa, unlike in Europe, high birth rates persisted, despite declines in mortality rates — causing escalating population growth rates. Whitaker (1988)demonstrates the impact of improved medical care on total fertility by pointing out that the average Kenyan woman had 6.2 children in 1960; 7.2 children in 1970; and 8.3 children in 1980.

Reduced mortality rates but stable birth rates

Reducing mortality rates is largely in the hands of professionals — engineers who provide clean water and effective sewage systems; doctors who provide vaccinations and treat diseases and agriculturists who produce cereals with improved nutritional values. All these professional services can and do benefit large numbers of people simultaneously, and may only need sporadic implementation. However, individuals (non-professionals) must decide on their family size and must continuously practise family planning or use birth control measures to limit their family size for the duration of their reproductive lives.

High infant mortality rates

According to Timberlake (1985), in Africa 15 out of every 100 children die before the age of five. Women are unlikely to have few children if they can realistically expect some of their children to die before the age of five.

It may seem contradictory, but birth rates are unlikely to decline until infant mortality rates have declined in specific geographic areas. However, the infant mortality rates will need to be substantially reduced for a sustained period of time, before it has an effect on reducing the number of children born.

Acquired immunodeficiency syndrome (AIDS)

There is no medical cure for AIDS. All healthcare attempts are directed at the prevention of AIDS by the regular use of condoms. This message is useless to AIDS sufferers (except to alert them to their responsibility for not spreading AIDS), and probably irrelevant to people who consider themselves and their sex partners to be healthy and who practise safe sex without condoms. However, continued health education about 'safe sex' and use of condoms has caused many people to regard the condom merely as preventing AIDS, not pregnancies. Research is required to determine whether AIDS education, promoting the use of condoms, has indeed resulted in the reduced use of condoms for family planning purposes among couples in stable relationships.

Women's status in society

Many efforts aimed at educating Africans about family planning matters are worthless because they are directed at individual women. Such efforts might meet with more success if they consider the familial, social and cultural environment within which the woman lives. Usually the husbands, sometimes the mothers-in-law, and sometimes the whole family group are the decision makers, not individual women. It seems useless to direct education efforts at women who have limited decision-making powers, especially concerning sexuality and procreation, if these are regarded as a family affair (AbouZahr *et al*, 1996).

Generally, African women's status is regarded as inferior to that of African men. Women cannot and do not make decisions affecting their own and/or their families' lives. Thus, uneducated poor women, dependent on their husbands for their livelihood, cannot oppose their husbands' wishes concerning the number of children, for fear of losing their only source of financial support for themselves and for their children. The issue of women's status in society is very intricate. At the risk of oversimplifying, only selected aspects will be addressed.

Polygamy

This is still an acceptable practice in many communities. In polygamous marriages, the wife with the largest number of children is likely to be the husband's favourite wife. Consequently, a woman in a polygamous marriage is unlikely to practise birth control, thereby jeopardising her position of being or of becoming the husband's favourite wife.

Payment of bridal prize (lobola)

In many if not most African cultures, the husband has to pay a prize, formerly a specified number of cattle, but nowadays often cash. Having paid for his wife, the husband is inclined to regard her as any other possession he bought and legally possesses. Consequently, not only does the wife in such a traditional marriage have no status, but also no say concerning the number of children to be born. Indeed, in some traditional cultures, it is possible for the husband to reclaim the bridal prize if the wife is unable to bear children. In many cases the man can insist that the woman proves her fertility by bearing a child, or even children, before marriage. 'In African culture children are an anchor in a marriage relationship. They give dignity and status to the couple as parents, and also give them a purpose in life. As a result a marriage can never be complete without children' (Pretorius, 1994).

This problem is exacerbated in Kenya where girls marry as early as 12 to 14 years of age. Some girls are even betrothed at the age of six (Kadandara, 1994). This issue of 'proven fertility' of women makes adolescents wary of using birth control measures lest they should cause infertility. Adolescent pregnancies precipitate a vicious cycle of poor education, joblessness, poverty and often prostitution to survive. Effective use of family planning techniques can definitely help girls and women plan when to have their children and plan their lives so that they are not destined to poverty and hopelessness.

Promiscuity

Women who want their partners to use condoms have to rely on these partners' goodwill to do so. Female condoms are not yet freely available in many African countries. This facility could enable more women to practise safe sex because it allows the women to make and implement the decision about whether or not to use a female condom.

African men regard it as their marital right to demand sex without condoms from their wives. No research could be traced documenting the use of condoms among South African men of various races. However, it is common knowledge that unmarried women do accept condoms at clinics and say they insist that their partners use them. Married women generally refuse to be seen with condoms because that would give their husbands cause to doubt their fidelity. On the other hand, men generally do not seem to demand fidelity from themselves — only from their wives — because men do accept condoms at clinics. Pretorius (1996) reported that African men do by and large engage in extra-marital affairs because they claim that men have insatiable sexual needs. In cases of infertility, or even small families of one or two children, the husbands can engage in extra-marital affairs because they want more children. Within a traditional African framework, a man is never regarded as infertile (except perhaps when he is impotent); it is the woman who is infertile and who is made to feel unhappy, guilty and depressed (Pretorius, 1994).

An issue that warrants further research is whether the status of women could hamper nurses in their family planning efforts. If a female nurse offers condoms to a male client at a clinic, it could be interpreted as 'making sexual advances' to the man. This could cause problems, especially if the nurse's husband should become aware of this perception.

Female circumcision

It seems ironic that while society at large seems to condone men's promiscuity, many communities continue to practise female circumcision to 'dampen women's sexual desire and vulnerability to sexual temptation. . . Girls grow up knowing that circumcision is essential if they are to some day be considered fit to marry, find a man willing to marry them, and raise a family' (Morris, 1996.

Female circumcision takes on more and more significance as circumcised African women travel to and seek medical aid in western countries unfamiliar with this practice, and where it is usually considered to be abusive to the women concerned.

An estimated 6000 girls, aged between nine and 15 years, are circumcised daily in at least 26 African countries. There are basically three types of 'surgery' performed, depending on the specific culture. In the first type, practised in Kenya, the clitoral hood is excised, but the clitoris and labia minora are preserved. In the second type, practised in Liberia, a clitoridectomy is done and adjacent parts of the labia minora are removed. In the third type, a clitoridectomy is done together with the removal of the labia minora and the medial parts of the labia majora, and thereafter the two sides of the vulva are sutured together, leaving a small opening for the passage of urine and menstrual flow; this is practised in Somalia, Sudan, Mali and northern Nigeria. A most surprising fact is that women, especially elderly women, are proponents of the continuation of this practice (Morris, 1996).

Women who have been subjected to female genital mutilation, and who continue to subject their daughters to such treatments, to comply with societal expectations and please the men in their lives, are most unlikely to use contraceptives to control the number of children they bear *unless* their families and husbands approve of these measures. Circumcised women might refrain from visiting western health services, and especially family planning clinics, if they fear the reactions of doctors and nurses on discovering their genital mutilation.

Socioeconomic factors

> *The phenomenon of population momentum and the current inevitability of high population growth have serious socioeconomic implications. The requirement in terms of infrastructure, physical facilities and services are tremendous, so that the population explosion could be regarded as the main factor inhibiting development in African countries.*
>
> (Cornwell, 1996)

Socioeconomic factors influence women's decisions concerning the number of children they bear in all societies. In Africa, these socioeconomic factors may be compounded by the relatively low status of women, generally, in Africa.

Children as workers

Many African women, especially in the rural areas, perform laborious daily tasks to provide water supplies, fuel and food for their families. These women often have neither the time nor the energy to plan their lives or those of their families. They struggle to keep their families alive on a daily basis.

In many rural African communities women need their children, especially their daughters, to help them with the daily chores such as fetching water and firewood and milling grain. As the older children leave the home and the village, the mother needs to carry on producing babies to help with future chores. As firewood and water become scarcer, more time is used to collect these essentials and child labour becomes more essential to many families' survival. Usually the girls have to help with the household chores while the boys are sent to school. Girls are usually expected to assume greater and greater shares of the household chores, causing them to fall behind in school work and ultimately to abandon schooling, even in areas where schools are available. Because the girls are deprived of educational opportunities, they are also deprived of future jobs, and possibly of the ability to use contraceptives effectively to plan their families and their lives.

As the father's level of income rises, the need for his children's labour declines, and his ability to educate his children increases, thus ensuring better futures for them.

Education

Women with low levels of education and literacy have a low status and are unlikely to find worthwhile jobs. Their only hope for survival is in finding husbands who will support them. Consequently, they marry and perform the roles of housewife and mother while their husbands decide on the size of the families. Literacy and education change people's values and attitudes and enable parents to make proper use of clinics and hospitals and birth control measures. Unfortunately, there is no significant correlation between lower-primary education and fertility. The greatest decline in fertility occurs where both husband and wife have a high level of education (Cornwell, 1996). If this is correct, the seven years of free primary school education offered to the children of the Republic of South Africa cannot necessarily be expected to enhance their chances of making effective family planning decisions later in their lives.

In many African schools, pregnancy is a sufficient reason for permanent expulsion. Other schools are starting to adopt a more lenient approach, but the emotional and physical load on the shoulders of an adolescent schoolgirl mean that it is virtually impossible for her to achieve success. Preventing adolescent pregnancies can save adolescent girls much hardship.

Even if some African women succeed in gaining technical qualifications, 'they might end up selling chickens because the male dominated industries do not feel confident in giving women, who might be better qualified than men, jobs in the technical field like, for example motor mechanics' (Kadandara, 1994).

Effective use of birth control measures requires a knowledge of bodily functions that few African women, especially in rural areas, possess. Birth control, such as pills, injections and condoms, need to be readily available. This is often not the case in Africa where such facilities may only be regularly available in large cities and towns, and the majority of women live in the rural areas.

Security for old age

Many workers, especially married women, cannot manage to save money for old-age pensions during their productive years. Thus, they cannot make financial provisions for their days of dependency. Old people who do not have pensions must rely on their children to care for them financially in their old age. African women, who cannot legally possess land in many African countries, need to have as many sons as possible to maintain some claim to some land.

Tribal security

The populations of most African countries do not identify with the national political entity, but rather with their tribes. These tribes are sensitive about their relative power (measured in terms of numbers) in the political hierarchy. Therefore, there is tribal opposition to birth control practices among its women. Indeed, Gould (1984) claimed that some communities could regard family planning programs to be 'a disguised form of genocide'.

Tribal issues also affect healthcare workers, especially nurses, offering family planning services. If nurses from one tribe offer family planning services to women of another tribe, it could be interpreted as efforts to reduce the numbers of the other tribe. If nurses and clients are from the same tribe, they could fear retaliation from family or village members.

Religion

Religions disempower women further to make and implement decisions concerning the number of children they will bear. Islam tends to restrict the rights and status of women, leaving men to decide about the number of children for the family. Roman Catholicism, practised by many African communities, opposes modern methods of birth control. This religion approves of the rhythm method but this could be a most problematic method to practise effectively in Africa where large numbers of men are migrant labourers.

Age of the African population

The United Nations estimates that more than 45% of Africa's population is below the age of 15. Demographically, this means that a momentum for future growth is built into the population structure. Even if the fertility rate should be brought down to two births per female, the African populations will continue to grow for another 50 years. This implies that, even if fertility rates were to drop to replacement levels now, Africa's population will still grow by a further 80% to 100% as a result of the momentum generated by the youthful population structure (Goliber, cited in Cornwell, 1996).

Multiple languages

The International Planned Parenthood Feder- ation emphasised that more than 450 dialects are spoken on the African continent, severely hampering family planning educational campaigns (Timberlake, 1985). It takes one to two generations for any family planning program to take effect, and even more if family planning educators and clients cannot under- stand each other.

The abortion debate

This debate is generally divided between those who believe that abortion on demand is every woman's right and those who regard abortion as murder. Whatever position the healthcare services adopt in a specific country, it needs to consider the fact that the majority of gynaecology beds in most hospitals are occupied by incomplete abortion patients, mainly suffering from haemorrhage and septicaemia. What needs the most urgent attention is that almost all patients suffering from abortion complications, and adolescents especially, had not used an effective method of contraception prior to becoming pregnant. Reasons for not using contraceptives include fears about the safety of contraceptives, lack of knowledge about family planning techniques and facilities, and lack of access to services. Research about post-abortion contraceptions appears to be almost non-existent. If married women aborted because they became pregnant by men other than their husbands, post-abortion family planning practices might be regarded as continued infidelity on the wife's part (Benson, *et al*, 1996).

Access to safe abortions can help to enhance women's health and reduce the population growth rate.

Conclusion

Finally and fundamentally, the success of curbing the population growth rates in Africa depends on empowering African women to make their own decisions. Such empowerment will require socioeconomic upliftment; increased financial independence of women; improved education for women; and access to healthcare, including family planning (spacing) services. 'Perhaps the interests of women would be better served by promoting policies that are less vague, less idealistic and more attainable than empowerment' (Asthana, 1996).

The common challenge is for women to improve their health status and reach their full potential. Women should become aware of paternalistic influences in their healthcare services. Women should value themselves and other women, become aware of their rights and claim these rights for themselves and for their daughters in the predominantly male-defined healthcare systems prevailing in many African countries. Given the fact that it is men who define female sexuality in many African cultures, family planning education efforts and exhibitions should be directed at men as well as at women — preferably in separate sessions at the outset (Davies, 1983).

Many women are illiterate, unskilled and destitute. Women need education, healthcare, physical safety, social services, skills training employment and income-generating projects. Women do not attend courses because of a lack of child care, transport, too much work at home, lack of family support and programs seen as irrelevant to their daily lives.

The actual fertility rates of women decline with socioeconomic development. The way in which men view women's role in society is important. Population and development policies must emphasise women's equality and advancement, education, employment opportunities and access to health services. Improving the health status of women also enhances their decision-making capacity at all levels, in all spheres of life, especially in the areas of sexuality and reproduction. Population and development programs are most effective when steps have simultaneously been taken to improve the status of women. Education is particularly critical to empowering women in all aspects of their lives.

To conclude, a quotation from Margaret Sanger, a founding member of the International Planned Parenthood Federation, seems appropriate. She claimed that the basic freedom of the world is a woman's freedom: 'A free race cannot be born of slave mothers. Women enchained cannot choose but give a measure of that bondage to her sons and daughters. No woman can call herself free until she can choose . . . whether she will or will not be a mother' (Roberts and Group, 1995).

References

AbouZahr C, Vlassoff C, Kumar A (1996) Quality health care for women: A global challenge. *Health Care Wom Int* **17**(5): 449–67

Asthana S (1996) Women's health and women's empowerment: A locality perspective. *Health Place* **2**(1): 1–13

Benson J, Nicholson LA, Gaffikin L, Kinoti SN (1996) Complications of unsafe abortion in sub-Saharan Africa: A review. *Health Pol Plan J Health Devel* **11**(1): 117–31

Cornwell L (1996) *Development Administration 1: Study Manual* 2. University of South Africa, Pretoria

Davies M (Compiler) (1983) *Third world: Second sex. Women's struggles and national liberation*. Zed Press, London

Gould KH (1984) Black women in double jeopardy: A perspective on birth control. *Health Soc Work* **9**(2): 96–105

Kadandara J (1994). *Women's Health: A Must for Development*. WHO, Global Commission on Women's Health, Geneva

Morris R (1996) The culture of female circumcision. *Adv Nurs Sci* **19**(2): 43–53

Pretorius C (1994) Infidelity in African culture. *Siren News: Unisa Cen Wom Stud Newslet* **2**(1): 19

Pretorius C (1996) Women's vital role in culture, the family and socialisation. *Siren News: Unisa Cen Wom Stud Newslet* **4**(1): 25

Roberts JI, Group TM (1995) *Feminism and Nursing: An Historical Perspective on Power, Status and Political Activism in the Nursing Profession*. Praeger, Westport

Timberlake L (1985) *Africa in Crisis: The Causes, the Cures of Environmental Bankruptcy*. International Institute for Environment and Development, London:

Whitaker JS (1988) *How can Africa Survive?* Coucil of Foreign Relations Press, New York

World Bank (1994) *Better Health in Africa: Experience and Lessons Learned*. World Bank, Washington, DC

Zopf PE (1984) *Population: An introduction to Social Demography*. Mayfield, Palo Alto, CA

13

Variations in contraceptive behaviour among unmarried Irish women

Abbey Hyde

Introduction

The past two decades have witnessed a steady escalation in non-marital births in the Republic of Ireland. In 1992, when data collection for the study to be presented began, the figure represented 18% of all births that year (Department of Health, 1993). Although the proportion of *non-marital* adolescent births had risen dramatically over the preceding 20 years, the rate of *all* births (marital and non-marital) to teenagers had not increased over the same period (Central Statistics Office, 1972–1992). Contraceptives have become more accessible to unmarried people in the Republic of Ireland over the past decade; indeed, the most recent change makes Ireland's laws on contraceptive availability among the most liberal in Europe (Jacobsen, 1994).

This chapter presents qualitative data on the contraceptive practices of 51 unmarried pregnant women in the time-span just before they became pregnant. It is suggested that women's contraceptive practices varied by virtue of their age and class, and their differing social circumstances. In the discussion, it will be argued that women's contraceptive practices are mediated by patriarchal controls over the female body, and that socially normative childbearing is framed by patriarchal discourses. It will be further proposed that differing patriarchal discourses may impact on women's contraceptive practices in ways that produce contradictory outcomes.

No *a priori* assumption was made that non-marital childbearing was problematic. Rather, it was the stigmatisation of this style of mothering in the past, and the expropriation of women's domestic labour within marriage (Delphy, 1992; Smart, 1984; Walby, 1990) that made an investigation of the topic timely and significant.

Methodological stance

Fifty-one women were selected from the pre-natal clinic of a major maternity hospital in Dublin on a convenience basis. Entry criteria to the study were that potential participants be unmarried to the father of the foetus and be first-time potential mothers. All but four women were in relationships with the putative fathers before the pregnancy, although the duration and reported quality of these relationships varied enormously. At least 14 women were no longer in relationships by the time of the birth, and another couple separated shortly after the birth. The ages of participants ranged from 16 to 36 years, with a mean of 22.7 years. Twelve women were under 20 years when they gave birth. In terms of socioeconomic status, 18 were unemployed, 11 were in manual occupations, 20 were employed in non-manual occupations (the bulk of which were low-paid clerical jobs) and two were schoolgirls.

Participants were interviewed on two occasions: in the later stages of pregnancy and between weeks six and eight post-delivery. The interviews were conducted from mid-1992 to late 1993. Data were analysed using a style of qualitative analysis resembling a 'grounded theory' approach (Glaser, 1978; 1992; Glaser and Strauss, 1967), but this strategy was used selectively.

Contraceptive practices — variations among women

Seven categories were constructed from the data to capture variations in individual participants' experiences of becoming pregnant: fertility denial, destiny dependence, progressive remissness, occasional or intermittent risk-taking, calculated risk-taking, pro-active fertility management and contraceptive failure or misuse. For a summary of each, see *Table 13.1*. The categories were created by the researcher on the basis of descriptions reported by the women.

Fertility denial

The predominant feature here was for women to report that they did not use and had never used any form of contraception because the possibility of becoming pregnant in their cases was not entertained at that point in their lives. Women did tend to express the view that they wanted a baby sometime, and had an idea about the circumstances and timing of when they would like this to happen. Nonetheless, at least half of the 10 women in this group would have preferred to have become pregnant later in their lives.

Participants in this group shared some characteristics. Apart from two who were schoolgirls, all the others had left school prior to the Leaving Certificate (final secondary school examination), and some had no school qualifications at all. Those employed tended to be in unstable, seasonal, unskilled types of occupations, with a great deal of job mobility. They were also younger on average than the study population as a whole. Of the 10, seven had regular or occasional boyfriends at the time they became pregnant, while three putative fathers were one-time sexual contacts.

A common initial response from women in this group was to report that they 'did not think' about the possibility of a pregnancy and using a contraceptive. However, further probing suggested that they may actually have 'thought' about pregnancy as a possibility, but denied it in their own case as something that would happen to others and not to them. The following example (21-year-old, unemployed, first interview) epitomises this sense of denial:

> **AH**: Before you became pregnant, did you think about the possibility of becoming pregnant?
>
> **Norma**: *It never dawned me mind. It never dawned on me at all. I never even thought of it.*
>
> **AH**: Were you using a contraceptive?
>
> **Norma**: *No. I just thought, "It wouldn't happen me." That's what I used to say, "It wouldn't happen me."*

(**NB**: The age of women is given as their age at birth of the baby. Employment status in all cases is that at the beginning of the pregnancy, although a number of those in seasonal or temporary employment became unemployed during the pregnancy and a small number of women resigned from stable employment in view of the pregnancy. Some occupations have been changed to similar ones within the same socioeconomic group according to the current Irish six-point scale. This is to protect the anonymity of participants.)

Some reported a belief that a pregnancy would not arise until they themselves were socially ready for it, even in the absence of contraceptive usage (19-year-old factory worker, first interview):

> **AH**: Before you became pregnant, did you ever worry about becoming pregnant?
>
> **Clare**: *No, I never thought, like, that it would happen to you. Like it wouldn't happen. I didn't think it would happen that night. I never thought it would happen until I was about twenty-five or twenty-six like me dad was always saying, "You never think."*

Table 13.1: Categories of pregnancy experience

Category	n	Characteristics of participants	Defining features
Fertility denial	10	Younger than average; most without a Leaving Cert; many unemployed or in unstable, unskilled jobs	View that 'it won't happen to me'. Seven had either regular or occasional boyfriends at the start of the pregnancy. Three were one-time sexual contacts.
Destiny dependence	8	Younger than average; most without a Leaving Cert; many unemployed or in unstable, unskilled jobs	View that 'if it happens, it happens', although some would have preferred to become pregnant at a later point. All were in relationships at the start of the pregnancy.
Progressive remissness	7	Average age; most with Leaving Cert and most employed at the start of pregnancy	Previous regular use of contraceptives had become increasingly less regular; more risks were bing taken, but participants reported they did not want to become pregnant. All were in stable relationships at the start of the pregnancy.
Occasional/ intermittent risk-taking	7	Average age; some with Leaving Cert; some employed at the start of pregnancy	Occasional risk-taking, but likely to be considering using a contraceptive. Putative father usually a new or infrequent sex partner
Calculated risk-taking	5	Older than average; most with Leaving Cert; most employed at start of pregnancy	Prior to becoming pregnant most felt they would like to become pregnant in the near future, but did not abandon all measures of pregnancy prevention; took risks that they were aware might result in pregnancy. Four out of the five were cohabiting.
Proactive fertility management	5	Older than average; most with Leaving Cert; most employed at the start of pregnancy	Women here perceived their situations to be conducive to childbearing, having achieved, for the most part, alternative goals in life that they had sought. All were cohabiting at the time they became pregnant. Almost all had experienced regular contraceptive use prior to making a decision to attempt to become pregnant.
Contraceptive failure or misuse	9	Average age; most with Leaving Cert; most employed at the start of pregnancy	Contraceptives either failed or were not used appropriately. Seven were condom users, two were pill users. Varied types of relationships; some long-standing, others new or occasional.

Destiny dependence

For this category of eight women, fertility was primarily governed by destiny; if a pregnancy happened, it happened. There was a tendency for women to report that their social situations were not as they would wish for the purposes of child-rearing, but they were prepared to accept a pregnancy if it occurred, regardless of circumstances. This group is distinguished from the first group above primarily in the acknowledgement that a pregnancy might occur in their case. Women in this group resembled those in the fertility denial group in terms of socioeconomic status, educational levels and age.

Participants tended to be in stable relationships at the start of the pregnancy, and this was found to be significant in how the pregnancy was perceived for some women, as the following example (19-year-old machinist, first interview) suggests:

> ***Emma:*** *We talked about it and about [pause], of babies. From the start I kind of knew that I'd be staying with him, so like we didn't worry as much as someone saying, "Jasus, if I get pregnant!" Like we kind of said, "If it happens, it happens." But I think after this we'll have to start thinking of using something.*

Although participants here took the view that if a pregnancy 'happens, it happens', there was evidence that the pregnancy was also construed as a mistake to varying degrees.

Progressive remissness

A predominant feature of this group was that previous consistent use of contraceptives had become increasingly less regular, and more risks were being taken as the relationship each participant was in at the time of conception progressed. All seven women in this category were in long-term relationships when they became pregnant, yet all conveyed that they *did not* want to become pregnant at that point in their lives. All had formerly used oral contraceptives, but for various reasons discontinued the pill. The majority took alternative precautions for a while, and this was usually followed by a higher level of risk-taking, such as coitus interruptus or isolated episodes of unprotected intercourse.

The socioeconomic positions of participants in the group varied, but, for the most part, they were better educated than participants in the previous two groups. Most had completed secondary education, and some had training in skilled occupations such as clerical work. The majority were in relatively stable jobs at the time they became pregnant. The age profile of this group was average for the study population as a whole.

In two cases, participants were spatially apart from their partners for longer than usual around the time of conception, and the relative infrequency of intercourse prompted the decision to discontinue the pill. Others abandoned the pill because of side-effects, and followed this with condom use, and later still with unprotected sex (26-year-old cleaner, first interview):

> ***Susan:*** *I was on the pill about four or five years, and I didn't know that you're supposed to come off it for a break.. .. The only part of the leaflet I read was how to start taking the pill, and that was it, so I sat down and read it one day, and it was all this "tumours on your liver, and breast cancer," and I was saying to him [partner], "I'm not taking that, look what you can get." And as the doctor says to me, "You haven't had a break from the pill since you started."*
>
> *. . . so I said [to partner], "If you want nukies [sex], you'll just have to do something else!*
>
> *. . . I came off the pill then, and that was only a couple of months before I got pregnant, and we were kind of careful at first, but you know yourself.*
>
> **AH**: When you say you were careful, what do you mean?
>
> ***Susan:*** *We used condoms. They were horrible though . . . Well we weren't, like, really sexually active anyway. That's how I got caught out. He was too frisky around Christmas!*

This shows the vulnerability of those in established relationships to the risk of unanticipated pregnancies, an issue that has received little attention in research reports to date. While most women in this group were aware that they were at risk of becoming pregnant, here again there were elements of a sense of invincibility to pregnancy in evidence, frequently associated with previous 'escapes'.

Occasional or intermittent risk-taking

This group of seven was characterised by women who occasionally or intermittently had sexual intercourse without using contraceptives, and who (apart from one) had used contraceptives previously, either with the putative father or another man. Women in this group were more likely to be considering a more reliable method of contraception, and had become pregnant by new or infrequent sex partners. The prospect of a pregnancy at the point in their lives when it occurred was generally experienced as undesirable by all but one woman.

The socioeconomic positions of women in this group resembled those in the progressive remissness group above in terms of educational qualifications and age.

Some participants here had plans to commence oral contraceptives, each having recently begun to have sex with her partner. This highlights a vulnerable area for pregnancy to occur during the time span between first intercourse with a partner, and the stabilisation of the relationship. The infrequency of sex, along with excessive alcohol intake, was a factor in not using a contraceptive for some women.While there appeared to be some disquiet about becoming pregnant among women in this group, there was a tendency to suppress the real possibility of pregnancy once the sex act was over. As in the case of participants in other groups, previous sex acts without the outcome of a pregnancy reinforced feelings of impregnability.

Calculated risk-taking

In the period leading to the pregnancy, a feeling of social readiness to mother was experienced by the five women in this group. They believed that pregnancy would not pose a problem because they had achieved, for the most part, what they had set out to do in life. Their contraceptive pattern resembled the practices of the progressive remissness group insofar as contraceptive use had become increasingly more lax in the period preceding the pregnancy. However, prior to becoming pregnant most participants in this group had experienced a fairly recent feeling of 'broodiness', or a feeling that they would like to become mothers in the near future, in contrast to those in the progressive remissness group who did not want to become pregnant. Women here did not, however, abandon all measures of pregnancy prevention, but took risks that they were aware could result in a pregnancy. A sense of 'If it happens, it happens', identified earlier in relation to the destiny dependence group, was to some extent noted among members of this group, but women here felt their social circumstances were now suitable for childbearing. Apart from one participant who had a fairly casual (although long-standing) relationship with the father, women in this group were cohabiting with their partners.

Four out of the five participants had completed secondary schooling, and women tended to be in higher socioeconomic groups and older than those in the previous groups.

A predominant pattern for this group was a hesitancy about removing barriers to a pregnancy totally, but also a sense that pregnancy would not constitute a problem (28-year-old musician, first interview):

> **AH**: How long had you been trying to conceive? [Participant had already said the pregnancy was planned.]
>
> **Sile**: *Not that we had really been trying either. You take a risk, and if it happened, it happened, but we knew like what we were doing, that I could have conceived at that time. . . . We were using condoms before this. The last two months we decided to take a risk, whereas before I definitely didn't want to get pregnant. So it happened quite quickly.*

As was the case in other groups, some sense of invulnerability to pregnancy because of previous 'escapes' was evident.

Proactive fertility management

Compared to the previous group, the five women in this group went a step further in that they relinquished all attempts to prevent a pregnancy, yet did not frame their sexual behaviour as 'risk-taking'. As in the case of those in the previous group, women here perceived their situations to be appropriate for childbearing, having achieved, for the most part, alternative goals in life that they had sought. All of the women were in stable relationships and cohabiting. All but one had experienced regular contraceptive use prior to attempting to conceive.

The socio-demographic profiles of women located in this group was similar to that in the calculated risk-taking group. The distinction between the two groups is highlighted in Lorna's account (29-year-old salesperson, first interview) of her approach to pregnancy:

> **Lorna**: *I was on the pill and I remember we were going away for our Christmas do, and I forgot it. I left it, and [partner] said to me, "Look leave it. If it happens, it happens." And I thought, "No, you don't plan it like that, 'if it happens it happens'." I sort of pictured this real romantic, "Yeah, we'll have a baby," and all this. Like I wouldn't have gone near him because he had just said, "If it happens, it happens." But then, it was around January and we went for a drink, and he said, "I'd love a child now," he said, "I really would," and that was so much better.*

The overriding characteristics of this group, in summary, were a self-perceived social readiness to mother and the pregnancy being preceded by a decision to forfeit all contraceptive methods.

Contraceptive failure and misuse

For the nine women located in this group, contraceptive measures had either failed, or were not used appropriately. Participants were in various types of relationships with the putative fathers, from long-standing to new or occasional. None of the women wished to conceive at that point in her life, although this was more so for some than for others.

Most women had completed secondary schooling and gained further training in a skilled occupation, predominantly clerical work. Almost all were in stable employment when they became pregnant. The mean age of women here approximated the average for the sample as a whole.

Fearing infertility

Before attempting to develop theory from the above data, a brief note is necessary on the assertion by some authors that women may attempt to test their fertility without particularly wanting to become mothers at that point (Bury, 1984; Rainey *et al*, 1992). They have suggested that fertility testing may occur because of women's doubts about their physiological capability to become pregnant. However, in the present study, disquiet about an inability to conceive tended to be more often expressed by participants in the calculated risk-taking and in the proactive fertility management groups who, for the most part, reported that they *did* want to become mothers at the stage in their lives around the time of conception. A small number in the destiny dependence category, and a few across other groups expressed similar concerns, which may partly explain their willingness to embrace a pregnancy in less than appropriate circumstances by their own estimation. However, most women indicated little or no concern about the possibility of infertility.

Discussion

Data obtained for the present study has revealed a diversity of contraceptive practices among a sample of unmarried participants. Variation was noted in relation to class position, age, the stage of a relationship and social circumstances. Of central importance in theorising from the above data is the extent to which participants *wanted* to be pregnant. It has been noted elsewhere that issues surrounding the how wanted or otherwise a pregnancy was are nebulous; there are degrees to which pregnancies may be wanted or not (Finlay *et al*, 1994), and unplanned pregnancies are not necessarily unwanted (Finlay *et al*, 1994; 1995; Macintyre, 1977; Macintyre and Cunningham-Burley, 1993). For the most part, though, data suggest that the majority of pregnancies in this study were not intended, and the notion of whether or not women wished to become pregnant (that is of concern here) becomes redundant in instances where a considerable proportion reported that they had not even entertained it as a possibility.

The author proposes that variation in data is likely to relate to women's experiences of the conflicting patriarchal discourses that influence different women to varying degrees. In the Republic of Ireland, a dominant set of discourses elevates the two-parent heterosexual family above other family formations. Although it is often commented that unmarried women with children receive proportionately more generous welfare benefits than married couples with children, and can circumvent the public housing queue, non-marital motherhood is still socially controlled by stigmatising discourses. Evidence of such discourses may be found in recent media reports of public and political opinion on non-marital motherhood, in which young mothering (*Evening Press* Oct 4, 1993; *Irish Independent* Mar 13, 1989; Oct 1, 1990; Nov 13, 1991; Sept 9, 1993; *Irish Times* May 5, 1987; May 25, 1989; July 26, 1990; Mar 4, 1994; Nov 13, 1994; *Sunday Independent* July 20, 1987; *The Star* Apr 13, 1989) and non-marital mothering (*Evening Herald* Sept 10, 1987; Dec 18, 1987; *Evening Press* Sept 9, 1989; Aug 13, 1992; Oct 4, 1993; *The Examiner* May 14, 1996; *Irish Independent* May 23, 1987; Feb 10, 1988; May 25, 1989; May 1, 1992; June 13, 1992; *Irish Press* Jan 25, 1992; *Irish Times* Sept 10, 1987; July 26, 1988; Jan 28, 1989; May 25, 1989; Oct 19, 1993; *The Star* Sept 23, 1992; Apr 13, 1989; Sept 28, 1993; Apr 11, 1996) continue to be considered as problems. (The newspaper search here was not comprehensive, but a range of press articles was consulted from both conservative and liberal elements of the press.)

Even the more positive media reports buttress the norm of the two-parent heterosexual family and normative age prescriptions in highlighting the high proportion of dual-parent non-marital families (*Irish Independent* Sept 9, 1993), the transient nature of welfare dependency (*Irish Times* Oct 19, 1993) and the stabilisation in the numbers of adolescent pregnancies (*Irish Times* Mar 7, 1994). Although these endeavour to dispel the myths surrounding non-marital childbearing, focussing on the high proportion of two-parent non-marital units reinforces the norm of dual heterosexual parenting. Highlighting the stabilisation in adolescent births imparts a view that youth and childbearing together are problematic, but a problem that is being contained. While such accounts strive to frame non-marital motherhood in a more positive light compared to those that overtly criticise it, they are also covertly suggesting that single (without a partner) and adolescent parenting are problematic, but represent only a relatively small proportion of the growing number of non-marital births. In effect, the public is being reassured that the social organisation of reproduction around the nuclear-style two-parent heterosexual family is not being undermined to the extent they might assume, and alternatives to this style of organisation are a minority. Thus, although non-marital and adolescent pregnancies are still considered to be problems, there is evidence of a level of acceptability of non-marital childbearing provided that the circumstances in which it occurs approximate those of marital situations. This level is a changing form of patriarchy (Walby, 1990) insofar as even the more liberal version still propels women towards specific ends, that is towards affiliation with individual men in the organisation of reproduction. The interests of patriarchy are served by such discourse in view of their potential to place women in exploitative positions through economic dependency and the expropriation of female domestic labour in marital and quasi-marital situations. Evidence that female domestic labour continues to be expropriated in marital situations is found in both Irish (Kiely, 1995; Market Research Bureau of Ireland, 1992; Second Commission on the Status of Women, 1993) and international research (Cowan and Cowan, 1992; Croghan, 1991; Richardson, 1993). Evidence in the case of quasi-marriages comes from an expanding body of international studies (Blair and Lichter, 1991; McRaie, 1993; Phoenix, 1991; Shelton and John, 1993; South and Spitze, 1994).

This is not to suggest that all marriages are necessarily patriarchal, but there is overwhelming evidence that even in modern marriages and quasi-marriages, women's domestic labour is expropriated. Chandlier (1991) has argued that family forms developing around quasi-marriage and non-marriage require examination, since they do not occur in a social and economic vacuum. She refers to the notion of 'degrees of marriage/non-marriage' in the organisation of reproduction, with cohabitation varying from a *de facto* domestic relationship to a non-hierarchical commitment (Chandlier, 1991).

That a number of women in the current study became pregnant outside of a quasi-marital situation (although most women were in relationships, a number of these were either casual, new or unstable; just a third of the women were cohabiting by the time of the second interview) might suggest resistance to dominant discourses referred to above. However, data presented here do not support this proposition; very few women actively defied established social relations of reproduction through deliberately choosing non-marital motherhood without aligning themselves with individual men. However, some resisted the more traditional patriarchal position by choosing not to marry where this was an option (because of the prohibition on divorce, marriage was not an option for some women if either they or their partners were separated), and others continued in relationships without cohabiting, although this was the long-term plan of almost all if the relationship was to be sustained. In a few instances, women were content without a partner, albeit they had not sought to become pregnant (Hyde, 1996). Overwhelmingly, however, pregnancies tended to be inadvertent to varying degrees other than some of those arising in quasi-marital circumstance. The majority of women drifted into becoming pregnant rather than choosing to become pregnant (even if some were happy to become pregnant). The author argues that patriarchal discourses in addition to those referred to above were also affecting women's contraceptive behaviour, namely those discourses that render women passive in controlling their own bodies.

On the one hand, therefore, women are being drawn through dominant discourses into marriages and quasi-marriages for the purposes of childbearing, which demands agency in terms of contraceptive use, and negotiation in heterosexual relations beyond marriage and quasi-marriage. [Considerable empirical evidence (Holland *et al*, 1990; Pollock, 1985; Wight, 1992) exists to indicate that female agency is demanded in negotiating contraception because gendered norms prescribe responsibility for contraception as a female rather than male responsibility. As indicated, discussion of this issue is beyond the scope of this paper.]

This assumes an acceptance of non-procreative sexual relations outside of marital-type circumstances. While more traditional patriarchal thinking would disapprove of this, there is evidence of a growing acceptance within Ireland of sex before marriage (Hyde, 1996; Whelan and Fahey, 1994), although not, as indicated earlier, of childbearing outside marriage, or at least outside of quasi-marital situations.

On the other hand, the female body is rendered passive through medicalisation, lack of education about the body, sexual harassment, rape, domestic violence and the threat of violence in public places. Thus, different sets of discourses can make varying demands and have contradictory outcomes. Some women are likely to be influenced to a greater extent by particular sets of discourses over others. The data indicated that the most actively planned pregnancies were those of better educated women (in the proactive fertility management group), whose circumstances most closely resembled the marital situation, while arguably the most passive in terms of planning were pregnancies of young working-class women (in the fertility denial group), who had not even considered pregnancy as a possibility in their cases.

This is not to suggest that particular discourses predominate (Cooper, 1994), with working-class women influenced by one set of discourses and middle-class women another. Rather, there was evidence that both sets of discourses influenced women across the board to varying degrees and at different times. For example, invulnerability to pregnancy was noted among some women in groups other than the fertility denial group, while some women in the latter believed that they would become pregnant when the time and circumstances were right for them (indicating the influence of discourses on general prescriptions for child- bearing). For those in the destiny dependence group, being in a stable relationship was particularly important in their acceptance of the pregnancy, indicating their internalisation of dominant views about alignment to individual men in the social organisation of reproduction. Thus, discourses about childbearing can be fissured around different themes.

Among women who were passive in terms of fertility management, yet did not want to become pregnant, the extent to which their bodies were disciplined through social regulation may simply be different rather than greater than their effectively contracepting sisters. In the case of the latter, under the guise of a sense of agency, the possibility that their bodies are controlled according to a discourse which disciplines them to produce two children, when they are at least over 20 years old, and married to (or in a quasi marriage with) a male partner is as plausible as the notion that they are agents of their own destiny. Those proactively contracepting to conform to social and gender prescriptions for motherhood may be viewed as having acted to fulfil socially constructed gender expectations. The proactive fertility management group came closest to this, in that all were in quasi-marriages.

Hyde argues that women in general are operating within the wider context of power and patriarchy, in which a language of 'control' over their bodies in the face of contraceptive 'choices' masks the overall context of control in which social arrangements of reproduction are defined. This difficulty relating to 'choice' has been noted by others (Katz Rothman, 1994; Morgan and Scott, 1993), in that 'choices' become transformed into pressures to choose the most socially endorsed possibilities.

The notion that what apparently manifests itself as female agency may simply be the effect of power remains unresolved and rests uncomfortably with feminist politics. Where layers of patriarchal discourses are seen to impinge upon gender roles in diverse ways, there is a danger that any notion of female agency is theorised out of existence, because female needs, desires and so forth are seen to be socially constructed on male terms (Cooper, 1994). Such an issue extends beyond the scope of this chapter. Nonetheless, many non-marital pregnancies in the present study, whether intended or not, presented a challenge to the institution of marriage; a significant site of patriarchal power.

References

Blair SL, Lichter DT (1991) Measuring the division of household labour: Gender segregation among American couples. *J Fam Iss* **12**: 91–113

Bury J (1984) *Teenage Pregnancy in Britain*. Birth Control Trust, London

Central Statistics Office (1972–1992) *Report on Vital Statistics*. The Stationery Office, Dublin

Chandlier J (1991) *Women Without Husbands: An Exploration of the Margins of Marriage*. Macmillan Education, London

Cooper D (1994) Productive, relational and everywhere? Conceptualising power and resistance within Foucauldian feminism. *Sociol* **48**(2): 435–54

Cowan CP, Cowan PA (1992) *When Partners Become Parents: The Big Life Change for Couples*. Basic Books, New York

Croghan R (1991) First-time mothers' accounts of inequality in the division of labour. *Feminism Psychol* **1**(2): 221–46

Delphy C (1992) A theory of marriage. In: McDowell L, Pringle R, eds. *Defining Women: Social institutions and Gender Divisions*. Polity Press in Association with the Open University, Cambridge: 138–9

Department of Health (1993) *Vital Statistics Fourth Quarter and Yearly Summary, 1992*. The Stationery Office, Dublin

Finlay A, Shaw N, McKeever M, Whittington D, McWilliams M (1994) *Adolescent Sexuality, Teenage Pregnancy and the Notion of an Underclass: Reflections from Northern Ireland*. Paper presented at the BSA Annual Conference, Sexualities in Social Context, University of Central Lancashire, Preston, England, March 28–31

Finlay A, Shaw N, Whittington D, McWilliams M (1995) *Adolescent Reproductive Behaviour in the Western Health and Social Service Board Area: A study carried out by the Centre for Health and Social Research, University of Ulster* (executive summary). Western Health and Social Services Board, Northern Ireland

Glaser B (1978) *Theoretical Sensitivity*. Sociology Press, Mill Valley, CA

Glaser B (1992) *Emergence Versus Forcing: Basics of Grounded Theory Analysis*. Sociology Press, Mill Valley, CA

Glaser B, Strauss A (1967) *The Discovery of Grounded Theory: Strategies for Qualitative Research*. Aldine Publications, Chicago

Holland J, Ramazanoglu C, Scott S, Sharpe S, Thompson R (1990) Sex, gender and power: Young women's sexuality in the shadow of AIDS. *Sociol Health Illness* **12**(3): 336–50

Hyde A (1996) Unmarried Women's Experiences of Pregnancy and the Early Weeks of Motherhood in an Irish Context: A Qualitative Analysis. Unpublished PhD Thesis, Trinity College, Dublin

Jacobsen H (1994) Multiple Meanings: Young Women's Experiences with Contraception. Unpublished MPhil dissertation, Trinity College, Dublin

Katz Rothman B (1994) *The Tentative Pregnancy: Amniocentesis and the Sexual Politics of Motherhood*. Pandora, London

Kiely G (1995) Fathers in families. In: McCarthy IC, ed. *Irish Family Studies: Selected Papers*. The Family Studies Centre, University College, Dublin: 147–58

Macintyre S (1977) *Single and Pregnant*. Croom Helm, London

Macintyre S, Cunningham-Burley S (1993) Teenage pregnancy as a social problem: A perspective from the United Kingdom. In: Lawson A, Rhode D, eds. *The Politics of Pregnancy: Adolescent Sexuality and Public Policy*. Yale University Press, Yale

Market Research Bureau of Ireland (1992) *Mna nah Eireann*. MRBI, Dublin

McRae S (1993) *Cohabiting Mothers: Changing Marriage and Motherhood?* Policy Studies Institute, London

Morgan DHJ, Scott S (1993) Bodies in a social landscape. In: Scott S, Morgan D, eds. *Body Matters: Essays on the Sociology of the Body*. The Falmer Press, London: 1–21

Phoenix A (1991) *Young Mothers*. Polity Press, Cambridge

Pollock S (1985) Sex and the contraceptive act. In: Homans H, ed. *The sexual Politics of Reproduction*. Gower, Hants: 64–77

Rainey DY, Stevens-Simon C, Kaplan DW (1992) Self-perception of infertility: A deterrent to effective contraception among female teens? *J Adolesc Health* **13**(3): 42

Richardson D (1993) *Women, Mothering and Childrearing*. Macmillan, London

Second Commission on the Status of Women. (1993). *Report to Government*. Stationery Office, Dublin

Shelton BA, John D (1993) Does marital status make a difference? Housework among cohabiting men and women. *J Fam Iss* **11**: 115–135

Smart C (1984) *The Ties That Bind: Law, Marriage and the Reproduction of Patriarchal Relations*. Routledge and Kegan Paul, London

South SJ, Spitze G (1994) Housework in marital and non-marital households. *Am Sociolog Rev* **59**: 327–47

Walby S (1990) *Theorising Patriarchy*. Basil Blackwell, Oxford

Whelan C, Fahey T (1994) Marriage and the family. In: Whelan C, ed. *Values and Social Change in Ireland*. Gill and Macmillan, Dublin: 45–81

Wight D (1992) Impediments to safer heterosexual sex: A review of research with young people. *AIDS Care* **4**(1): 11–21

14

The importance of predecessorship in childbirth

Maureen G G Laryea

Introduction

The concept of predecessorship is not new: it is an integral part of any status passage. Weeks (1972) defined a status passage as 'the moves which individuals make in and out of various social positions during the course of a career'.

When an individual moves from one social position to another, invariably there will be other people who had previously occupied the same position. Strauss (1962) referred to these individuals as predecessors because they have been through most of the experiences likely to be encountered by the incumbent of the position. The availability of predecessors allows for continuity of specific experiential information about a particular social position. Strauss (1962) described the way predecessors perform their role:

> *In a host of ways, you are prepared for what is to come, you are made aware of the immediacy of the next transition, are reminded that you have made a passage . . . The more subtle of the preparation include prewarning you that certain events will soon happen, that you will experience certain feelings, and when you do the predecessors will stand by with interpretations of such predicted events. Their interpretations embody the special language of the group. Post fact explanations are also at hand, so that when a person encounters situations for which she has no definitions, she will be offered ready made ones . . . We went through this . . . It means . . .*

This kind of preparations is possibly intended to give the individual a realistic perception of events, adequate situational support and coping strategies, as long as others do not give the individual numerous contradictory explanations about a particular event. The concept of predecessorship is applicable to the process of childbirth.

When a woman becomes pregnant for the first time, she moves from a status of childlessness to motherhood, while a woman who has previously given birth moves from being a mother of one child to being a mother of two; each position has its unique experiences. The latter is a predecessor to the former. There are two groups of predecessors in childbirth. The first are healthcare professionals who have been legally designated to look after expectant women. Within this group are three categories:

- male doctors by virtue of their training and practical experience gained from their work. They possess a wealth of esoteric knowledge, but have no personal experience of birth and cannot relate to the experience of the women they look after
- women who have not yet given birth or may not wish to. Like the male doctors, they have a wealth of knowledge and experience
- women who have given birth and can, therefore, relate to the experience of childbirth. They also have knowledge of birth as a result of their training, but because their professional training encourages social distance and discourages self-disclosure, they do not always share their personal experiences openly with expectant women. Furthermore, the heightened awareness of birth diminishes over time.

The second group of predecessors is made up of women who are not healthcare professionals, but who have previously given birth. They readily share their experiences with other women; their knowledge is usually considered by healthcare professionals as subjective, dangerous and sometimes obsolete. Women who hold a predecessorship role have, among other things, personal experience of birth and a knowledge of the rules, ceremonies, procedures and some of the difficulties that may occur during childbirth. It is the first group of predecessors who organise classes to prepare expectant women for labour and birth because they have been socially and professionally assigned this responsibility.

Selected literature review

It is important to view preparation classes for birth as a way of facilitating the process of birth. The class content is intended to make women have confidence in themselves, in their ability to cope with labour. Over the years, in some western societies, lay participation in teaching the younger generation about childbirth issues has been minimal. More reliance has been placed on the expertise of healthcare professionals. Therefore, first-time expectant women missed out on the experiential knowledge of other female members. Over-reliance on healthcare professionals' expertise has been due in part to a number of factors, such as:

- **geographical mobility**: young married couples tend to move away from home shortly after marriage or before the birth of the child. As a result, the expectant or nursing mother has no close relatives to teach or reassure her
- **the generation gap**: each generation has its own views, practices and knowledge of childbirth
- **the use of technology** in childbirth may have increased over-reliance on healthcare professionals since they have technological skills. Technological knowledge cannot be mastered by family members and friends
- **the belief that medical knowledge** about parenthood and reproduction comes from experts and is, therefore, 'proper' knowledge (Pendergast and Prout, 1990).

Studies have criticised the content of preparation classes (Oakley, 1981; Perkins, 1979; Rees, 1982). They cite poor preparation of teaching sessions, lack of realism about the burdens of parenthood, conflicting advice and wrong impressions. These criticisms are levelled at the people considered to have expert knowledge about childbirth, and who are supposed to guide the women through the period of childbirth.

In the last two decades, criticism has been levelled at the way healthcare professionals prepare women for labour and birth. Sargent and Stark (1989) showed that the emphasis during preparation in some parts of America is focussed explicitly and implicitly on hospital policies. Similarly, preparation classes in New Zealand consist of procedures and policy matters; women are not given the information they need to challenge the establishment (Gilkison, 1991). It is apparent that these approaches do not empower those expectant women who want to participate in their childbirth experience and make decisions about it.

In the last decade, there has been an increase in the number of preparation classes for childbirth organised by groups that are not healthcare professionals. There are no figures to show the number of women who attend these classes. The class content incorporates what parents-to-be wish to learn. Classes are also intended to increase women's belief in themselves and their ability to give birth, and to give them knowledge so that they will be empowered and able to participate in decision making.

The study

The purpose of this study was to establish the reasons why some expectant women choose to prepare themselves for labour and birth by using the services of people who are not healthcare professionals, when they will deliver in hospital attended by healthcare professionals. The term *predecessor* as used here refers to an individual who has been through the experience of childbirth. The study was carried out in two Canadian provinces and three cities in the UK.

Study design

A descriptive exploratory design was used. The aims were twofold:

- to explore the reasons why some expectant women choose to attend preparation classes run by women who are not healthcare professionals
- to describe the strategies and activities expectant women engage in at the preparatory classes.

Sample size

Ninety-five Caucasian expectant women who were attending preparation classes not run by healthcare professionals took part in the study. Sixty were from two Canadian provinces and 35 from three British cities. Because the membership of each class was small, a number of locations were used in order to obtain a reasonable sample. Since there was no exclusion criteria, the sample was made up of first, second and third-time expectant women.

Methods of data collection

Observational techniques

Two techniques were used. The author adopted the participant-as-observer role throughout the course of preparation classes. In this role she was free to move, mingle and talk with participants, and to read some of the books and academic papers made available by the teacher. She also listened to the content of the discussions and noted who participated.

Laryea also used the complete participant stance when the women engaged learning relaxation techniques. Although this was an activity from which no data was required for this study, she needed to be present afterwards to find out the kinds of issues women talked about during refreshments.

Interviews

Respondents were interviewed twice in their own homes. After the discussion series, each woman who attended was interviewed to obtain information about demographic characteristics, reasons for attending the group, views about her pregnancy, the kind of supportive behaviour/activities she received from the leader and/or members of the group, and the kind of supportive behaviour/activities she considered helpful. The investigator prepared for the interview by reading each respondent's profile, which had been developed over the five to eight weeks of group meetings. The interviews lasted 50 to 60 minutes and were audiotaped. The women spoke freely because the investigator was known to them.

The second interviews were carried out within two weeks of delivery. These interviews proved more difficult to arrange in some cases, so 10 women were interviewed by telephone. The interviews lasted 45 to 60 minutes and were taped. Data collected included the women's views about labour and birth, what they considered to be supportive behaviour/ activities and the extent to which they perceived they were able to help themselves during this time. Information on the early postnatal period was gathered, including what the women considered helpful behaviour during this time, decision-making on issues concerning the baby, and difficulties they confronted and how they solved them.

Data analysis

Quantitative analysis was performed on structured interview questions as well as numerical and frequency counts of the range of topics discussed. Questions were copied onto cards, which were sorted according to categories before relationships between categories were established. The qualitative data from open-ended questions were analysed using the constant comparative method to identify major categories. These were reviewed by a panel of experts. Frequencies were calculated for the number of responses in each category.

The findings

Tables 14.1 to *14.3* show the demographic profiles of participants.

Table 14.1:Differences in age of the Canadian and British women

Age (yrs)	Canadian	British
less than 20	1 (2%)	—
20 to 30	35 (58%)	19 (54%)
30 to 40	23 (38%)	16 (46%)
40+	1 (2%)	—
Total	60 (100%)	35 (100%)

Table 14.2: The different gestational stages of pregnancy of Canadian and British expectant women

Weeks of Gestation	Canadian	British
28 to 30	12 (20%)	21 (60%)
31 to 34	48 (80%)	14 (40%)
Total	60 (100%)	35 (100%)

Table 14.3: Differences in parity of the Canadian and British expectant women

Parity	Canadian	British
First pregnancy	40 (67%)	27 (77%)
Second pregnancy	15 (25%)	5 (14%)
Third pregnancy	5 (8%)	3 (9%)
Total	60 (100%)	35 (100%)

Reasons for choosing preparation classes

In search of detailed information

All respondents in both samples said that their reason for attending the classes was to obtain detailed and balanced information to enable them to ask the right questions of caregivers, challenge decisions made by them and speak to them as equals during negotiations. They also wanted detailed information in order to make informed decisions and be active participants throughout the process of childbirth.

The respondents believed that information from healthcare professionals lacked detail and was sometimes based on what they thought mothers should know. The women said that detailed information would increase their ability to analyse and rationalise pregnancy issues for themselves, would minimise feelings of panic and would ultimately reduce the number of visits to the doctor for minor issues. The women maintained that when an individual is given balanced information, she will select what she considers appropriate for her situation. In the process she becomes self-reliant. But when little information is given, she is unable to make decisions and often has to refer to someone else for guidance, thereby becoming over- dependent.

The women who were new immigrants to Canada gave an additional reason for attending the preparation classes: they wanted to learn from Canadian mothers the expected behaviour in labour.

Listening to the experience of others

Most of the Canadian (37 or 62%) and British (23 or 66%) first-time mothers indicated that the literature on childbirth written by healthcare professionals was informative. However, their analysis was that it was more focussed on procedures during pregnancy, labour and birth, conveying the notion that in labour women were passive recipients of care. In their view, the literature was written from the medical perspective. Recent personal accounts of individuals during pregnancy, labour and birth and how they responded and participated in the process were omitted. Therefore, one of the most frequently cited reasons for attending the classes was to hear other women's positive and negative reactions to childbirth. They referred to this as the 'gut reactions'. For these women, formal and informal knowledge was considered important since it offered a fuller picture of childbirth. Thus, it can be argued that predecessors are useful in providing the experiential knowledge that might help expectant women prepare themselves for the birth event. In accordance with Strauss (1962), this type of preparation gives the individual a realistic perception of events.

Seeking confirmation from experienced mothers

The women said they attended the classes to be in the company of those who had previously given birth. They also wanted the benefit of being prepared for labour and birth by someone who had been through it and knew about the hospital system. The teacher/leader was seen as a person who was aware of some of the common difficulties facing women during this time, someone who would be able to advise on how best to avoid or overcome them. Because of her knowledge on issues relating to birth and the readily available personal accounts of other group members, expectant mothers were at ease discussing with others their feelings, sensations, nutrition and personal views. The women believed that receiving confirmation from others was vital in building self-confidence. This was always expressed as 'It's good to know that all I feel and think is normal'.

Seeking support from the leader/teacher

The majority of the women (89 or 94%) joined the classes because they wanted the support of the leader/teacher. Support in this context was defined as giving advice, information and/or confirmation of the woman's actions and/or giving emotional support. Women who wanted a home confinement came to ask advice on how best to approach doctors to negotiate for at-home delivery. They also wanted to know the available alternatives if their doctors refused to deliver them at home.

The four young unmarried Canadian women affirmed that they joined the classes to get to know the leader/teacher, befriend her and ask her to be their labour coach and support person. To them, the leader/teacher was the most appropriate individual for this role because of her personal birth experience and assertiveness, which was defined as 'her ability to argue and make requests clearly and insistently'. Boyfriends were ruled out as unsuitable for this function since they were not conversant with the intricate issues of birth. These young women were also uncertain of their partners' ability to resist healthcare professionals' dominance when decisions had to made during labour.

Choices available

Sixteen women (17%) who were pregnant for the second or third time said that one of their reasons for joining the classes was to obtain information on choices available in childbirth because in their earlier pregnancies they were not made aware of the choices available. To these women, this information was important to have, since it enabled them to enter into meaningful discussion and put forward sound arguments when negotiating with their doctors for the kind of delivery they wanted.

Seeking coping skills

Sixty-nine women (37 Canadians, or 62%; and 32 British, or 91%) believed that because childbirth is a personal experience it is the right of each individual to be actively involved rather than being just a participant. Active involvement was considered to include learning the techniques to minimise the effect of pain in labour. In their opinion, learning these techniques required expert coaching before they could be perfected.

Seeking a conducive atmosphere

Several reasons were given by Canadian (43, 72%) and British (30, 86%) women why they wanted their husbands or partners to be well-informed about childbirth. First, their partners needed to be knowledgeable because they had important roles during labour and birth. The roles required them to possess information about and insights into some of the problems faced by expectant women during this time. The women believed that a better understanding is formulated when both partners work and learn as a team. Moreover, in labour they expected their partners to act as advocates and perform the role effectively. A number of partners had children from previous marriages, but had not accompanied their wives to classes because it was during the time when to be seen at such gatherings was considered unmanly. Therefore, for them, involvement in the classes was a new experience. Part of the reason for choosing to attend was because the women heard from others that the size of the classes was smaller compared to the classes run by the healthcare professionals; and the couples and expectant women received individual attention. They assumed that in a small group it would be easy to open a discussion and to encourage active participation. They were confident that their partners would join in the discussions. *Figure 14.1* shows the patterns of interactions between participants during group discussions.

More than half (49, 52%) of participants said they wanted their husbands to be in the company of other expectant fathers so that they could listen to

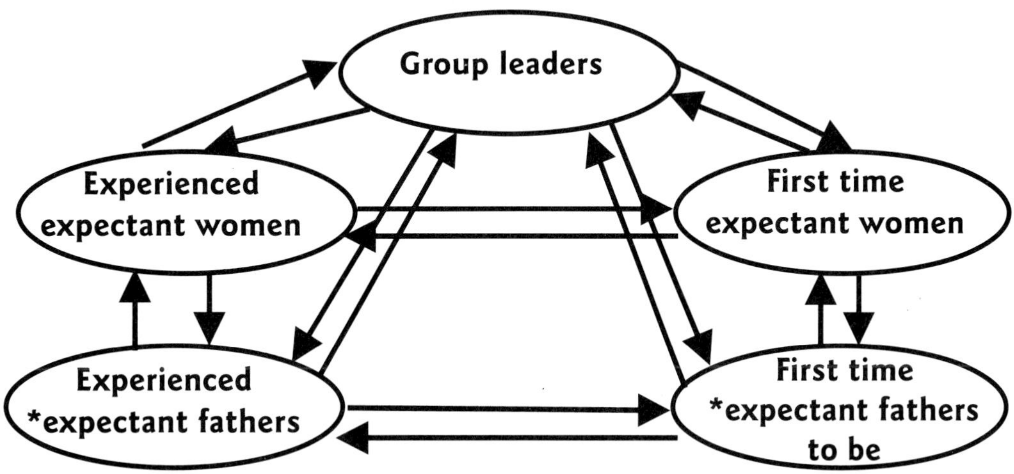

*The expectant fathers are included in this diagram because they participated in the discussions and activities. As relevant participants they supported their partners throughout childbirth.

Figure 14.1: Patterns of interactions between participants during the group discussion meetings (Canada and Britain)

their accounts, personal views and feelings about birth, and possibly learn from them. The women also held the view that husbands or partners needed to be in the presence of other expectant women to hear them talk about physical discomfort and emotional feelings. The rationale was to make husbands realise that their wives were not malingering.

Resource person

Having a resource person to turn to was considered by all respondents to be the most important supportive action during pregnancy. A resource person in this case was someone who had been through the experience of giving birth or was knowledgeable and familiar with the experience. She needed to be available and accessible.

Canadian and British women pregnant for the first time (30, 45%) said that, as pregnancy advanced, new physical and emotional changes occur that they found puzzling. It was during such times that the detail of their pregnancies and also certain issues do not need medical attention, but rather someone who knows how an expectant woman feels and can guide her through the process, or clarify issues that puzzled her. Not only was the resource person expected to be knowledgeable on matters pertaining to childbirth, she was also expected to have the ability to create an environment that allowed women to feel relaxed and free to discuss matters that troubled them. One mother said:

> *'It's been hard for me being single. There are a lot of things I had to find for myself. I needed someone to answer my questions, someone to walk along side me, point me to the right direction. I needed a person who would not think that I was stupid, but had a good idea of what I was going through. Someone who was accessible, available and who understood my pain, and knew my need. Someone who was non-judgmental, and would not reject me as my family had done'.*
>
> [a Canadian woman]

A resource person was expected to keep confidences. One Canadian first-time mother in her early 40s reported that she always felt embarrassed by her age. She had never discussed the matter with her husband, who was much younger than she. During a routine visit to her doctor, he made reference to her age by explaining to her in the presence of her husband that because she was an 'elderly' first-time expectant woman she might not be able to cope well with the stresses of labour and birth and might need surgical intervention. According to her, not only was the doctor's statement embarrassing, but, most important of all, it eroded her self-confidence. She needed to discuss with someone her fears of being a potential failure in labour, which, in her view, was tantamount to being condemned long before labour started. To retain her confidence, she spoke to her leader privately. She said:

> *'Because I look at my group leader as my resource person, I could not hide my anger and frustration with my doctor. I discussed with my leader what strategies I could use to make my doctor see that I wanted a vaginal delivery, not a c-section because of my age. I just poured out my heart to her, I cried and cried as I was telling her this. She did not think I was crazy or hysterical and I'll tell you something else, she didn't think it was my hormones making me feel like this either. I felt she understood me. I would not have done this anywhere else. I did not mind telling her that I was sensitive about my age. She listened to me and pointed out that women of my age group in the past, were usually given the chance to go into labour. She suggested that I go back to my doctor and discuss with him other available options.*

Inherent in this statement are three important issues that can boost or destroy maternal confidence. First, it is important for an expectant woman to have someone to confide in, who is able to listen to her and offer encouragement. Second, a pregnant woman needs to feel that her point of view is understood; she needed to know that all available options had been discussed with her. Third, a casual remark can destroy the maternal confidence. It is debatable whether age alone should be used as the determining factor in the management of labour. It is usual practice to take other factors into consideration.

Timing of meetings

One of the important reasons that participants were attracted to the group was the timing of the meetings, most of which were held at a time convenient to participants. In Canada the evening classes allowed working fathers to attend and be actively involved. Their active participation was said to enhance the feelings of joy, tranquillity and togetherness. Furthermore, the fathers' active involvement in pregnancy was considered to be a factor that encouraged family-centred care throughout childbirth. Because of the active part husbands and partners played during this time, they also needed to be well-informed about childbirth.

Discussion

In childbirth some women may be uncertain and apprehensive about the outcome of birth; giving them relevant information will help reduce these emotional reactions, which in turn contributes toward the women's well-being during this time. Therefore, the principal reason why women attended these preparation classes was to obtain detailed information they could use to help themselves during childbirth. The information required by a woman at any point in the nine months may be adequate or inadequate to meet the demands of the new situation. In childbirth, regardless of the number of times a woman has given birth, she still needs some information about various aspects related to it. This could be attributed in part to two main factors. First, the uniqueness of each childbirth experience may produce different body sensations and feelings that require new coping strategies. Second, the rapid changes in techniques, procedures and policies all generate new information that some expectant women might not know about, since the information exchanged between women, their doctors and other healthcare professionals is often controlled and mainly focused on preparing them for the birth of their babies. While it is essential to enlighten women about policies and procedures, the information given should be directed toward meeting women's needs. It is not surprising that all respondents came to the meeting seeking detailed childbirth information.

Preparation classes can be viewed as a vehicle for promoting women's health, since information and education are prerequisites for making informed decisions. The emphasis should be on enabling women rather than disenabling them. This approach is time-consuming because it requires that women be given time to explore and discuss issues related to health in childbirth and others that are central to their interest. The goal should be to increase their knowledge by giving balanced appropriate information to enable them to make their own decisions, achieve self-determination, understand events and ask appropriate questions. Simmons and Parsons (1983) said that empowerment starts when individuals are encouraged to develop a critical awareness of their situation. Similarly, Wallerstein and Berstein (1988), in their discussion of empowerment education, commented that it is intended to primarily help individuals to participate actively and gain control over their life events. Expectant women attending preparation classes for childbirth need to be exposed to this approach if they are to negotiate their care with doctors and gain a balance of control in childbirth.

Negotiations

Negotiations are discussions between two or more individuals with apparent intention to resolve (Pruitt and Carnevale, 1993). Because of the divergence of interests between some women and healthcare professionals over the management of childbirth, women's wishes about the way they want their childbirth managed are often in conflict with doctors; this sometimes leads to maternal dissatisfaction with some aspects of their care.

Since healthcare professionals are 'gate keepers' to esoteric knowledge and give access to maternity services, women have to negotiate with them the place where they wish to be confined, the way they wish to have their labour managed and the number of people they want to be present at delivery. Successful negotiations are in part based on a sound knowledge of the issues to be discussed and the availability of choices. There is evidence to show that expectant women are not always informed of the available choices in terms of the place of confinement (Crookston *et al*, 1994; Department of Health, 1993).

Women engaged in negotiating aspects of their care not only need to be persistent with their requests, they also need to have a resource person to provide encouragement and additional information when necessary. Successful negotiations help increase the women's self-esteem and confidence. It is also possible that the negotiations help increase the women's level of trust in their caregivers.

This leads to four implications. First, empowerment education during pregnancy is paramount in helping women develop critical awareness of the way childbirth is managed. Second, care of expectant women requires healthcare professionals to adopt a flexible approach to accommodate individual wishes; this would change the way childbirth is practised. Third, the presence of a resource person who is able to discuss with women their concerns and available choices may be invaluable to some women during this time. Fourth, successful negotiations contribute to the women's feelings of well-being, which is crucial to women's health, their families and community.

Social support

In most status passages there are relevant participants whose task is to ensure that the status passage is accomplished. These people also give support to the individual. It is generally acknowledged by healthcare professionals that women attend preparation classes for childbirth primarily to obtain information; this view is indisputable. However, the women in this study also attended the classes to receive different types of support from members of the class and from the leader/teacher. Cronenwett (1985) said that support involves a provider and a recipient; the provider must be available and accessible. These two components are essential because, as the individual moves through the status passage, new puzzling events unfold. Thus, a woman who is a primigravida confronted by fears and doubts may need to talk about them, but healthcare professionals are not always available and accessible, so expectant women tend to use their predecessors and peers.

In conclusion, women who choose to prepare themselves for birth using groups not led by healthcare professionals are empowered by such groups through dissemination of professional knowledge and the sharing of experiential knowledge from predecessors and peers. The availability of predecessors provide particular information that is not readily available in some of the health professionals' textbooks.

Limitations of the study

The findings of this study must be interpreted with caution because the sample was not representative of the total population. It consisted primarily of middle-class, well-educated women. Their needs may be different from those of expectant women from other social classes.

References

Cronenwett L (1985) Parental network structure and perceived support after birth of the first child. *Nurs Res* **134**(6): 347–52

Crookston L, Harrisson SP, Sharp G, Vamplew C (1994) *Review of Maternity Services in South Cleveland: A Survey of Clients, Midwives and Auxiliary Staff*. Health Care Research Unit of Durham with Women and Children's Division. Durham University Press, South Cleveland

Department of Health (1993) *Changing Childbirth: Report of the Expert Maternity Group*. Part 1. HMSO, London

Gilkinson A (1991) Antenatal education: Whose purpose does it serve? *N Zeal Coll Midwives J* 4, May: 13–15

Oakley A (1981) Adjusting to motherhood. *Nurs Times* 1: 899–901

Pendergast S, Prout A (1990) Learning about parenthood and sex education in English secondary schools. In: Garcia J, Kilpatrick R, Richards M, eds. *The Politics of Maternity Care Services for Childbearing Women in the Twentieth Century Britain*. Clarendon Press, Oxford

Perkins ER (1979) *What do Clients Need? Toward a Responsive Health Education Programme*. Leverhulme Health Education Project Occasional Paper No. 19.

Pruitt DG, Carnevale PJ (1993) *Negotiations in Social Conflict*. Open University Press, Buckingham

Rees C (1982) Antenatal classes: Time for a new approach. *Nurs Times* **78**(48): 1446–68

Sargent C, Stark N (1989) Childbirth education and childbirth models: Parental perspectives on control anesthesia and technological intervention in the birth process. *Med Anthropol Q* **3**: 36–51

Simmons C, Parsons R (1983) Empowerment for the alternatives in adolescence. *Adolesc* **18**: 193–200

Strauss AL (1962) Transformation of Identity. In: Rose AM, ed. *Human Behavior and Social Process: An Interactionist Approach*. Routledge and Kegan Paul, London

Wallerstein N, Berstein E (1988) Empowerment education: Freire ideas adapted to health education. *Health Educ Q* **15**(4): 379–94

Weeks D (1972) *Self, Society and Social Interaction. Social Interaction: The Sociological Perspective*. Unit 5–8, Social Science, 2nd level course, unit 6. Open University Press, Milton Keynes

15

Breast-feeding in feminine routine

Ana Márcia Spanó Nakano and Marli Villela Mamede

Introduction

The last national research on breast-feeding in Brazil revealed that 97% of women start suckling and, of those, 43% discontinue before the child is three months old (Brazil, 1995). Mixed suckling is widely done and the most frequent cause of early weaning mentioned by the women studied is hypogalactia. Women rarely admit to deciding not to suckle the child of their own will and have ready stereotyped answers adapted to what seems to be accepted and expected in their social environment, for in our society breast-feeding is valued and demanded of mothers.

Arguments used by campaigns to encourage breast-feeding have had little effect. The campaigns stress the importance of suckling for the child, focusing on the biological, nutritional and economic aspects, but disqualifying women's real wishes and positioning women as objects in the process, or instruments to achieve the campaigns' goals. They also assign to women alone the responsibility and blame for the social problems that lead to infant morbidity and mortality.

The problem we discuss now, that of early weaning, is very old. History shows that women have always sought a way of getting rid of breast-feeding or delegating the suckling function. Historical reports about breast-feeding, like the ones presented by Badinter (1985), demonstrate the variability of the social behaviour of feeding from the breast at different times, and shows the social relationships of women to man and child in each historical context.

We understand that breast-feeding is a complex and multidimensional practice, and so cannot be reduced to its biological determinants, the main reference for health professionals. This is because breast-feeding does not concern only the female body, but also its articulation with women's social reality.

We focus our analysis on the woman who experiences the suckling process, in terms of a social act, considering as a starting point the meanings she herself attributes to the practice. The aim of this study, therefore, is to understand women's ideas about breast-feeding, with a view to identifying:

- the amount of information they have, their beliefs and values about breast-feeding
- the relationships they make between the maternity and breast-feeding
- the relationships they see between the suckling process and other functions they perform in their everyday lives
- the meanings they attribute to the experiences and demands related to breast-feeding.

Methodological theoretical reference

The theoretical choice for analysis in this study was feminist theory that understands breast-feeding as a practice articulated to social reality, where the roles women and men play contribute to the building of gender and, according to which gender, is seen as an analytic category.

Gender, in contrast to sex, is a social product that is learned, represented, institutionalised and passed on from generation to generation, as pointed out by Sorj (1992). Therefore, it should not be seen as a simple, natural and indisputable fact, but as a social and relational process, mediated by power.

The concept of gender suggests immediately the idea of relation, since subjects are produced through relation and in relation. Thus, gender is a social construct and, as such, historical.

We understand that women's decisions and actions in their suckling routine are guided by their representations. According to Moscovici (1978), to represent something, or a state, does not only mean to unfold it, repeat it or reproduce it, but also to reconstruct it, to renew it, or modify it. He elaborates a dynamic and explicative concept when he introduces the term 'social representation'.

The concept of social representation is widely discussed by researchers. Jodelet (1994) proposed the following general concept of social representation, which is shared by the authors: 'Social representation is a form of knowledge, socially elaborated and shared, having a practical approach and contributing to the construction of a reality common to a social group'.

In our investigation, representations of the women studied constitute the empirical data we resort to in order to understand the construction of the postulates they use, elaborate and communicate about the suckling act.

We assume that the representations the women have about feminine identity include their representations about breast-feeding, with a possible overlapping of meanings about being a woman (mother, wife, worker and citizen), and suckling.

Investigation process

The research methodology selected for this study was a qualitative approach. The study setting was the population of women attending at a health unit in Ribeiro Preto, State of Sao Paulo, Brazil. The social actors in the study were women who were experiencing suckling for the first time, not necessarily being primiparae, and who were willing to talk about their experiences. These women were engaged in either exclusive or mixed suckling, their children being between 1 and 12 months of age at the time of contact.

Since this was a qualitative study, our main concern was with the saturation of data, although some quantification was necessary to clarify the sample. Twenty-two nursing mothers participated in the study, with ages varying from 18 to 24 years. Most (17 or 77.27%) lived with their sexual partner. More than half (13 or 59.1%) had gone to primary school. Most (12 or 54.5%) were housewives who only worked at home; of the others, 55.56% were economically active, earning between one and two times the monthly minimum wage (the Brazilian minimum wage was equivalent to $108 US per month at the time). Most (17 or 77.3%) were Catholic. Sixty-four percent were engaged in exclusive suckling and 35% in mixed suckling.

The interviews were carried out in the subjects' homes; were recorded with their permission — it is important to mention that all nursing mothers approved of the procedure. The instrument for data collecting was the semi-structured interview, based on a guiding script and observation of context constituents.

The data were transcribed and analysed according to the Bardin (1977) technique of content analysis. We performed a thematic analysis, in which utterances were taken as register units and grouped according to theme contents.

Based on the empirical data about breast- feeding and after identifying the study's problem or object, we organised the discussion into three topics.

Data analysis

Subjects' social representations about breast-feeding

What we tried to gather was the women's level of information, values and beliefs about the topic of breast-feeding. Breast-feeding was represented as being responsible for the children's physical and emotional well-being, and human milk was said to be high in nutrition and immunisation value, as can be seen in the following quote: 'They say it is healthier for the child, [it] develops more quickly, so I have to suckle because of that' (interview subject no. 20).

The women investigated also had a wider conception of health, in that they associated breast-feeding with subjective conditions for the child's well-being: 'the child seems to be happier when it sucks at the breast' (18).

The women studied considered mothers' milk the ideal kind of food because it is complete in terms of the nutrients necessary for the child's nourishment, because it is healthy and pure. They opposed artificial milk as impersonal, unnatural and impure: 'My milk is much stronger than powdered milk or the milk in the box, I believe it's stronger, what is going to satisfy it is my milk. I think there is a difference in terms of food between one kind of milk and the other because the rest makes the baby to feel full, but not well nourished, you have to give other things to complement' (16).

Such women demonstrate that they have a wider notion about what nourishment means, artificial milk being only 'food', not 'nourishment' for the child.

When comparing different kinds of milk, they would even equate human milk with vaccines or a medicine to cure diseases, in contrast to artificial milk, which would cause disease or be a pathogenic agent: 'Breast milk is important because if you give the other, the baby can get more diseases . . . Breast milk has formed antibodies, so it doesn't have any health problem' (11).

We noticed that, if on the one hand women recognised the superiority of human milk for the baby, on the other they saw artificial milk as a resource to alleviate mothers of the burden of full-time dedication to the child. Ease of use of a nursing bottle is evident when women are faced with the reality of routine and, when work and lack of time overlap, they tend to develop an appreciative view of the use of nursing bottles: 'The baby bottle is very good from the point of view of her getting full quickly because in ten minutes she suckles and goes to sleep, now the breast no, she takes a lot of time' (6).

We can see that the content of the campaigns to encourage breast-feeding has been crystallised in the investigated women's imagery, although sometimes they lack the vocabulary to express it. Because their social role is so defined by biological determinants, breast-feeding is taken for granted as part of women's 'nature'.

Breast-feeding as an exercise of maternity and social gender relations

Breast-feeding is presented by the interviewees concurrently with pictures of beauty, affection and nature. Some women interviewed implied that breast-feeding was something sanctified, while showing that at the same time they hold it as 'natural' for the feminine gender and equate it with elevated standards of motherhood:

> *'Suckling is important for the baby. I think it is a factor that is part of the mother . . . It is natural really'.*
>
> [1]

> *'It is a form of caress, the mother gives love when she suckles . . . To suckle is something divine, it is something that came from God himself [who], besides giving us the gift of having children, gives suckling too'.*
>
> [10]

Reviewing the history of breast-feeding, such statements reflect the incorporation of discourses that involved women in the seventeenth century, picturing maternal love as instinctive and natural to all women.

Once the suckling act has the connotation of something sacred and pure, the breast becomes asexual, sometimes losing sensitivity and sensuality:

> *'The breast, I think it is only good for this, here, to suckle, I don't know what else it could be used for? Of course it has other uses but the child needs the breast a lot.'*
>
> [13]

Dignifying maternity embodies for women the experience of happiness, but also of sacrifice, giving, pains and suffering that, for Badinter (1985) is still widely undergone by many women.

> *'I am very worried about him. I don't like to see him cry, so I don't mind myself very much, or my body, now it is more part of suckling . . . I don't get much sleep, have to stay awake, am worried about him, I know I shouldn't be like that.'*
>
> [12]

In their representation of giving and sacrifice, women see themselves as turned away from themselves, disposing of themselves for the benefit of others. They sacrifice themselves for the children who demand immediate attendance of their needs, so revealing the devaluation of their own bodies and regarding it as inferior to their children's.

The idealised picture of a donating and sacrificing motherhood creates the image of the masochist mother, as Badinter (1985) calls it, according to which all suffering coming from motherhood should be well coped with, since it is inherent to the function of a mother.

> *'I'll suckle in spite of the breasts aching . . . When she suckled I wanted to take the breast out, but I insisted, felt a great pain, but went on suckling her.'*
>
> [16]

Pain, seen as something 'natural', must therefore be restrained, since it connotes being a mother and integrates the 'normal' process of breast-feeding that all women go through and bear. On the other hand, exaltation of pleasurable feelings when breast-feeding a child is expected by the social environment.

The concept of motherhood, to which the women studied refer, is the one they assume as a priority, of full-time dedication and exclusive responsibility. It cannot always be followed strictly, thus changing the feeling of responsibility into one of blame, as can be seen from this interviewee's discourse:

'When I go out I get some milk for him, but I get worried, thinking if he is not hungry, it's such a hurry . . . I feel stuck, it is a lot of work, I feel annoyed and when this feeling comes I regret it, to think this way, I blame myself.'

[20]

The women's representations of the act of breast-feeding supports the concept they have about what it means to be a woman: to be immersed in suffering, their freedom cut off, overburdened with the responsibilities and duties of motherhood. The suckling act is framed on the model of romantic and altruistic motherhood that constitutes a source of distress and conflicts for women since that model is difficult to fit into the present context.

The nursing woman's everyday routine

Analysis of the last topic makes it possible to gather the meanings the interviewees attribute to the demands from breast-feeding, as well as the relationships they establish with the other functions they perform in their daily routine.

Breast-feeding, represented as a normal process in the reproductive cycle, may generate expectations of a phase easily overcome by women, but when they actually experience it, women ask for guidance or reference models, uncovering the difficulties they meet, and their frustrations and suffering.

'I thought it was easier, I hoped it would be so . . . that when I had a child, for the time it suckled I would find it easy, that the milk would not get hard, that it would stop only when one wished.'

The issue of expressing milk is relevant for the women as well as for their relative environment, as a determinant of their capacity for being good nursing mothers and qualifying them as mothers:

My mother-in-law, chiefly, I think because she didn't suckle, kept saying that I would not be able to manage it because the baby was very greedy, that my milk was not enough, I got worried.'

[12]

We observed that it is the woman herself who makes the decision about what to do in face of the problem of milk shortage, especially regarding milk complementation.

'I have little milk, I said to the doctor that she became nervous as the milk took too long to come, so of my own account I started to give her NAN, then he told me to give her one hundred twenty grams, as I didn't have much milk.'

[4]

The image of the physician is a powerful one, as she represents the knowing authority and is seen as a strategic element to legitimate hypogalactia by prescribing milk complementation.

As Meyer (1996) puts it, the production and organisation of social life, especially the production of knowledge by the subjects involved, is through the productive dimension of multiple and widespread powers that act on the areas of relationships, symbolism and skills.

Thus, through the representations by the nursing mothers in this study, it can be see that they turn themselves into subjects in a continuous process of discipline, regulation and self-regulation, which for Foucault (1986) constitutes the centre of operations of the power networks.

Expectations about suckling as a 'natural' process lead to disguising signs and symptoms of mammary discomfort:

'. . . any problems? No, no . . . only the nipple, after that none, I used ointment, massage, cocoa butter on the nipple, my mother-in-law gave me, she said it was like that . . . at the beginning it was very hard, I suffered, the nipple cracked, the wound even opened, when she suckled it bled, I had fever a couple of days but went on suckling, I had to suckle her.'

[13]

We could assume, therefore, that mammary injuries are regarded as associated with the female body, which is attributed a lesser value than the child's, and which bears the stigma of being 'naturally' submitted and plundered. Thus, pain, a sign indicating abnormality, is disqualified by reason of the sacrifice established and expected in the role of mother. This helps us to understand why mothers seek care for mammary injuries too late, when the condition worsens.

By adding suckling to their other duties, mothers become overburdened by the overlapping activities and responsibilities. This reveals the women's represented omnipotent and omnipresent character, wishing to cope with everything, as can be seen in the following:

'When I cook I start thinking: Oh! I have to suckle, I have to do the washing, I have to tidy the house, it is too much trouble . . . I can't do everything, so I'm losing weight.'

[12]

In demanding a lot more of themselves, women try to shift indefinitely from one activity to the next, and thus have the illusory perception of being omnipotent. As a consequence, the drop in the quality of how women perform their multiple roles cannot be avoided, and raises feelings of incompetence, creating conflicts and demands within family relationships (private space) and on the job (public space).

'My mother, when she drops in and the house is in a mess, she says: it's because you idle away . . . What have you done until now? Why haven't you cleaned the house? I say it's because with the child I'm busy the whole day. I won't leave him aside to take care of the house.'

[9]

It is obvious that the social dimension is a framework for how women perform their roles, and it is frequently the women themselves who reproduce and maintain this inequity and discrimination:

'I'm exhausted, going to work the next day is not easy, but I'm trying to manage. This is the worst month in my job, there are income tax declarations to do for lots of clients. I'm going mad. I should have scheduled better, so I blame myself . . . My client has already phoned four times. He doesn't want to know [about my problem].'

[7]

When they assume that their larger responsibility, specifically motherhood, lies in the private sphere, they also incorporate the values constructed for women in this sphere, which do not allow for renunciation without feelings of blame or restriction.

Overlapping functions becomes a factor of discrimination in the job market, which is structured by the hegemonic male universe and becomes an illegitimate space for women.

Within family relationships, women defer to the male image. Men, even though they detach themselves or are detached somewhat from breast-feeding, since it is considered part of the female experience, have a significant influence on how women see themselves in relation to the suckling role. Male participation is represented as encouraging breast-feeding:

'He supports me a lot. He says: she's crying, she wants to suckle . . . [and he] warns [me] when it's time to change the breast.'

[1]

Although husbands' demand that their wives suckle, it is possible to see the subtle or sometimes direct exercise of power over women by means of the consequences resulting for the baby:

'My husband demands a lot that I breast-feed. I wanted to start weaning the baby and he disagreed . . . chiefly when the baby had diarrhoea when I gave him the other milk. He said, did you see? You wanted to wean him away. See what happened?'

[11]

Men's influence over women can also be an obstacle to breast-feeding, since it may raise feelings of insecurity in women. It can effect their body image, due to the consequences attributed to breast-feeding, such as causing the breasts to drop and making women feel less attractive to their partners (see *interviewee 10*), or when the partner demands more attention from the woman because he feels remote from the process (see *interviewee 21*):

'My friend told me not to suckle because the breasts drop, get flaccid and men don't like it . . . but what shall I do, I have already made my life, I am already married, what should I want beautiful breasts for?'

[10]

'He felt put aside and said, "You don't pay attention to me, you only mind the work, the child and yourself. You don't care for me, you forgot me!" I said to him, "Be patient with me, I think I'll learn with time . . . I saw I was wrong.'

[21]

In this way, women bear the blame for not being able to cope as they were meant to. They strengthen the social construction of the feminine gender as circumscribed within the private space, with maternity as the major role.

The difficulties experienced by the women studied, in the face of the overlapping of breast-feeding with other roles, are assumed by them as a typical female problem, not a social one, since the ideological discourse does not allow women to be aware either of the lack of social structure to support motherhood or of the lack of respect for gender differences.

Final considerations

We understand, from these women's statements, that breast-feeding is not only a biological phenomenon, but also includes a culturally constructed body of ideas and values, constituting a social practice that is historically legitimised and places women in a specific place within the set of social relationships.

In their representations on breastfeeding, women focus their attention and purpose on the child, which is an effective way of instituting breastfeeding as a maternal obligation, transferring to women the solution of more complex problems of infant disease. Their representations identify their feelings and values about breastfeeding and their behaviour discloses how they either accommodate to it or resist it.

The women studied demonstrate accommodation in their discourses when they represent breast-feeding as a process demanding patience, dedication, sacrifice and deferred compensations. They reveal, in practice, their resistance when they perform actions, such as mixed suckling and early weaning. They ally themselves with the same biological determinant that defined them as nursing mothers, declaring themselves unable to suckle their children; that is, milk production is accepted by the social environment, not condemned, and they obtain support from the community in which they live.

With the resistance movement, women create and recreate another kind of power. This is expressed more subliminally and subtly, since it takes place in the blurred field of emotionality and affectivity, which are more frequently a feature of the female's, rather than the male's powergame. Foucault (1986) refers to this specific kind of power as discipline or disciplinary power. In this context, discipline or disciplinary power is not an apparatus or an institution, but a strategy or a device that is a mechanism and an instrument of power. Therefore, for Foucault, it means the methods used by individuals to control their bodies' operations, insure the constant subjection of their forces.

The data in this study show the appeal of placing suckling within women's scope. It commits health professionals to promoting the view that suckling will be seen, not only from its biological aspect, but placed in a wider context that involves what it means to be a woman, a mother, a wife and a worker. They make it clear, however, that this new approach, for which women have asked, does not deny the child its rights and needs, but seeks to achieve a balance between the demands of both parties. Opening women's space so they can feel free and emancipated to express their real wishes in regard to suckling their children may be an important strategy for understanding breast-feeding as a process reaching beyond its biological determination.

It is urgent that strategies are explored that encourage women to be aware of their condition. It implies that professionals should assume an educational function, acting not only on the here and now of nursing women, but also on previous stages, when the feminine and masculine identities are being constructed. This relates to the phase of maternity and to the socialisation process.

References

Badinter E (1985) *Um Amor Conquistado: O Mito do Amor Materno* [A Conquered Love: The Myth of Maternal Love], 5 edn. Trans. Dutra W. Nova Fronteira, Rio de Janeiro

Bardin L (1977) *Análise de Conteúdo* [Content Analysis] 7 edn. Ediçoѕ Lisbon: 70

Brazil, Ministry of Health, National Institute of Food and Nourishment (1995) *Aleitamento Materno e Municipio* [Breast-feeding and Municipality]. UNICEF, Brasilia

Foucault M (1986) *Microfisica do Poder* [Metaphysics of Power] 6 edn. Graal, Rio de Janeiro

Jodelet D (1994) Représentations sociales: un omaine en expansion [Social representations: An expanding area]. In: Jodelet D, ed. *Les Représentations Sociales*, 4 edn. Presses Universitaires de France, Paris: 31–61

Meyer DE (1996) Do poder ao gênero: uma articulaçao teórico analíca [From power to gender: A theoretical-analytical articulation]. In: Lopes MJM, Meyer DE, Waldow VR, eds. *Gênero e Saúde*. Artes Médicas, Porto Alegre: 41–55

Moscovici S (1978) *A Representaçao Social da Psicanálise* [The Social Representation of Psychoanalysis. Zahar, Rio de Janeiro

Sorj B (1992) O feminismo na encruzilhada da modernidade e pós modernidade [Feminism at the crossroads of modernity and post-modernity]. In: Costa A de O, Bruschini CA, eds. *Uma Quest o de Gênero*. Rosa dos tempos, Rio de Janeiro: 15–23

Section IV

Traditional cultures and women's health

Women's social situations and the norms and expectations society places on them at a particular point in time have much to do with how they achieve their aspirations and their hopes for the future. Gloria Geller's longitudinal study looks at the aspirations of a group of women 20 years after they wrote their 'diaries for the future', and a portion of the same group of women 10 years after they wrote such diaries. She draws on life-course analysis to consider the women's aspirations and subsequent experiences with respect to the social, economic and political context of the 20-year period from the 1970s to the 1990s in Canada. Geller traces the women's well-being from their dreams in high school and through their life-course experiences.

Yoshiko Uchiyama discusses the place of women in Japanese society, and the class and sexual discrimination they experience in this highly industrialised yet paternalistic society. Although Japanese women made some strides in obtaining access to higher education and better-paying work, most companies in Japan are still reluctant to hire and promote women to well-paid jobs. Her chapter addresses the issue of changing cultural imperatives for Japanese women at the dawn of the twenty-first century by focussing on the evolution of traditional values that have gone towards structuring female roles in traditional Japanese society.

As the population ages and women are living longer than men, a large body of literature appears to focus on the health problems and social demands of the elderly, especially women. The resilience and strength of older women and their contributions to society, as well as their quest for knowledge to keep themselves as healthy as possible, has not been given much attention in the avalanche of literature on old age. Vicki Torsch's ethnographic study of older Chamarro women in Guam demonstrates the motivation of these older women to educate themselves and their families about self-help measures for leading healthy lives. Americanisation and social, political and economic change have transformed the traditional life-style into a more sedentary one, with more consumption of processed food. The tradition of caring and sharing, a basic value in Guam's society, has been overtaken by individualism and materialism. Chamorro women have a life expectancy of 76 years, and this population also has a high percentage of chronic illness, but they are highly motivated to learn self-help measures to keep themselves as healthy as possible. Torsch discusses the positive impact of integrating the elders' viewpoints in planning health delivery to these women.

Mollyn Bohnen and Deanna Balantac present the Personal/Professional Origins Model (POMelo) to assess the micro-origins/identity of the individual. Using POMelo to study Filipina-American nurses, they found that no two nurses drew a totally similar identity; rather, using cultural descriptors, all subjects drew models that represented their individual portraits of cultural identity. The authors present POMelo as a sensitive instrument to assess women's identity within their own culture.

Zohar Nir's and David Galisky's study explored the differences between two ethnic groups — Ashkenazi and Sephardi Jews — in relation to socio-economic background, family instrumental support during hospitalisation and family relationships. The study population consisted of 157 Ashkenazi and 161 Sephardi in a geriatric rehabilitation unit in Israel. In both groups, children were the most frequent source of support during hospitalisation. This chapter addresses the differences and similarities between the two groups and the implications for both the patients and care-givers.

Taiwan's culture, like most of the world's cultures, is patriarchal, and daughters-in-law are expected to care for their parents-in-law. With the increasing care needs of the frail and sick elders, the care-giving responsibilities of daughters-in-law are a major burden. Shu-Yuan Chao and Patricia Roth studied a group of Taiwanese women care-givers, and discuss the cultural factors that influence the care-giving constraints and impact of care-giving on the care-giver against the backdrop of Taiwan's male dominant culture.

Domestic violence, ie. wife abuse, and its effect on women has only been systematically studied recently. In Taiwan, with a strongly traditional patriarchal culture, women and children legally belong to men/husbands. The men's power and abuse of women sometimes lead the wife/women to attempt suicide. Often, victims who fail in their suicide attempts are seen in the hospital by medical professionals, but little attempt is made by medical people to diagnose or treat the social emotional needs of the women. The treatment is centred solely on the physical aspect. Yow-Hwey Hu, Shu-Chen Kua and Jeffrey J H, Tsai studied the records of women who came to the emergency services of a teaching hospital in Taiwan after suicide attempts. More than half were misdiagnosed or underdiagnosed as 'poisoning by accident'. Many were young wives living in abusive situations and trying to end their miserable lives by suicide. The authors discuss the gendered nature of the problem, the oppressed condition of women, the lack of understanding by medical personnel and the implications of the study.

Traditional Korean society is very patriarchal and dominated by Confucian ethics, both of which define the man as the head of the family; women's functions are to be good wives and good mothers, and to care for the household. In a society that prefers sons, merely tolerating daughters, being female limits opportunities. What is the situation for disabled women? Margaret Storey and Sang Soon Choi, in a case study of several disabled Korean women, identify some of the strengths, difficulties and struggles the women face in today's highly industrialised Korean society.

16

Women's well-being and the life-course: findings of a longitudinal study

Gloria Geller

Introduction

The past fifty years have seen great changes in the lives of women in many countries of the world. Although there were contradictory and conflicting messages in this country for women to return to the home and to 'nest' immediately post-war, as the economy changed and women's participation in the labour force was required there was an increase in the proportion of women involved in the labour force. By the late 1990s over 50% of undergraduate students in many Canadian universities were women and 52% of Canadian women were in the labour force (Statistics Canada, 1995).

The changes wrought by the restricting of the labour force during this era has profoundly affected the lives of women, men and children within the context of the family. Our very notion of what constitutes a family has changed greatly, becoming a highly politicised area of controversy. Family size has decreased over the past half-century. Many couples are living common-law rather than marrying. Divorce rates have increased. The traditional nuclear family of father as breadwinner and mother as homemaker with two or more children living in a home of their own is very much in the minority. Family types include single parents (especially mothers) and children, two working parents and children, two working people without children, blended families, and same-sex partners, often with children.

We might well ask how have these changes affected the lives of those who have grown up during this era of phenomenal change. How have young people negotiated the terrain carved out for them by their elders? How have these changes affected their life opportunities? What obstacles do they experience during their transitions from one stage of life to another? What experiences do young people have in common as a generation living in the latter part of the twentieth century? What differences do they experience because of gender, class, race and ethnicity?

These questions, among others, are considered in this chapter, which is based upon longitudinal research conducted with 20 women who were part of a larger group of women. This group wrote 'diaries of the future' about their hopes and dreams for their own futures, as high school students in 1973 in and around the city of Toronto. Follow-up interviews have been conducted on two occasions; 10 years later in 1983 and 20 years later in 1993. The women's dreams as young women in high school and their subsequent experiences are discussed within the context of a life-course approach, and findings that focus on the women's well-being are emphasised.

Women and the life course

As noted by Hareven (1980), 'the life course encompasses the pathways by which individuals fulfil different roles over their lives, sequentially or simultaneously. . . The life course concerns itself with the process of transitions under different historical conditions'. Hareven specifies the three features of life course analysis as including: a) the timing of transitions over an individual's career, which entails the balancing of entry into and exit from different roles; b) the impact of historical processes on the timing of transitions, including the socio-economic and cultural forces characteristic of a specific time period that impinge directly on life course timing; intra-cohort variation, due to differences in exposure to events lead to important differences between members of the same cohort; and c) the direct consequences of earlier life course experiences on subsequent development. The life course approach links individual biography with collective behaviour as part of a continuum of historical change.

In this research, the transitions between school and work and work and family life are shown. The dilemmas confronted by the respondents are indicated through the women's reflections on intimate relationships and on roles of wife, mother and housewife as compared to views while in high school. The historical context of this research, conducted over a 20-year period between 1973 and 1993, is evident from the fact that the respondents have lived through a time in which women's roles have been changing profoundly, particularly with respect to the significance of education for women, and expectations with respect to women's involvements in both public and private spheres of activity. The economic context has had a significant effect on women's opportunities. There was a recession in the early 1980s around the time of the first interview, followed by an economic boom in southern Ontario in the late 1980s, followed by a recession in the early 1990s. With the advent of a global economy, the downsizing and cutbacks of this latter period had implications for these women as well. Social class differences are apparent among the women with respect to aspirations as well as achievements. Educational opportunities influence occupational choices. Decisions to marry and to raise a family have implications for women's life-course as well. Placing this research within the life-course model provides us with a context within which to place the experiences of the 20 participants in this study.

Women and well-being

Women's sense of well-being encompasses physical, emotional, spiritual and social components (Gold, 1993). The elements required to ensure a sense of well-being includes such things as: 1) support by family and friends; 2) positive self-esteem; 3) the ability to identify problems, search out solutions and develop actions, and 4) availability of opportunities to exercise personal control. In considering the life-course of women, it is important to recognise these components of well-being. Considerable evidence from around the world indicates that the low status of women in many countries contributes to a lack of well-being for many women. A report by the Pan American Health Organization (PAHO) noted that:

> *'Significant improvements in women's health and well–being can be achieved only if there are general gains in the status of women in education, employment and representation in decision making roles.'*
>
> [Women and Mental Health Committee, 1987]

The authors of this report indicated the relevance of the PAHO plan of action for Canadian women.

Of particular significance to the well-being of women is the issue of poverty. The ongoing problem of poverty, especially among single-parent women, remains a national shame (National Council of Welfare, 1995). In this work, we focus on women's life-course and the well-being of women from a range of different social class backgrounds. In the final portion of the article we consider the well-being of the women who participated in this study.

Research methodology

The schools

In 1973, 'diaries of the future' and demographic questionnaires were collected from about 240 high-school-aged women students in the Toronto area. The results of the demographic questionnaires indicated significant social class differences among the students in these Toronto schools. Toronto Private School is a school for girls and young women within the city of Toronto that has a predominantly upper middle-class student body. Toronto City School is a commercial high school with a predominantly working-class student body. Located on the outskirts of the city of Toronto, Toronto Suburban School is a composite high school with both academic and commercial streams. The social class background of the students in this school is predominantly middle-class (Geller, 1973; 1984; 1996).

Data collected

Students at the beginning of their high school careers in Grade 9 and those at the end of high school, in grades 12 or 13, were the population sampled. In high school the young women wrote 'diaries of the future' about their hopes and dreams for their futures through to old age. Demographic data obtained from each of the students included information about the country of birth of the student and her parents, ethnic background, and the education and occupation of parents.

Most young women wrote about the future with respect to such issues as education, occupation, intimate relationships, marriage and children. Many of the women wrote about their desire to travel or to participate in some activity such as sports or the arts. Often they would indicate a desire or wish for their own good health and/or happiness, and that of family members.

In 1983 and 1993 follow-up interviews were conducted with a subsample of the original group. In cases in which the women were not available to be interviewed, they were sent the interview questionnaire and asked to complete it and mail it back. This chapter presents findings based upon data gathered from 20 women who responded to our questions on at least one occasion. It summarises the findings on educational, occupational and family aspirations and achievements, and presents respondents' reflections on intimate relation- ships and roles as wife, mother and housewife. Issues of well-being are considered by focussing on what is most important for their personal satisfaction and their aspirations for the future. Women's caring work and well-being are discussed; so, too, are differences between schools as they appear relevant to the women's life-course opportunities and experiences.

Research findings

Profiles of respondents

Twenty women wrote 'diaries of the future' in three schools in the Toronto area. Eleven women were interviewed or completed follow-up questionnaires twice and nine were interviewed or completed a follow-up questionnaire once.

Nine of the women interviewed were from Toronto Private School, two from Toronto City School and nine from Toronto Suburban School. Twelve of the women were in first year high school at the beginning of this project and eight were in grade 13. The women in high school were about 14 to 16 years of age, while those in grade 13 were 17 to 19 years old. At the time of the interviews in 1983 the age spread was 24 to 29 years of age; 10 years later it was 34 to 39 years of age.

Educational aspirations and achievements

Most of the women aimed to go on to post-secondary programmes, particularly university. Very few aimed only to complete high school. Many of the women did go on to further education beyond high school, either college or university as can be seen in *Table 16.1* (note: pseudonyms are used). Social class differences are apparent. The working-class women in City School were in a program that was meant to lead them to job opportunities after high school. The young women at Private School had opportunities for further education by virtue of their greater economic and social privileges. Suburban School shows somewhat greater diversity. A number of women in this school chose community college programs to give them credentials in particular occupations, such as social service worker. On the other hand, several took general arts programmes at Ontario universities.

There is a fairly high level of congruence between aspirations and achievements, especially in the case of women who were in grade 13 at the time of the initial study. These students were planning their futures at the time the research was conducted in the late spring of 1973. On the other hand, the students who were at the end of their first year in high school had a long way to go before they would be making these decisions.

Occupational aspirations and achievements:

Table 16.2 presents the occupational aspirations and achievements of the respondents at the three stages of the study. Also shown are the salaries they earned.

As is the case for the women's educational aspirations, the young women who were grade 13 students were likely to have more realistically identified an occupation than those in grade 9. However, aspirations and achievements often differed considerably. Decisions about occupation are influenced by such factors as educational, work and recreational experiences as well as opportunities available within the social, economic and political context.

Marital and family aspirations and achievements

In *Table 16.3* we depict the young women's aspirations with respect to marriage and children and their achievements in these areas. The information below includes both interview periods and indicates the women's status at the time of the second interview.

Most of the women had aspired to marry and to have children when they wrote their 'diaries'. A couple

Table 16.1: Educational aspirations and achievements

Name	Aspirations	Educational achievements, 1983	Educational achievements, 1993
City School			
Betty	Bible school	Grade 12	—
Joan	High school	Grade 12	—
Private School			
Ruth	University	Honours BA; BEd, Queens	MEd, OISE, PhD, in progress
Rosemary	Study nursing or social work	Diploma in nursing; social work	—
April	University	Waterloo and Western Ontario Urban Planning; in progress	—
Janice	No mention	No response	American Academy of Dramatic Art
Melinda	University	Switzerland, Gr 13 Columbia University, Speech Pathology Degree	University of Toronto & McGill, BA
Heidi	France or Switzerland Finishing School	Gr 13, Ontario McGill, BA, MA	no response
Loretta	University	University of Toronto, BEd, MA	no response
Audrey	University	Queens, BA	no response
Lynne	Tulane University, New Orleans	no response	University of Maine, Math/Computer Sci, degree not completed
Suburban School			
Diana	no mention	Western Ontario & Carlton Honours, BA, MA	—
Theresa	University	Concordia Jr College & University of Toronto, BA	—
Maggie	University	Guelph, Honours, BA	—
Frances	University	University of Toronto, Medicine	—
Mary	Nursing school	Sheridan College, correctional worker's diploma	no response
Brenda	Medical school	Sheridan College, nursing	—

of Private School women did not mention marriage and these same women as well as a couple of Suburban School women did not mention children in their 'diaries'.

There is a considerable social class difference between the groups with respect to age at marriage and having children. It would seem that Private School women were likely to marry and have children at a somewhat older age than the women from the working-class and middle-class schools. Private School women focussed on establishing themselves in their careers prior to settling into marriage and family life.

Reflections on the life-course

Intimate relationships

In the interviews the women discussed their views about intimate relationships and their experiences of being wives, mothers and housewives. Some of the women said their views about intimate relationships had not changed. Several indicated that their comprehension and experience of such relationships deepened.

Betty had rethought her own relationship six years before. She said:

> *'Separation, being single would be better than the situation at that time. I was the more ambitious person. The stress of holding down career and family, the process of 'maturation and commitment to family and job caused problems in my marriage . . . Now long–term relationship is very important.'*

Ruth, who was single, wrote about the changes in her views. Her parents' divorce had a profound effect on her views. She wrote:

> *'In 1973 my mother was my biggest role model. I wanted to do just what she did. In 1983 she and my dad separated and divorced. My world was shattered. I then experienced an abusive relationship for a year and an abortion. I ran away to* [another country]. *I was alone, adrift and very, very disillusioned. I think I was very naive in 1973 and thought my mother was perfect and happy. She wasn't. I have experienced so much shit with men that I no longer think I'll find a life partner with compassion, strength, intelligence and commitment to social justice so I have given up. If it happens, it happens. I've decided to look after myself and not 'wait' for anyone else. I also don't see myself necessarily 'ending up' with a male anymore. I might easily find emotional intimacy with a woman partner.'*

Frances, who was a divorced, single parent, stated that her views had not changed, but as her marriage eventually led to her divorce, she learned:

> *'I have no control over another person. Within the first month of marriage I learned he was only interested while he was having fun. I was busy with my [medical] practice and children and he had no sense of commitment. I know what is important, am a Christian person, not a wishy-washy person, which he was. He was having problems. It was a shock when he left. I have experienced good and bad times.'*

Janice, who was single, said her views had changed. She said.

> *'I look at my partner's past relationships. I look at their honesty, their values, their ideas. I have been in a number of relationships and found I would not want to spend the rest of my life with these people, but some others were just not interested in having a family.'*

An important part of the transition to adulthood is the development of intimate relationships. Early life experiences, especially within the family of origin, plus experiences in relationships in adolescence and early adulthood, are significant components of these women's life course. In the next section we consider the situation of those women who have found a male partner and started a family.

Roles of wife, mother and housewife

We asked those who were mothers to reflect upon their experiences of being wives, mothers, and housewives as compared to their views in high school. Eight of the women were mothers and one was a stepmother. The mothers worked outside the home. Most of them made use of day care centres. One woman's mother babysat her children while she worked, another woman had a live-in nanny and another had a babysitter in her home. Four of the women stated that housework was shared between herself and her husband, one said she did most of the work, one was divorced and in one case the nanny did the housework. Five of the women were satisfied with their husband's involvement in child-care and housework and three were not satisfied. Several women were more satisfied with their partners' involvement with child-care than with the amount of housework they did. The women appreciated the fact that their husbands spent time with and took care of the children which was the primary basis for their satisfaction.

Most of the women said they found that having children was much harder than they thought when they were in high school. Betty said:

> *'Like night and day. I was very idealistic in high school. Thought I would live a comfortable life with a picket fence and no trials and tribulations. I am a career person and also give a lot of importance to family. I spend more time talking and doing things with my daughters than my mother did, more like what my father did. We go to the zoo, to parks, on hikes, bird watching, to museums and art galleries and see plays.'*

April's comments were:

> *'I wish I had thought more carefully about the possibility for part–time work in the future. Now I have reached career success with a good income, yet I am stressed out with all the conflicting pressures. I feel guilty leaving my son every day.'*

Brenda's comments were somewhat different from many of the others. She said:

Table 16.2: Occupational aspirations and achievements

Name	Aspirations	Occupational achievements and salary, 1983	Occupational achievements and salary, 1993
City School			
Betty	Stewardess	Manager (Bell, Canada) $12–15,000	Manager $35–40,000
Joan	Secretary	Secretary $12–15,000	Secretary, $35–40,000
Private School			
Ruth	Researcher	Outdoor instruction, under $5000	Graduate student and lecturer, $24,000
Rosemary	Nurse or social worker	Nurse, $20–25,000	Nurse, $50–55,000
April	Day care worker	Urban planning, $12–15,000	Planning director, over $60,000
Janice	Architect; interior designer/enviromental law	No response	Actress, model US$35–45,000
Melinda	Actress	Antique dealer, $10–12,000	Speech pathologist, US$35–45,000
Heidi	Dentistry; teach languages	Public relations, $12–15,000	no response
Loretta	clinical psychologist	High school teacher, $20–25,000	no response
Audrey	No mention	Actor, bicycle tour leader in Europe, $5–8000	no response
Lynne	Doctor	no response	Manufacturing project leader, $45–50,000
Suburban School			
Diana	Law; teaching	Policy, plann & developt, over $25,000	Vice-president, pub opin res company, over $60,000
Theresa	Drama-theatre	Course developer (Bell Canada), over $25,000	Computer manager, over $60,000
Maggie	Drama-theatre	Job creation, Dept of Employment & Immigration, $20–25,000	General manager, theatre, $55–60,000
Frances	General practitioner	Doctor, over $25,000	Family practitioner
Mary	Nurse	Social worker, $20–25,000	no response
Brenda	Paramedic	Nurse, over $25,000	no response
Joyce	Folk singer/soc worker	employment counseller, $25,000 +	no response
Pat	Occupational therapist	Employee benefits consultant, over £25,000	no response
Carol	Self-employed	Manager (Bell Canada), $25,000 +	Grad Student (on leave from Bell Canada), $50–55,000

> *'More fun than I thought it would be. I had a strict father and now I don't have to follow orders, I can make my own decisions. I enjoy being on my own. I do more work, have more responsibility than my husband. I am more aware of what needs to be done than he does, cleaning and emotional needs. Men are brought up to have stuff done for them, they aren't aware of what needs to be done.'*

And Carol found things to be pretty much as expected:

> *'Pretty comparable to what I expected. I still pay relatively little attention to housework. The house is organised and kept tidy but I don't have any compulsion to have a spotless house. I have more important things to do with my time.'*

Table 16.3: Marital and family aspirations and achievements

Name	Aspirations to marry	Marital status last interview	Age married (yrs)	Children	Aspiration children
City School					
Betty	Marry	Married	23	2 girls	Children
Joan	Marry	Married	23	2 girls	Children
Private School					
Ruth	Marry	Single	—	—	Children
Rosemary	Marry	Single	—	—	Children
April	Marry	Married	29	1 boy	Children
Janice	No mention	Single	—	—	No mention
Melinda	Marry	Single	—	—	Children
Heidi	No mention	Single	—	—	No mention
Loretta	Marry	Single	—	—	Children
Audrey	Right man	Single	—	—	Children
Lynne	Marry	Separated	27		Children
Suburban School					
Diana	Marry	Married	22	2 boys, 1 girl	Perhaps
Theresa	Doubts she will marry	Course developer Engaged	—	Fiancé has 2	No mention
Maggie	Doesn't know	Common law	—	Partner has 3	Not clear
Frances	Marry	Divorced	28	2 boys, 1 girl	Children
Mary	Marry	Married	24	Pregnant	Children
Brenda	Marry	Married	22	—	Children
Joyce	Marry	Married	22	1 boy	Children
Pat	Marry	Single	—	—	Children
Carol	Marry	Married	24	2 boys, 1 girl	Children

Up to this point, we have presented findings on the aspirations and achievements of our respondents within the context of education, occupation and family. We have identified some significant social class differences among the respondents in these areas. The women who were from working-class backgrounds completed school, married and had children at an earlier age than most of the other women, especially those from the private school. This latter group of women went on to further education, and held off marriage and having children presumably in order to establish themselves in their careers and/or to pursue other interests. Several of these women pursued graduate education. In the final section of this chapter, the women's well-being based upon their aspirations for the future are considered. The women's well-being is then considered within the context of a woman and life-course discussion.

Most important for well–being:

In *Table 16.4* the women's personal needs and satisfactions are presented. Health, happiness, family, children, relationships, knowledge and accomplishments are among the things they identified as being important for their well-being. Relationships are, as we would expect, a very significant aspect of these women's well-being. They also emphasise satisfying work, achievements and financial security as being important to their well-being. For these thirty-something women occupational achievement seems somewhat less significant than relationships. Many of the women do, however, clearly expect to have satisfying careers.

The fact that several of the women have children and others hope to have children in the future is an important issue at this stage in their lives. What they once 'dreamed' about in high school is a current reality in their lives. While in high school, it was difficult for many of the women to envision 'both lives' of raising a family and holding down a career. Once this situation becomes a reality or they are considering how to make it a reality, they confront the complex issues faced by contemporary women of juggling their lives and in most cases, having to alter their priorities.

Future aspirations

In *Table 16.5* we present the women's aspirations based upon the most recent interview. Family life was important for most of the women we interviewed. Those who had not yet had children tended to emphasize a desire to have children. The women's interests, hobbies and desire to travel continue to remain a significant part of their future aspirations.

Devotion to family life and jobs remains evident, but some of the women want more time to themselves to focus on other interests. More flexible hours, part-time work and self-employment were options that a number of the women were considering. There was also an emphasis on personal development. Some women who had been in the labour force for a number of years, cited time to pursue other interests as well as more time for others as quite attractive. More freedom for themselves was expressed by some of the women in their hopes for the future.

Women's well-being and the life course

At the beginning, this chapter discussed the changes that occurred in women's lives in the past 50 years. In considering the life-course experiences of the women in this study, the significance of these changes is apparent. Compared to women of earlier eras, these women placed a considerable amount of emphasis on education, due in large measure to their expectations that they would pursue a career for at least some of their lives. Most women in the study intended to continue their education beyond high school and most did so. Class differences were apparent with respect to aspirations and achievements in the sphere of education. Working-class women from City School did not, in high school, aspire to higher education, compared to the middle- and upper middle-class women.

All the women in our study sought employment, and those who had children continued to work once they had children. These women were subject to a considerable amount of stress in their efforts to juggle jobs and careers. The women who were slowest to marry and start a family were the private school women who were the women who also held the highest status professional occupations. The women who married and had children at the youngest ages were unable to pursue further education.

The women who continued on to post-secondary education were also among those most likely to be affected by the economic changes of the early 1980s, including a recession that had a considerable impact on jobs. After a period of economic buoyancy, there was another recession in the early 1990s, a time when corporations 'downsized'. Some of the women in our study were concerned about retaining their jobs at the time of the interview in 1993.

The women in this study were clearly affected by the economic and social changes of the last quarter of the twentieth century. As modern women, they both expected and had to work. This latter situation had serious implications for family life. While in high school, most of the women had aspired to marry and have children, and continued to aspire to marry and have children throughout the 20-year period, they all had to confront the complexities of how they would handle a job or career and a family. Several of our respondents spoke of the difficulties they had carrying the double burden, and some were reconsidering their

Table 16.4: The women's well-being

Name	Year	Personal needs/satisfaction
City School		
Betty	1983	Doing something she enjoys; well her career, watching her daughter
	1993	Grow; recognition she receives at work; taking on responsibilities she is given; watching daughter develop to be open-minded person
Joan	1983	Her family; her health
	1993	Her family; children's and her own health
Private School		
Ruth	1983	To love and be loved; to create; nature; to live in a community
	1993	To nurture and sustain relationships that are important; a fabric of friends; people she can be with unconditionally and who look forward to hearing from her
Rosemary	1983	Be happy at work, in family life; job — financial security so she can travel
	1993	Being close to family — more important than ever
April	1983	Boyfriend and family is important; finding a job that is fulfilling; stable job, relationship and friends
	1993	Business is quite fascinating; having a child much more wonderful than anticipated
Janice	1993	Family, friends, work
Melinda	1983	To be liked, loved and respected
	1993	Open communication; time; confidence
Loretta	1983	Writing; being happy doing what she does to earn a living
Audrey	1983	Thirst for more knowledge; meet people who stimulate her interests in other areas of knowledge; career — to do something in which she is able to see her accomplishments; to feel that what she is doing is helping other people; drive to help with basic needs of people
Lynne	1983	Accomplishment in work; self-discipline; something interesting to do every day; creative outlets in music and design; physical fitness
Suburban School		
Diana	1993	Be happy
Theresa	1983	Knowing everyone she cares about is happy
	1993	Job satisfaction; family; immediate circle of friends; take care of her own family's 'behinds'
Maggie	1993	Comfortable, honest relationship, supportive and respectful; balance personal life and work; health
Frances	1993	Being happy; profession on track; maintain her house; go to Florida on her own; that her kids be happy and that they live with her, remarriage; be happy and content where she is
Mary	1983	Achieving the best that she can; have goals so as not to become stagnant
Brenda	1983	Work; feeling good about herself; her marriage
Carol	1993	Maintain strong marital relationship; family relationships; continue her search for job satisfaction

* No comments from Heidi and Joyce

responsibilities, with the options of part-time employment and self-employment being given consideration. Another option exercised by many of our respondents was to put off having children until they were established in their careers. In a time of economic downturn undoubtedly decisions about having a first child or more children become a consideration. Family size remained relatively small, although several of the women interviewed had three children.

Responsibility for childcare remained a personal consideration. At a time of reprivatisation of the family and devolution of responsibilities of caring for family members to the 'community', these women appeared to seek personal solutions and answers to their dilemmas. The women whose husbands did childcare were satisfied with their partners' involvement with the work of the home. Societal responsibility to the women and families raising the next generation of citizens was not addressed by our respondents. It is important, however, to raise concerns about the lack of social support offered to families and to the failures of social policy to respond to their needs, such as a universal childcare policy, that have long been identified as essential for women's equality and, therefore, women's well-being in Canadian society.

There are different approaches to how we might consider the question of women's well-being in contemporary society. In this study, responses to questions about personal needs and satisfactions clearly emphasised a need for affiliation through relationships. Other aspects of their lives were important and several women said that both career and family are

Table 16.5: Future aspirations

Name	Year	Aspirations
City School		
Betty	1993	Self-employment in catering; art, painting — look into this; take care of herself and her own interests; travel; when house is paid for buy more property or move up — be more financially secure
Joan	1993	Stay at home — work part-time for spending money — not to have to work full-time; sew, continue education — take day classes; do gardening
Private School		
Ruth	1993	Stay in career — steadily gain competency as university lecturer; work her way back to Canada; own her own house; live in an earth-friendly way with a loving relationship
Rosemary	1993	Keep job; thinking about having children
April	1993	Build her business so she can quit her job; have another child; continue to be happy with her husband; travel more
Janice	1993	Have a family
Melinda	1993	Find a soul-mate and get married; have children; continue in speech pathology in private practice
Heidi	1983	Be successful in career, respected by peers; have a long, happy marriage with a 50th anniversary party
Loretta	1983	Write something of significance and be noticed; be happy; live with husband
Audrey	1983	Have a career in international affairs
Lynne	1983	Establish international flying school in the Caribbean
Suburban School		
Diana	1993	Stop working; pursue things she doesn't have time for — read and learn; live in the country; make preserves
Theresa	1993	Retire at 50; spend time with nieces and nephews, mom and dad; paint; have full control over how alarm clock is set; be involved with dying people and their families as a volunteer'
Maggie	1993	Continue to work in her field; do something of value in theatre; commitment to her relationship; have a cottage in Nova Scotia
Frances	1993	Kids stay with her; deal with ex-husband; look after children and practice; have vacations — take breaks
Mary	1983	Have a family, continue self-growth
Brenda	1983	Work part-time; have children and a dog; travel to Florida and Hawaii
Joyce	1983	Complete grade 10 piano
Pat	1993	Take law course; continue to think about marriage and family
Carol	1993	Pursue finding career satisfaction; marriage and family are extremely important as is career — it is difficult to juggle all aspects and difficult to plan

important. Betty, for instance, stated that she had reconsidered her relationship, since she found her family life and career were in conflict. In the end she decided the family life was more important to her and that she would need to make some changes in how she approached her job. Like so many other women, emotional connections are a significant aspect of Betty's identity.

Women's caring relationships and need for connection as a significant aspect of women's well-being have been discussed to a great extent since Gilligan (1982) identified 'women's different voice'. As Gilligan maintains: 'By changing the lens of developmental observation from individual achievement to relationships of care, women depict ongoing attachment as the path that leads to maturity'. Miller's (1991) work also follows this train of thought. She notes: 'women's senses of self and of morality revolved around issues of responsibility for, care of and inclusion of other people, participating and fostering the development of other people as sources of growth, satisfaction and empowerment, the wellsprings of true inner motivation and development'.

On the other hand, women's focus on relationships over their own needs has been shown by some authors to be detrimental to women's well-being. Guberman (1990) notes: 'many would question whether women's well-being is being assured in the family, violence against women, comparative well-being of single and married women, the concrete amount of work assumed by women in the family'. Authors, who recognise the detrimental aspects of women's caring, maintain that women's roles as the primary care-givers in the society are socially constructed rather than something that is inherent to being a woman. Baines *et al* (1991) state: 'the gendered division of labour creates a socially constructed dependency that is the consequence of providing care for others rather than the outcome of receiving care'. They continue: 'the obligations and expectations embodied in the imperative of caring shapes women's opportunities and has significant costs and consequences for them'. Further, they say: 'the notion that caring comes naturally to women fails to consider the significance of socially patterned roles and process of socialisations, women learn to take their place in society as informed caregivers to children and elderly relatives and transfer this to the public sphere and provide caring services as cleaners, child-minders and teachers'. They further discuss the fact that policies to diminish the inequalities women face in the labour force will not be effective until there are changes in their domestic and child-care responsibilities. They also note that caring work which is largely visible and lacks validation in the society is also a labour of love involving relationships of profound importance to those who do the caring as well as those cared for .

As long as this is the case and as long as women are socialised to be the caring members of society, girls and women will have to determine how to live the 'two lives' with which they are confronted. This research shows that women continue to have to make hard choices, including whether or not to have a family, if they are to pursue a career. While women in this study appeared to think they still had the option to have a family if they chose to, it may well be that this option will narrow considerably within the next few years. On the other hand, some of them may decide not to have children, but were not ready to say this at the time of the interview. Those who had families, generally had to limit their careers at the time while devoting time and energy to raising children. It is evident that women's well-being is compromised if they have to make the difficult choice between a satisfying career and a family life.

The findings of this longitudinal research raises questions about the well-being of the younger women growing up in our society. We cannot expect them to return to an earlier time, when they were expected and able to focus upon their caring role in society without also having to hold down full-time employment. However, now that women are expected to carry double and often triple loads, surely society has some responsibility to give recognition to women's very crucial care-giving work, without which our society would be a much less pleasant place in which to live.

References

Baines C, Evans P, Neysmith SM (1991) Perspectives on caring. In: Evans P, Neysmith S, eds. *Women's Caring: Feminist Perspectives on Social Welfare*. McClelland and Stewart, Toronto

Geller G (1973) Role aspirations and life-style orientations of high school women. Master's thesis, University of Toronto

Geller G (1984) Aspirations of female high school students. *Resource Fem Res* **12**(1): 17–19

Geller G (1996) Educational, occupational and family aspirations of women. In: Galaway B, Hudson J, eds. *Youth in Transition: Perspectives on Research and Policy*. Thompson Educational Publishing, Toronto

Gilligan C (1982) *In a Different Voice: Psychological Theory and Women's Development*. Harvard University Press, Cambridge, Massachusetts

Gold M (1993) *Women's Wellness Project: Final Report*. Hamilton-Wentworth District Health Council

Guberman N (1990) The family, women and caregiving: Who cares for the caregivers? In: Dhruvarajan V, ed. *Women and Well-being*. McGill-Queen's University Press, Montreal and Kingston

Hareven TK (1980) The life course and aging in historical perspective. In: Back KW, ed. *Life Course: Integrative Theories and Exemplary Populations*. Westview Press, Boulder, Colorado

Miller JB (1991) The development of women's sense of self. In: Jordon JV *et al*, eds. *Women's Growth in Connection*. The Guilford Press, New York

National Council of Welfare (1995) *Priority Profile 1993*. Minister of Supply and Services, Ottawa

Statistics Canada (1995) *Women in Canada: A Statistical Report*. 3 edn. Minister of Industry, Ottawa

Women and Mental Health Committee (1987) *Women and Mental Health in Canada: Strategies for Change*. Canadian Mental Health Association, Toronto

17

Changing cultural imperatives for Japanese women

Yoshiko Uchiyama

Introduction

The Seventh Maternal Health Conference of Kanagawa Prefecture was held in Japan in 1994. The issue of procedures for female genital examination was raised, and one American woman complained about the examination procedure as conducted in America: 'The doctor did not consider my privacy. I was mortified by the examination procedure'.

In Japan there are two kinds of procedures for examining female genitals. In the first, a curtain may be used to separate the examiner from the woman, so she is thereby unable to see the examiner. The curtain thus acts as a metaphorical blindfold. when an American woman experienced this method of examination, she thought that communication between patient and doctor was very difficult. She felt that the examiner could not fully divine the patient's reaction to the procedure since the examiner could not see the patient.

The second type of procedure is to use a sheet to cover the patient's abdomen and legs. in this way, the patient is kept warm during the examination, yet can communicate directly and easily with the examiner. The examiner is able to observe the patient's behaviour and facial expressions, and is able to explain the procedure and necessary treatment during the examination. Some foreign women request the sheet when undergoing genital examination in Japan. Japanese women, however, tend not to show any preference, nor do they complain.

This chapter addresses some possible cultural influences that may help in understanding Japanese women's reactions to and compliance with medical procedures that might appear isolating or invasive to others. From this example, explanations for other socio-cultural imperatives for Japanese women may emerge.

Japanese cultural heritage

The Japanese have historically expressed two cultural streams. One is the heritage of 'ritualism', which is similar to that practised by Chinese, Taiwanese and Koreans. Ritualism has been influenced by Confucianism, and formed the basis of the military (Buke) community in which there was a clearly defined social stratification. The 'boss' in each military community imposed a set of social rules that were promulgated within a hierarchy of social organisation. People at the bottom of the social hierarchy were, in general, suppressed and repressed. Within each level of the social strata, people developed a set of ceremonies, rites and formalities. This helped them to maintain pride and perpetuate a social conservatism. People tended to marry within the same social stratum, and the desired mate for a man was to become a good wife and wise mother. When a man went into battle, his wife managed the house and took care of child-rearing. Confucianism taught that a woman did not have a house of her own as a child, as a wife or in her old age. This meant that the woman had no distinct identity beyond that of wife and mother. Confucian ritual thought and practice continues to affect Japanese women in many aspects of their lives, including attitudes of subordination and acceptance. In this manner, Çonfucianism is an influencing factor on the everyday lives of Japanese women, even in their acceptance of intrusive medical procedures.

The second stream of Japanese cultural heritage is 'Retreatism', originally formed as an indigenous cultural pattern of social organisation in rural Japan by farmers living in the mountains. These farmers practised a type of shifting agriculture, moving from plot to plot, burning their fields in rotation cropping. They referred to themselves as 'the guest of the mountain fields'. These traditional farmers formed themselves into self-administrating groups and were very democratic. However, in time of need, they pooled their resources to help each other and to maintain public order during times of natural disaster, disease or for distribution of resources. These groups were always associated with high-level decision making.

These farmers followed an animistic form of spiritualism, praying to the natural phenomena found in nature. Their life-style remained primitive as they sustained themselves in their mountain villages. They tried to maintain their cultural traditions while adopting and assimilating cultural features from outside, including the use of Chinese characters for recording their life experiences. In this way, they became familiar with new, interesting and often strange things. They thought the lives of people were very important. They believed that humankind lived naturally and that man was an integral part of nature. They married freely within their group, but also married people from other groups. We often hear of interesting episodes, such as *'Yobai, Ashiir, Wakasyuyado'*, which imply free sexuality before marriage. This, then, reflects part of the cultural expression for the traditional farming people of Japan.

The modern structure of Japanese society

The two main cultural streams, Confucianism and Retreatism, have moved into today's society, and influence the everyday lives of Japanese people. However, these two cultural streams have undergone change over time, and have been especially influenced by three major events: the end of the Civil Wars, the Meiji Restoration and the Second World War.

Before the Tokugawa era, which followed the Civil War, people lacked basic security. There were many kinds of leaders following the Civil War, such as *Daimyou:Tonosama*, who were eager to unify the countries in Japan. If any one leader could unify Japan, that leader would be able to become the head of all the other significant figures as a *Shobun: Seitaishougun* and would get special credit from the Emperor for achieving unity. Ieyasu Tokugawa was appointed to this position of Shobun, unifying all Japan. The Emperor did not have any power; he was a symbol of the people who respected him like a God King. During this era, about 300 years ago, other leaders (daimyou) who were not under Tokugawa had their own territories and managed the local population and regional production. However, they needed a great deal of money since each leader travelled throughout his own territory in his administrative role. Furthermore, each leader was obliged to travel to Edo, modern-day Tokyo, to visit his wife, since leaders' wives were kept at Edo by order of Lord Tokugawa. This meant that each leader remained for three years moving through his territory and visiting Edo. The trip from a leader's territory to Edo was called the procession of *Daimyou-Gyouretu*, and was seen as a great demonstration of the leader's power and authority. This demonstration of power was such that any people or animals crossing in front of the procession would be killed on command by *samurai*. Ordinary people sat beside the road and bowed, and could not raise up their heads until the procession had passed. However, midwives were permitted to cross the path of the procession in case of a medical emergency. Because the procession required a great deal of money, people were heavily taxed in terms of money or rice. Their lives were, in consequence, very difficult and miserable. As tenants on the land in a peasant economy, the masses were poverty-stricken. They sought salvation by way of insight and acceptance of Buddhism, as the philosophy of Buddha fitted into their lives. Buddhist teachings included:

> *Human life is suffering in sickness, old age and death.*
>
> *The cause of suffering is lust or desire. Freedom from this is seen in the quest of personal fulfilment.*
>
> *To overcome human misery one need only find the cause and the means for eliminating it.*
>
> *The noble eight paths are illuminated as right thinking, correct motive, correct speech, correct action, correct livelihood, right exertion, right concentration and right meditation.*

It seems that people did not resist suffering, nor did they have any problem behaving correctly. They required strong patience to persevere; this characteristic is referred to as *Gaman*. Nakane (1978) said that Japanese society is structured vertically in a hierarchical manner. Maintenance of a social hierarchy requires acceptance, and social order is preserved by correct behaviour and ritual. Today, ritualism continues to play an important role in Japanese society.

Hierarchical social structures are prevalent in Japanese society and go towards maintaining social order in a traditional cultural framework. Hierarchies are found within the family, within communities, within institutions and in the work place. It seems as if each social unit is like a *Koma*, a popular Japanese toy. The toy, a spinning top, is made of wood with a large core. For the top to start to revolve, it needs an independent source of power. Once the core is balanced, it revolves in a powerful, quiet, useful, secure and very smooth manner. This analogy explains how the social group has sound function and shape, and through good organisation will continue to thrive. The ideal family, within the extended family unit, continues, with the father as head as motivating power, his wife and children respecting the authority of the father and behaving according to the family structure and the ideals of Koma. This is how some schools, communities, companies and often the nation operates. These Koma also strive for harmony, like the family, and the most successful Koma works with usefulness and stability. If they are oppressed from outside or internally, some Koma would stop, topple over and cease to function. Each person who is in a Koma tries to be tied to the core of the group, supporting the group and defending each other within the group. Being tied to the core requires some compliance to the group purpose in order to sustain the core and those who make it up. Koma is, therefore, an important characteristic in understanding Japanese social patterns and the individual's place in Japanese society.

In the Meiji period, Japan wanted to become a developing country, and the Japanese endeavoured to make a strong country. They achieved expansion of armaments and the development of industry. The Meiji period was significant because the people of Japan enacted civil laws and recognised the rights of the family and obligations of preserving the alliance of kinship. The present definition of family was created and the man's authority as head of the household and his power as husband and father was increased. The woman retained the role of wife and mother and did not have the vote or the right to own property. She was expected to accept her role and position in the family and in society. In Japanese there is a saying: *Gamansuru*, which means 'stick it out'. Through *Gamansuru*, the wife was able to persevere.

After the Second World War, the people of Japan adopted a new constitution. The family again changed and the woman achieved suffrage and was able to hold general property. She felt more liberated.

Recently, the Japanese economy has expanded and people now have access to higher education. The average person expresses his or her feelings, beliefs, opinions and thoughts more freely. However, the boss as head of the group is almost always a man. Yet the man has always depended on others. It seems that men remain, in this regard, rather immature, and if a man does not get good results, no one complains or asks for an accounting. People think that if a man fails he must be suffering from some evil force or is experiencing bad luck, either from inside or outside of his group. This rationalisation is referred to as *Amae* or, as noted by Doi (1987), it is a dependence.

The woman's role continues to be one of support, and she is expected to contribute to the Japanese system by caring for her man; this is known as *Keisyukanpaku*.

Private decision-making

In discussing decision-making, we can identify three ethical choices with which Japanese women are faced. The first is love as self-sacrificing commitment. This is love. People die for love, and this reflects the ancient ideals of Retreatism. The most attractive example of this comes out of the Second World War when young Japanese men said, 'We should die to become a shield for our family and country'. The second ethical choice for Japanese is a moral choice external to self and part of a public morality. The next ethical choices are *Tatemae* and *Honne*. These are formalised expressions in the home, the school or at the work place in speech, styles, gestures and postures that go to reinforcing the nature of *Tatemae*. Women, both within and outside of the home, do not express *Honne*. However, when women are alone with female relatives or close friends, they may release their feelings. If a woman directly expresses her emotions and desires, other people would frown on her. She must endure shame or *Hagi*, which is a strong criticism; Japanese severely dislike being criticised.

Conclusion

Through these ethical choices with consideration for traditions of hierarchical authority and the submissive, supportive role of women in Japanese society, women have not been encouraged until recently to be self-expressive and critical. These cultural values and traditions, although under pressure for change, are reflected in role relationships, and women often continue to remain non-critical and passive in their relationships to male authority figures. This extends to all levels of social interaction, including the relationship between a woman and her doctor, where a woman must endure for the sake of family, community and society.

References

Doi T (1987) *Structure of Amae*. Koubundo Tokyo

Nakane C (1978) *Dynamics of Vertical Society*. Koudansya-gendaisinsyo, Tokyo

18

Empowering women toward health in later life: The health of Chamorro women

Vicki L Torsch

Introduction

Empowering women toward health in later life requires an awareness of their health status, combined with an understanding of their socio-cultural conceptions of health and health care needs. In the past and the present, health programmes are often begun with the goal of improving health among the elderly in a community, only to fail because the programmes have been hastily conceived without understanding the social and cultural values of the elders to be served. It has been documented by Ma (1996) that in the absence of an understanding of a cultural group's socio-cultural beliefs and traditions, the goals of healthcare are likely to be jeopardised.

It is the objective of this paper to elucidate the socio-cultural perspectives on health and healthcare needs among the elderly Chamorro women of Guam. By integrating their socio-cultural perspectives on health with pertinent historical and biocultural factors, implications for healthcare delivery will be elucidated.

Research methods

Field research was carried out on Guam during 12 months of 1994–1995. Participant observation and semi-structured interviews were used to gain an understanding of socio-cultural conceptions of health and healthcare needs. Using a life history format, 50 elderly Chamorro women and 10 men were interviewed; their selection was based on age, education, social and economic status, and residence. Participant observation included participation at two senior centres and various cultural activities, including *novenas* and fiestas. Towards the end of the fieldwork, a focus group was held with elders at the Mangilao Senior Center to review the themes of interviews and define their priorities for problem resolution. The author conducted a demographic analysis of the biocultural factors affecting the elderly Chamorro women's health status. The integration of the demographic analysis with the women's socio-cultural concepts served to validate the information gathered and augmented the attempt to elucidate the implications for delivery of health services.

Aging and health

In an anthropological analysis of health and aging, health is conceptualised as enmeshed in biological, psycho-social, politico-economic and cultural contexts (Millard, 1992). In this theoretical framework, health is defined in a broad, holistic sense to include biocultural features of physical and mental health and well-being (Henderson, 1990). As such, the health of a population is reflected in such quantitative dimensions as life expectancy, mortality and morbidity as well as in the qualitative dimensions embedded in personal and socioeconomic characteristics. Further, health and disease are perceived to exist in the context of culturally based meanings and value systems.

Various studies indicate that after age 60 years, people's capabilities as well as impairments seem to be closely related to the effects of their particular environments and their own individual choices and patterns (O'Neill and Sorensen, 1991; Staats *et al*, 1993). Health problems are related to multiple issues of language, culture, and social, environmental and economic factors (Gaw, 1975). In focussing on various cultural groups, Kleinman (1975) reported that culturally constructed health and health beliefs result in a wide range of unique patterns in health-seeking and maintenance behaviours in different societies, concluding that illness and healthcare are directly woven into the cultural fabric. The findings of these various research efforts validate the importance of understanding the socio-cultural conceptions embedded in the Chamorro's perspectives on health.

Historical contexts of health among elderly Chamorro women

In reviewing the historical contexts of health among the Chamorros, we find that their health deteriorated during the Spanish colonial period (1668–1898), which is well documented in the historical, archaeological and physical anthropological records (Pietrusewsky *et al*, 1995; Rogers, 1995). However, the Chamorros in the twentieth century regained an adaptive standard of living and surpassed the life expectancy of the pre-contact Chamorros.

In the process of Americanisation, elderly Chamorro women, indigenous to the Pacific island of Guam, have experienced rapid cultural changes, affecting their health status, cultural traditions and beliefs, as well as their concepts of health and healthcare needs. Health delivery programs, based on American models, have been developed to serve their needs. These have historically ignored the Chamorros' traditional health beliefs and practices.

The historic demographic record indicates that, associated with the Americanisation of their social, political and economic structures, has also been the Americanisation of their health status and illness patterns. As Guam's society began changing from a subsistence economy to a cash economy, wage labour jobs meant less physical activity for many, along with changes in the diet towards imported processed foods. These shifts in behavioural and nutritional patterns, along with the stresses of rapid westernisation, set the stage for a demographic change in the health status of Chamorro women.

Biocultural contexts of health status

Quantitative dimensions

In exploring the biocultural contexts of the elderly Chamorro women's health status, Torsch found two major demographic trends in the twentieth century. The health consequences of improved health delivery, sanitation and the general standard of living on Guam have meant a longer life expectancy for its people as well as a change in the primary causes of mortality and morbidity.

Longer life expectancy in general means that more people are living in better health and at a higher functional state. With an improved standard of living, life expectancy among Chamorros (both sexes) has risen from 34.5 years in 1902 to 69 years in 1993. Their extended life spans are manifested by demographic indicators such as the increased number and percentage of elderly, increased median age, gender differences, and functional states and disability rates.

Life table analysis (1994) presents a significant gender difference in life expectancy at birth, with Chamorro women exhibiting greater longevity than men (73 years versus 65 years). This is similar to the US pattern, though life expectancy at birth is lower for Chamorro women than for US women (78.8 years).

The second major demographic change in the twentieth century has been the shift in the leading causes of mortality and morbidity from infectious to chronic diseases. When Americans gained control over Guam in 1898, they initiated a systematic public health campaign to eliminate infectious and parasitic diseases, which were rampant. By 1980, the transition from infectious to chronic diseases was complete; since 1980, chronic diseases have been the three leading causes of mortality among all age groups on Guam.

Inspection of the 1992 cause-specific mortality data among the Chamorros presents the developed society cluster of heart disease, cancer, cerebro-vascular diseases and diabetes, echoing the leading causes of death in the US among all ages, including the elderly (*Table 18.1*). When considering the rates among Chamorro women aged 65 years and over, a population at risk for each of these chronic diseases as well as for pneumonia is found.

Table 18.1: Cause-Specific Mortality Rates for Chamorros (per 100,000), 1992

Disease	All age groups	Women aged 65+
Heart	95.4	1559
Pneumonia	12	205
Diabetes	32	492
Cardiovascular	32	492
Cancer	70	862

Source: Guam Department of Public Health and Social Service, 1992 text

Just as in other developed societies, Chamorro elderly women represent an increasing percentage of the Chamorro population as well as an increasing percentage of those with chronic health problems (Guam Department of Public Health & Social Service, 1992). Major health problems among elderly Chamorro women include diabetes, high blood pressure and obesity (Kasperbauer *et al*, 1985). These reflect genetic predisposition, behavioural risk factors and culturally specific factors, such as diet and tolerance for obesity, as well as the extended life spans of the Chamorros (Guam Department of Public Health and Social Service, 1991; Pinhey *et al*, 1994). Among elderly Chamorro women is found a high-risk group requiring diligence in preventive and therapeutic interventions for chronic illnesses.

Qualitative dimensions of health status

The health of a population is also reflected in qualitative dimensions embedded in personal and socioeconomic characteristics. Significant factors affecting the health of elderly women include income, marital status/widowhood and living arrangements. Exploration of these factors reveals that a larger percentage of Chamorro women aged 65 years or more live in poverty than do women in the same age range in the US (18% versus 12% in 1990). This is significant on Guam, where the cost of living is about twice that of the US mainland, and serves to disadvantage the elderly economically (Economic Research Center, 1990).

Marital patterns are similar to US patterns, showing a large percentage of widows and more women widowed than men. The greatest difference is in living arrangements. The majority of elderly Chamorro women live in intergenerational extended family households and compounds, while the usual living arrangement in the US is the nuclear family. In looking more closely at the implications of the differences in living arrangements, it is noticed that about 4.9% elderly Chamorro women live alone, compared to 42% of US women aged 65 years and over (1990). The living arrangement dictated by Chamorro tradition has historically served as a 'social insurance' for elders in time of need, allowing for the sharing of resources, mutual support and care of frail elders. As for those elderly Chamorro women who are not able to live in extended family units (owing to the death of their children; outmigration or divisive family feuds) they are left to fend for themselves, often in impoverished circumstances. These circumstances present implications for social and healthcare delivery to supplement or replace family support.

Sociocultural conceptions of health

Just as the health of elderly Chamorro women is mirrored in their personal and socioeconomic characteristics, their health is also reflected in their sociocultural conceptions of health and well-being. Sociocultural conceptions include their health beliefs, customs and traditions, as well as attitudes about health and well-being in late life. Elucidating the attitudes of persons on complex concepts, such as health and well-being makes simple consideration difficult; however, an understanding of what is culturally meant by good health, poor health, old age and so forth is required for ethnically sensitive healthcare assessment and delivery.

Through the qualitative medium of inter- views and participant observation, Torsch attempted to gain an understanding of the elderly Chamorro women's sociocultural conceptions about health in late life and their perceptions of their healthcare needs. When asked about the characteristics of later life, the majority of those aged 65 years and over responded positively about the elderly experience, tending to regard later life as a normal part of the life cycle, continuous with their earlier years. A 66-year-old, Teresita, relays this attitude in her response:

> *'I have many years of experience in life. They were full. but I don't think of myself as "old." I think I have many more years of life, and I look forward to them. I am the same person as I always have been. It's true that my body is showing "wear," but my mind still thinks like I am a young person.'*

Only 3% of elderly Chamorro women identified chronological age as a marker of old age, compared to 40% of the men. Elderly Chamorro women described the continuation of being the same person in spite of having crossed the 'timeline' for old age, and they expressed an acceptance of the changes involved in the life course.

The elderly women also discussed many positive messages that their culture communicates to them about being elderly, including respect, the inclusion and participation of the elderly in the family and community, and the important roles of the elderly as conveyors of traditions as well as head of the extended family system. Bernadita Dungca, a native Chamorro and author of *The Chamorro- English Dictionary*, described the traditional Chamorro world-view towards the elderly:

> Saina is the Chamorro term for respected elder. It has positive connotations in Chamorro thinking, including wisdom to share, having respect, being active and a 'power' in the family and community. The eldest *saina* is the authority over her siblings; also authority over [children]. The *saina* sees to it that those under her authority have their needs met. She cares for them as long as she's able. When she is no longer able, she turns over this responsibility to a sibling, who then cares for the *saina*. The *saina* have no fear about not being taken care of. The nature of the interaction is reciprocity.

The description of the *saina*'s role indicates that the Chamorros perceive two stages in the elderly experience. In the first, the elder continues to perform activities of daily living in a relatively disability-free state. They continue their social and family activities as well as meeting the reciprocal obligations of Chamorro culture. In the second stage, the elder becomes frail with health disabilities impeding the performance of activities of daily living.

In keeping with their focus on functionality in dividing late life into two stages, the Chamorro women aged 60 years and over tend to focus on functional abilities when describing the changes in late life. They depict changes in physical health, mental health, social and family relationships, and work roles. It is impressive that 72% of the Chamorro women interviewed identify increased physical health problems as a significant change in late life, as compared to 30% of the men. Maria describes her experience with arthritis:

> *'When young, we could do whatever we wanted, go wherever we wanted to go. But now, we are getting old; and you know, it's . . . different because I am getting tired. Physically, I am starting to feel aches and pains. I have arthritis and that can slow you down quite a bit. I wish I had the strength I had before. I love to work in my garden and tend my flowers. [But] when a person reaches the age of 60 to 100 years, they start to get sick and aren't able to do as many things as they used to do before.'*

The emphasis by the elderly Chamorro women on increased physical health problems coalesces with the demographic analysis of their health status, in which they present high rates of chronic illness.

In their general descriptions of health in late life, they also describe the experience of 'getting close to death' and often experiencing the death and illness of a loved one. Lydia, at 94 years of age, depicts this experience in her life:

> *'My two sisters were sick from stroke. Juanita died already. My mother died. I took care of her. All my life, I'm very happy because my husband was very good to me. Then he became ill and died. It's peaceful being old; but I don't want to be old so I call St. Mary. And I pray to join her, but sometimes she doesn't hear. All the time I pray.'*

The spiritual dimension of their lives is an element that affects the elders' perceptions of health and well-being. The majority of Chamorros are Catholic, and the interviewed women feel that their faith assists them in their adjustment to the functional changes as well as the losses in late life.

Changes in mental health are another category that they present as occurring in late life. Worry and stress about one's family, about one's financial situation and about the possibility of no longer being self-sufficient are identified concerns. The opening of Guam's first nursing home has created a feeling of uncertainty among the women interviewed. They express hope that their family will care for them at home in the traditional Chamorro way, but they describe feeling anxious about the future.

Becoming forgetful or mentally incapacitated by dementia are also mentioned as mental health changes in late life. Ramona, a 65-year-old retired teacher, explains her opinion about mental changes in old age.

> *'As you age, your life changes, your health changes, you change. I believe old age is when people lose the ability to think rationally. When they develop mental incapacity, they are old. When people get old, they sometimes lose memory so they don't remember things.'*

The focus on becoming forgetful or developing dementia coalesces with the demographic indicators of their health status, in which Chamorro women over age 75 years present a greater frequency of central nervous system diseases than men (1990). It also meshes with the large amount of media and research attention that is given to the occurrence of amyotrophic lateral sclerosis/Parkinsonism (ALS/PD), which is a disabling condition known as *lytico/bodig* and is unique to Guam.

The elderly women also depict changes in their social role and relationships in later life. Included in this category are the new role of being a grandparent, changes in relationships between themselves and their spouse, and the opportunity for leisure and freedom from the responsibility of maintaining the household.

Sociocultural conceptions of health needs

The Chamorro women describe an increase in physical health problems and certain mental health problems as significant health changes in late life. These identified changes tend to coalesce with the quantitative and qualitative dimensions of their health status. The elder Chamorro women's health status, conceptions of health and well-being in later life, and their cultural values are instrumental in their sociocultural perspectives on their healthcare needs.

Owing to increased health problems in late life, the elders believe that availability of medical and health services is very important to the elderly. They identify the importance of health insurance in making health services available and affordable. The elders also express gratitude for social security and medicare, which assist them in being financially secure. Many elders compare their security with their own parent's experiences without such financial security or healthcare.

The elderly Chamorro women also stress the importance of health education, preventive measures and treatment in maintaining quality of life. They describe their lack of education as a significant problem affecting them. Of Chamorro females aged 70 years and over, 84.5% had six or fewer years of school (1990). They believe that they could make better life choices for themselves and their families if provided with pertinent information. Some of their recommendations include education on how to stay physically fit, on healthy nutrition and on ways to exercise safely.

Those who attend the island's senior programs advocate participation in social activities to stay mentally and physically sound. The women discuss the increased opportunities for more leisure time as a major benefit of being an elder today as compared with their own parent's experiences. The senior centres are described as places where social support and health-related education and screening could be coordinated for elders.

The elders not only want educational opportunities to learn, they also want to put the new knowledge into action in their lives. For example, in response to learning about the benefits of a heart-healthy diet, the elders at the Mangilao Senior Center recommended nutritional changes in the lunches served at the Center. They had learned that it was better to broil chicken than to fry it and not to cook fish in coconut milk because of the coconut oil's high cholesterol level. Therefore, they wanted their lunches to reflect this health information. Their motivation to learn and apply self-help measures reflects their desire to improve the quality of their lives.

In addition to the decline in health and physical strength with age, numerous sociocultural factors are delineated as significant to the health and well-being of the Chamorro women in late life. Having a productive, participatory role in the family along with a strong family support network is perceived as a significant health need. The elder women discuss their roles in caring for their frail parents at home and express the desire to be cared for at home by their families. They equate removal from their family to an institution, such as the new nursing home, as equivalent to dying.

In the focus group dialogue, the elders rank sociocultural factors, such as the Americanisation of attitudes and values, as their main priorities for change. As described in the historical review, the Chamorros have witnessed the modification of many traditions and values; some have been advantageous, some not. A tradition of caring and sharing has been a basic value in Chamorro culture. It is perceived as being weakened by American values of individualism and materialism. The maintenance of this value is perceived as a significant health need, affecting family cohesion and support as well as eldercare.

Even though elderly women cite decline in health most frequently as a problem, in focus groups they listed the health category last among priorities for change. The importance of cultural values reflects their significance to the Chamorros' perceptions of well-being and reinforces the importance of understanding a cultural group's sociocultural conceptions.

Implications for healthcare delivery

The significance attached to their cultural values indicates that the goals of healthcare for this cultural group will be augmented by designing healthcare programs that respect their cultural heritage. The elders portray the value they as Chamorros have toward intergenerational extended family bonds, community caring and sharing, education and respect for elders. Therefore, it seems that health benefits can be optimised through the design of family-inclusive health regimens and education programs. Home-based care programs will be more in tune culturally with their values than institutional care. In addition, bringing healthcare into their everyday natural settings, such as the senior centres or local places of worship, will assist in making healthy living a part of the cultural fabric of their lives. When dealing with health problems, the goals of healthcare will be augmented by considering culturally specific factors that affect the ability or willingness to follow therapeutic regimens. For example, among the Chamorros, one must consider the effect of the feasting complex and their tolerance of obesity when developing programs to combat diabetes, heart disease and stroke.

Conclusion

Torsch's research is only the beginning phase of change and empowerment of Chamorro women toward health in later life. By integrating the historical and biocultural contexts of their health with their sociocultural conceptions, knowledge has been gained about their health and healthcare needs. Their motivation toward healthy living reflects the possibilities for empowerment in later life. The next phase of change will require an active partnership between the elders and the health professionals on Guam to develop a culturally sensitive health delivery system, which will empower elderly women toward health.

References

Economic Research Center (1990) *Guam Annual Economic Review and Statistical Abstract, 1976, 1975, 1981, 1982, 1985 and 1987*. Department of Commerce, Agana

Gaw A (1975) An integrated approach to the delivery of healthcare to a Chinese community in America: The Boston experience. In: Kleinman A, *et al*, eds. *Medicine in Chinese Cultures*. DHEW, Washington

Guam Department of Public Health and Social Service (1991) *Health Risk Behavior, Guam* Government of Guam & University of Guam, Agana

Guam Department of Public Health and Social Service (1992) *Statistical Report, Office of Vital Statistics*. Government of Guam, Agana

Henderson N (1990) Anthropology, health, and aging. In Rubinstein R, ed. *Anthropology and Aging: Comprehensive Reviews*. Kluwer Academic Publishers, Boston

Kasperbauer L, Rapadas L, Workman R (1985) *Health Status of the Population of Guam: Morbidity*. Vol. 3, Community Development Report no. 14. Goverment of Guam, Mangilao, Guam

Kleinman A, ed (1975) *Medicine in Chinese Cultures: Comparative Studies of Healthcare in Chinese and Other Societies*. DHEW, Washington

Ma G (1996) Cultural and Socioeconomic Dimensions of Healthcare Services in the Houston Chinese Community. PhD. dissertation, University of Oklahoma

Millard A (1992) The anthropological analysis of health. *Med Anthropol Q* **6**(1): 3–5

O'Neill C, Sorensen E (1991) Home care of the elderly: A family perspective. *Adv Nursi Sci* **13**(4), 28–37

Naval C (1994) *Life Table Analysis for Chamorros of Guam*. Office of Planning and Evaluation. Department of Public Health and Social Services, Mangiloo, Guam, Government of Guam

Pietrusewsky M, Douglas M, Ikehara-Quebral R (1995) An assessment of health and disease in the prehistoric inhabitants of the Mariana Islands. *Symposium on Current Status of Bioarchaeological Research in the Marianas Archipelago*, 64th Annual Meeting of AAPA, March 31, Oakland, CA

Pinhey T, Heathcote G, Rarick J (1994) The influence of obesity on the self-reported health status of Chamorros and other residents of Guam. *Asian-Am Pac Island J Health* (summer)

Rogers R (1995) *Destiny's Landfall: A history of Guam*.University of Hawaii Press, Honolulu

Staats S *et al* (1993) Subjective age and health perceptions of older persons: Maintaining the youthful bias in sickness and in health. *Int J Aging Hum Devel* **37**(3): 191–203

US Bureau of the Census (1990) *Census of the Population, Social and Economic Characteristics, Guam*. Government Printing Office, Washington, DC

19

Assessing women's identity within their own culture

Mollyn V Bohnen and Deanna D Balantac

Technological advances, changes in mores and population mobility have resulted in a dynamic evolving multicultural world society. Genetic engineering and test-tube babies, for example, are more commonplace than in the past. Intermarriage between races and religious groups has become more acceptable and frequent. Jet travel, world-wide unrest and relaxation of immigration quotas have allowed entry of multicultural peoples into the United States. These trends have resulted in societal changes world-wide.

Stereotypical characteristics previously common to cultural groupings are rapidly becoming a thing of the past. Pierce (1996) stated that there is increasing pressure to alter the four racial classifications that have been used by the census bureau since the 1970s: black, white, American-Indian/Alaskan native and Asian/Pacific Islander. He maintained that the census race statistics tell less of the true story of what we are as people. Increasingly, citizens of split races and ancestries have children. In describing this classification dilemma further, Pierce used the example of Colin Powell. Powell is classified as black, but his autobiography describes his ancestry as a mixture of African, English, Irish, Scottish and Arawak Indian. As we contemplate this phenomenon, to seek direction for the future we must ask some questions: What is an Asian/Pacific Islander? A Laotian refugee? A Filipino with Spanish ancestry? A Japanese Korean immigrant? A Hindu from Fiji? A Tibetan monk? How many individuals do we know in the United States who are 100% of a single ethnic group? The answers point out the fact that stereotypical groupings, as we previously knew them, are increasingly irrelevant.

In the last 20 years, nursing has taken giant steps to address healthcare consumers' cultural needs. Nurses have been educated and trained to be aware of their own culture in order to be more sensitive in developing care plans that address their clients' cultural diversity. Traditional cultural norms have been delineated for various cultural groupings that have guided nursing practice. As the population has become increasingly multicultural, the traditional nursing approaches are less and less applicable. Thus, the profession must find new avenues in addressing society's diverse needs. As a dynamic profession, nursing must venture into the twenty-first century and prepare to go beyond cultural awareness and sensitivity. Nursing care and interventions must reflect cultural competence.

In searching the literature for tools that have been used to assess an individual's perception of their own cultural identity, none were found. With the need to distance nursing care from the accepted stereotypical practices, a tool that captures the segments that form the whole person's cultural identity/origins needed to be developed.

The study asked the following research question: *Does the Professional/Personal Origins Model represent the personal perception of one's own cultural identity?* In developing the model, various objects that had segments or parts making up a whole were explored. Furthermore, easily identifiable objects were considered. The citrus fruits met these criteria. The pomelo (see *Figure 19.1*), a tropical citrus fruit, was chosen since it represented characteristics inherent to cultural assessment relevant to the tool being proposed.

Many inherent characteristics of the pomelo can be made to represent cultural identity and thus became the logical choice to represent the Professional/Personal Origins Model. The unique characteristic of the pomelo provides the rationale for why it was chosen as a cultural assessment tool.

The pomelo has a tough outside rind, representing a person's tough exterior with a hidden inner vulnerability. The rind also represents an individual's inherent personal tenacity. Finally, the rind represents the fact that culturally related practices and traditions, once incorporated into one's self, are difficult to change.

Pomelo sections or segments are more variable in size than sections of other citrus fruits. These variable segments represent the various facets of a person's origins. Additionally, the sections are difficult to separate manually, representing the clannish attributes of cultural groups. People feel safe and comfortable within their cultural groups and tend to stick together, much like the pomelo segments.

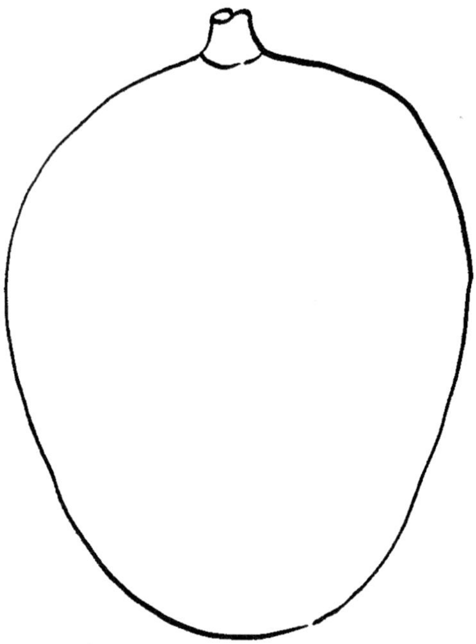

Figure 19.1: The pomelo (tropical grapefruit)

The sections are held together by a tough white membrane that must be carefully removed to fully expose and savour the edible fruit. This membrane represents the strength of character that binds the total individual together. The amount of membrane removed represents how much of the total person is revealed. In communicating and interacting with each other, people choose to expose portions of themselves depending on how comfortable they are and how much they wish others to see of themselves.

The edible portion (flesh) within the segments of a ripe pomelo may be either sweet or sour. Regardless of the taste, the fruit is enjoyed. Consumers familiar with it add salt to a sour pomelo and eat it; this is rarely done with sour oranges. This represents the fact that, despite variations in origins, people make unique contributions to a society. Furthermore, it reflects that people are neither totally good nor totally bad.

The ripe pomelo comes in a wider range of colours than other citrus fruits: various shades of green, yellow, gold and red — reflecting a person's varied ancestry, intermixed in a unique and valued individual. In addition, it represents colourful variations of people.

The seeds of the pomelo represent the continuity of culture. Values and traditions related to culture are passed from generation to generation. As cultural practices are passed on to the succeeding generation, individual experiences affect them so that they evolve, much like a pomelo seed growing into a new plant.

One must enjoy each segment of the whole pomelo to completely enjoy it. One cannot stop after eating just one section, so nurses must look at the 'segments' that make up the whole person to fully understand the healthcare consumer and promote holistic care.

POMelo: The Model

The POMelo cultural assessment model is a new approach to viewing cultural identity. Currently, an individual's cultural identity is assessed from other people's viewpoints rather than from their own self-perception. For example, an Asian postpartum woman asked the nurse if her family could bring her food from home. The nurse expected the family to bring traditional white cartons with Chinese food and was shocked when at lunch time she observed her patient enjoying two Big Macs. Similar experiences are increasingly encountered by practising nurses. Responding to the cultural needs of an individual requires that the nurse understand how that person perceives herself or himself rather than addressing the needs of the accepted stereotype that the nurse has learned.

P	**Personal/Professional**. One's origins, especially how an individual views oneself relative to these origins, determines the personal/professional self
O	**Origins**. One's origin is not determined by birthplace, skin colour or ancestry alone, but how the individual views oneself from each one or a combination of these perspectives
M	Model. The letters *elo* in the model are lower case since each represents the factors affecting the whole person's cultural identity/origin
e	eclectic, education (school), emblem, emigration, environment, essence, esteem, ethnicity, experience, expression. An individual's cultural make-up does not originate from a single source and is therefore eclectic. A person's culture is that individual's essence, which determines how the person expresses oneself and serves as an emblem for other people to see. Education or the lack of it, emigration, environment, ethnicity and experiences affect cultural identity, which in turn determines one's self-esteem
l	label, language, learning (life-long), limitations, lifestyle, lineage, location. Labels and limitations placed on people affect their cultural identity. The language spoken identifies one's origins. What a person has learned during a lifetime, the lifestyle one chooses to live, one's lineage and locations one has to be at, all enrich the person's cultural identity
o	occurrences, opinions, opportunities, options, orientation. Occurrences in life, other people's opinions, available opportunities and options as well as orientation to life as a whole affect cultural identity

A workshop was conducted for continuing education credits in southern California in August 1995. A sample of 31 Filipino registered nurses, alumni of the University of the Philippines, residing and employed in the United States, participated in the model development study. Subjects represented five regions of the Philippines. Using traditional, stereotypical cultural profiles for Filipinos and Philippine regions, all subjects individually completed a POMelo model representing their individual picture of their own cultural identity. Submitting a completed POMelo model for continuing education credits indicated that subjects consented to participate in the study.

The following is a sample of cultural profiles used:

Traditional Filipino/Philipino

- respect for elders
- strong family values
- strongly religious background (generally Catholic)
- education is highly valued
- speaks Tagalog

Traditional Ilocano Region

- industrious/hard-working
- migratory
- thrifty/frugal
- speaks Ilocano dialect

Traditional Western Visayan Region

- soft-spoken
- fun-loving
- generous
- speaks dialect
- good dancer, loves music, etc

Participants were given a picture of a whole POMelo representing their overall cultural self-identity. Subjects were further instructed to draw segments of their POMelos representing the culture(s) and subcultures that they perceived made up their total cultural identity. The number of segments may vary, depending on the number of cultural groupings subjects felt made up their overall culture. The sizes of the POMelo segments were determined by how much the person completing the model (using designed percentages from cultural profiles) conformed with or deviated from the stereotypical cultural profiles. Segment dividers were drawn in broken lines to indicate the fluidity of cultural identity, depending on the influences of the *elo* factors.

A descriptive analysis of all models com- pleted was performed. The findings showed no two models completed were alike, reflecting individual variation among subjects. Each model completed reflected a variety of cultural groupings (including regional subcultures) within the 'American-Filipino' person. No subjects perceived themselves as 'total' Filipinos, culturally. This finding suggested that, even though all subjects coming from a Filipino background, none identified their cultural selves as the Filipino stereotype. All were born in the Philippines, thus logically they should identify themselves culturally as totally Filipino. The finding was totally unexpected, but it did show the effects of emigration and the various degrees of acculturation on cultural identity. This further shows that in multicultural societies, individuals are in various stages of acculturation with needs that are variable and can not be met using one stereotypical strategy. Religion was subsumed within the subjects' cultural identities as Filipino and not separated. In a country like the Philippines, this finding is not unusual. The Philippines as a nation is predominantly (about 85%) Catholic, so their perception of themselves as being Catholic is identical with being Filipino when assessing cultural identity. Therefore, a nurse should recognise the importance of considering spiritual/religious influences when making a cultural origins assessment.

Another significant finding was that in several completed models, the regional and/or subregional cultural POMelo segments actually made up the subject's entire Filipino cultural identity. This suggested that not all Filipinos fit stereotypical pictures identified as Filipino. Filipinos come from 7000-plus islands, from various regional and subregional backgrounds and speak 86 different dialects that are totally dissimilar from the national language, Tagalog (which is one of the country's dialects and not necessarily understood by all Filipinos). In the same context, the American segment of the subjects' identity also specified southern California or the eastern US identity (which subjects adamantly considered separate from a stereotypical American identity), depending in which section of the US they lived.

The findings of this study indicate that the POMelo model may represent an individual's perceptions of her own cultural identity. It further indicates that the POMelo model probes deeper in assessing an individual's cultural identity. It traverses the macro-stereotypical traits or characteristics of the person's culture and allows insight into the micro-identity of the individual. The completed sample models show two Filipino individuals whose separate POMelos reflect segments that are totally different (Figures 19.2 and 19.3). Segments reflect that each viewed herself, for the most part, as American with Filipino segments reflecting regional variations.

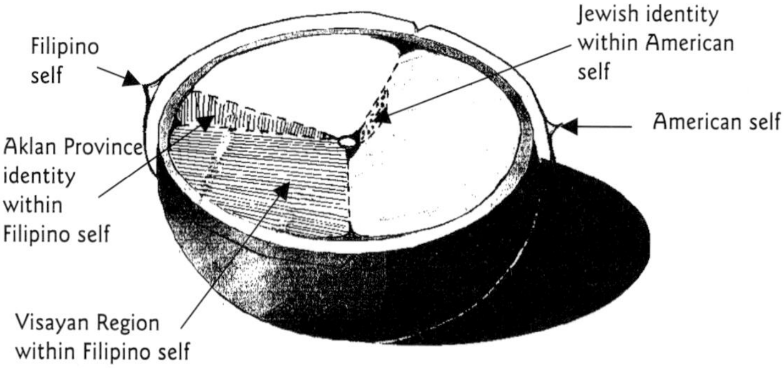

Figure 19.2: Completed model, subject born in the Philippines

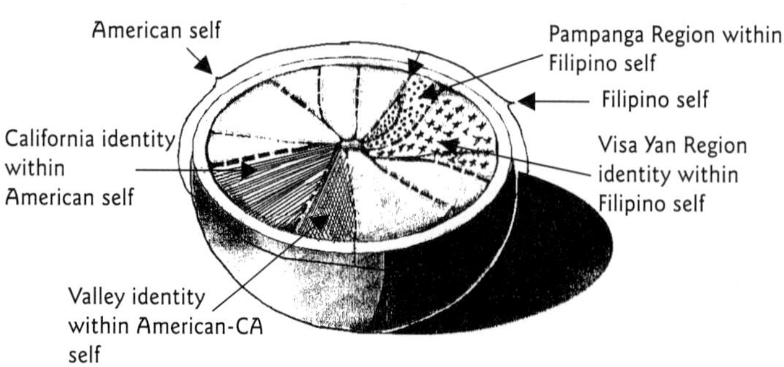

Figure 19.3: Completed model, subject born in America, parents born in Philippines

Further model development needs to be conducted to validate the POMelo model. A comparison study with Filipino registered nurses residing in the Philippines as subjects is recommended. In addition, completion of the model by various ethnic/ cultural groups in the United States and world-wide must be done. A study comparing the client's self-identity with that perceived by nurses should be considered.

The use of the POMelo model as a self-assessment tool of cultural identity has real potential. It is the initial step to move away from having care-givers assess clients' cultural identity using the caregivers' perceptions based on learned stereotypical characteristics or traits. Furthermore, the POMelo model provides nurses with a tool to more accurately assess clients' cultural needs.

The use of the POMelo model has implications for international nursing practice. It provides nurses with a tool to assess a variety of clients in various international settings, enabling them to personalise care, thus increasing their cultural competence in meeting the healthcare needs of a multicultural, global society.

References

Pierce N (1996, January 7) Economic segregation, not racial is the real issue. *Sacramento Bee*: A4

20

Sociodemographic differences between two ethnic groups in a geriatric rehabilitation unit in Israel

Zohar Nir and David Galinsky

Introduction

This study investigates the nature of two ethnic groups of chronic geriatric patients in their first phase of recovery in a geriatric rehabilitation unit (GRU). Particular attention was give to demographic background, family instrumental support, social roles before hospitalisation and perceived family relationship during hospitalisation.

Israel, as a modern western society, is highly pluralistic. It is composed of may subcultures that are not uniform in values and behavioural norms. There are, however, two main ethnic groups: Sephardi Jews who immigrated mainly from North Africa and the Middle East, and who generally demonstrate an Oriental tradition; and Ashkenazi Jews, who immigrated from western countries, mainly from Europe, and who generally tend to adhere to the values of western culture.

In the western view, becoming dependent means giving up many of the rights and responsibilities of adulthood (Diehl, 1989). The elderly are, therefore, encouraged to achieve a certain amount of independence (Farzan, 1991). The Oriental (eastern) culture promotes the value of aging. Older people are seen as valuable because longevity is viewed as a means of accumulating truth. Moreover, dependency and disability are considered to be part of fate, and are thus accepted with less negative emotions (Gaines, 1988; Helman, 1990; Perlmutter and Hall, 1992).

Chronic illness generates multiple needs that change over time, requiring ongoing adaptation on the part of both patient and family (Ben-Sira, 1991; Given and Given, 1991; McConnell, 1988b; Whall and Loveland-Cherry, 1993). Chronic bad health creates much stress on both the patient and the family, and may create negative family interactions (Farzan, 1991; Friedland and McColl, 1992; Friedman, 1993; Glass *et al*, 1993; Lieberman and Fisher, 1995; Mui, 1995; Reese *et al*, 1994). Such negative interactions may occur more frequently in families that are exposed to a greater number of stressful life events at the same time, such as aging, chronic illness, poverty and lack of resources (Krause and Borawski-Clark, 1995). Family response to chronic conditions has been identified as a significant influence on a patients's psychological and physical well-being (Anderson, 1988; Antonucci, 1985; Ben-Sira, 1991; Diehl, 1989; Farzan, 1991; Friedman, 1993; Evans *et al*, 1992; Given and Given, 1991; Glass and Maddox, 1992; Krause, 1987; Lindsey, 1988; Primomo *et al*, 1990). The way in which different families provide or seek care may be influenced by their cultural norms (Antonucci, 1985; Barker, 1991; Fong, 1985; Glass *et al*, 1993; Glass and Maddox, 1992; Helman, 1990; McConnell, 1988a; McConnell and Matteson, 1988a; 1988b; Perlmutter and Hall, 1992; Wray, 1992), as well as by their physical resources (socioeconomic class) (Krause and Borawski-Clark, 1995; Norbeck and Tilden, 1988). Their satisfaction with the amount of support that is provided to them may be reflected through their assessment of their perceived family relationships, which, in turn, is related more strongly to psychological than to other dimensions of well-being.

The family unit is the main source of emotional support, instrumental support and affirmation (Antonucci, 1985; Diehl, 1989; Friedland and McColl, 1992; Glass *et al*, 1993; House and Kahn, 1985; Lindsey, 1988). Although instrumental support has proven less beneficial to well-being than emotional support, there is some evidence that the former may relate to satisfaction with life, particularly in older adults, and to health outcome in several situations of health impairment (Friedman, 1993; Lenz *et al*, 1986; Primomo *et al*, 1990).

Instrumental support is generally seen as the provision of material assistance (eg. money, labour, goods and time, which includes taking over another's duties) and services to assist the person in need (Antonucci, 1985; Glass and Maddox, 1992; Gulick, 1994; House and Kahn, 1985; Lenz *et al*, 1986;

Ragasdale *et al*, 1993). The first experience of chronic illness in older adults may limit their functional and psychological abilities, which puts them, first and foremost, in greater need of instrumental rather than emotional support. In order of priority, then, basic physical and instrumental needs must be met before psychological needs can be approached.

Researchers have attempted to explore the ethnic differences with regard to health and illness (Fong, 1985; Gaines, 1988; Helman, 1990; Perlmutter and Hall, 1992) and in terms of mortality and stroke in northern Israel (Epstein *et al*, 1989). However, little data has been collected about the nature of these differences in the context of Israel's ethnic groups in terms of first-time chronic illness care, family instrumental support and family relationships throughout the first stage of elderly rehabilitation. This lack of knowledge means that healthcare professionals often overlook the norms of culturally different subjects during hospitalisation. The attention of the present study, therefore, was focussed on the ways in which key aspects of a cultural profile influence a family's behaviour during an elderly relative's hospitalisation.

Since sensitivity to cultural norms is essential to providing holistic patient care (Fong, 1985), and rehabilitation is a process of this holistic care (Diehl, 1989), studying different cultures may help professionals better understand family resources and behaviour in the rehabilitation unit, especially to understand the needs of the elderly in a multicultural society. It may also help to identify commonalities rather than differences between ethnic groups in order to effectively integrate the subjects' cultural backgrounds into the planning of the rehabilitation process.

Since social support is strongly related to cultural perception and the socioeconomic status of the social network, the goals of this study were:

1. to compare two ethnic groups with respect to their demographic background
2. to describe the possible differences between two ethnic groups of family instrumental support during the hospitalisation of their elderly relatives
3. to explore the variables that affected the elderly subjects' own evaluation of their relationships with families.

Methods

Sample

The study population of 336 elderly Jews – all immigrants – was obtained from a GRU located in a major hospital in the Negev, which serves as the headquarters of all medical services in southern Israel. About equal numbers of the sample were Ashkenazi (177) and Sephardi (159). Initially, the subjects had been admitted to the acute care service of the hospital. After treatment for the acute phase, which was, on average, about three weeks, they were placed in the geriatric unit. Of the sample as a whole, 201 (60%) had sustained a first-time stroke, 52 (15%) had hip fractures and 82 (25%) had various chronic physical health problems, with CIHD, DM and anaemia the most common. None had a history of psychosis or acute mental deterioration or global aphasia.

Instrument, and measurement of key variables

Within the first week of admission to the GRU, the Assessment of Dependency for Long-Term Care Benefits form (IDC-Brookdale Institute, 1989; Baich-Moray *et al*, 1994) was administered by a trained nursing student to all subjects in the study. In conformance with departmental criteria, informed consent was required from both the subject and his/her family.

The form has been used since 1989 by the National Insurance Institute of the State of Israel for every claimant for long-term care benefits. It encompasses a battery of scored structured sub-scales that determine and provide a profile of the subject's psychosocio-demographic data, as well as a scored, structured instrument for measuring dependency through activities of daily living. The main criteria for establishing eligibility is the dependency test. This battery assessment was found to be a reliable, accurate and valid tool for identifying the target population (Baich-Moray *et al*, 1994). Factor analysis and Cronbach's Alfa confirmed the theoretical structure and internal consistency of the form, respectively.

Data analysis

Statistical analyses were performed using the SPSS statistical package, with Pearson and Spearman correlations measuring associations between variables and the Pearson chi square to measure associations between frequencies of non-parametric variables. T-test and one-way and two-way analysis of variance (ANOVA) were used to explore the differences between two or more means.

Results

Sociodemographic characteristics

The first goal of the study was to explore the demographic variables of the sample. *Table 20:1* summarises these.

Table 20.1: The demographic characteristics of the sample (N=336)

Variable	%	Yrs	(SD)	Range
Ashkenazi group	51			
Males	47			
Age		74	(±9.6)	56–10
Females – age		75.1	(±9.1)	
Males – age		72.6	(±9.9)	
Length of residence in Israel		35.6	(±13.1)	2–75
Married	58			
Years of education		8	(±4.6)	0–20
Unskilled	32			
Blue collar	18			
White collar	20			
Religious	68			
Live near children	80			
Contact with formal services	68			
Contact with friends	17			
Volunteer activity	6			

Findings also revealed that a great many of the subjects had experienced contact with formal services (medical clinics, welfare registry offices and the National Insurance Institute — unemployment, welfare, etc), rather than socialising with friends, or in a volunteer activity prior to hospitalisation. Using an independent t-test (*Table 20.2*) and chi-square test (*Table 20.3*), the following findings were obtained. The Sephardi group was younger, poorer, less educated and less proficient in Hebrew, and held fewer social roles (*Table 20.2*). The Ashkenazi group was more likely to have better jobs and to be secular (*Table 20.3*).

Table 20.2: Characteristics of demographic variables by ethnicity

Variable	Ashkenazi (N=177) M (SD)	Sephardi (N=159) M (SD)
Age (in years)***	75.99(±10.0)	71.3(±8.99)
Proficiency in Hebrew***	3.8(±3.4)	2.6(±4.6)
Level of education (in years)***	10.2(±4.2)	6.4(±4.6)
Social roles*	5.2(±1.8)	4.6(±2.1)
Number of persons at home***	1.9(±0.93)	2.5(±1.4)
Income level***	3.26(±2.39)	2.64(±2.0)

t-test significant at: *p<0.05, **p<0.01, ***p<0.001

Table 20.3: Characteristics of demographic variables by ethnicity

	Ashkenazi	Sephardi
Ownership of dwelling***	124(70%)	79(50%)
Unskilled**	35(20%)	63(40%)
White collar**	56(32%)	17(11%)
Religious***	64(36%)	146(92%)
Dietary regimen***	39(22%)	56(35%)
Live near children*	71(40%)	95(60%)

Chi-test significant at: *p<0.05, **p<0.01, ***p<0.001

Generally, Pearson correlations indicate that the higher the level of education, the higher the level of proficiency in Hebrew (r=0.56, p<0.001) and the lower the level of religiosity (r=0.62, p<0.001).

With respect to a dietary regimen, Sephardi subjects were more likely to have dietary limitations than Ashkenazi subjects. No significant differences were observed between the two ethnic groups with respect to smoking and drinking habits, their co-morbidity condition, the use of domestic services or the severity of the present illness.

Living arrangements

Most subjects (84%) lived in their own home or apartment; 31% alone, 37% with a spouse or partner, 20% with children and spouse, 5% with children and 7% with non-family members (including nursing home). Ashkenazi were significantly more likely to own their own houses or apartments (*Table 20.3*). A higher proportion of elderly Ashkenazi lived with only their spouses (*Figure 20.1*) while elderly Sephardi were more likely to live with their nuclear family under the same roof — spouse and children (sometimes more than five people) — in multi-generational households (*Table 20.2*). Furthermore, when living separately, Sephardi were more likely to live near their children (*Table 20.3*).

Marital status

The chronological average age of widowhood for elderly Ashkenazi was 81.6 (±9.3); and 74.4 (±8.3) for Sephardi. Sephardi subjects faced widowhood at an earlier age than their counter- parts. When widowed, Ashkenazi were more likely to live by themselves, while Sephardi were more likely to live with adult children.

Main care-giver

Prior to hospitalisation, 12% reported having no primary care-giver, 39% had a spouse or partner as main care-giver, 37% had their children and 12% had a non-family member. Of the Ashkenazi elderly, 40% reported their spouses as their main care-giver and 27% their children; while the Sephardi elderly were more likely to have adult children (37%) and their spouse (37%) as main care-giver. Since there was a significant difference between the two ethnic groups and chronological age, the two-way ANOVA test was conducted to explore the role of age in type of care-giver before hospitalisation (*Figure 20.2*). Findings revealed that when Ashkenazi elderly reported that their children were their main care-givers, their mean age was 80 years, while when the Sephardi elderly had their children as main care-givers, their mean age was 72.8 years ($p<0.01$). These findings revealed that the Sephardi elderly received assistance from their children at an earlier age than the Ashkenazi elderly, and this may be consistent with the fact that the Sephardi subjects were more likely to be widowed at an earlier age. *Figure 20.2* also shows that, in the oldest age group, both ethnic groups were more likely to have non-family members as main care-givers.

Social roles

The Ashkenazi were more likely to assume higher scores than the Sephardi. There were no significant differences between the two groups with relation to

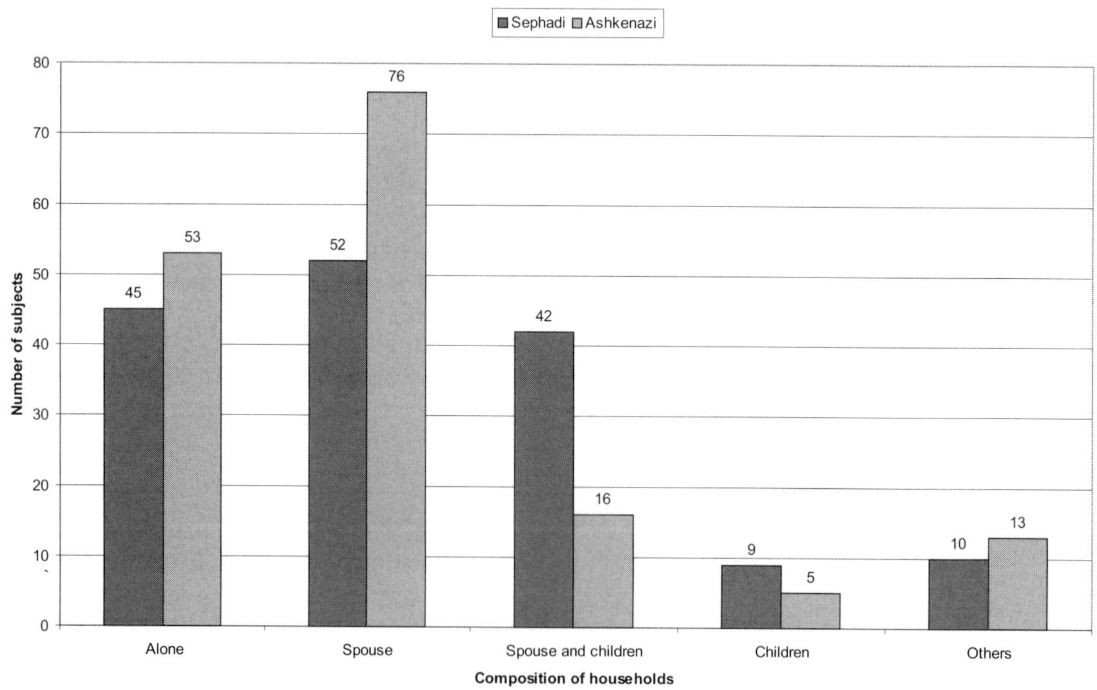

Figure 20.1: Ethnicity and its relation to subject's composition of households

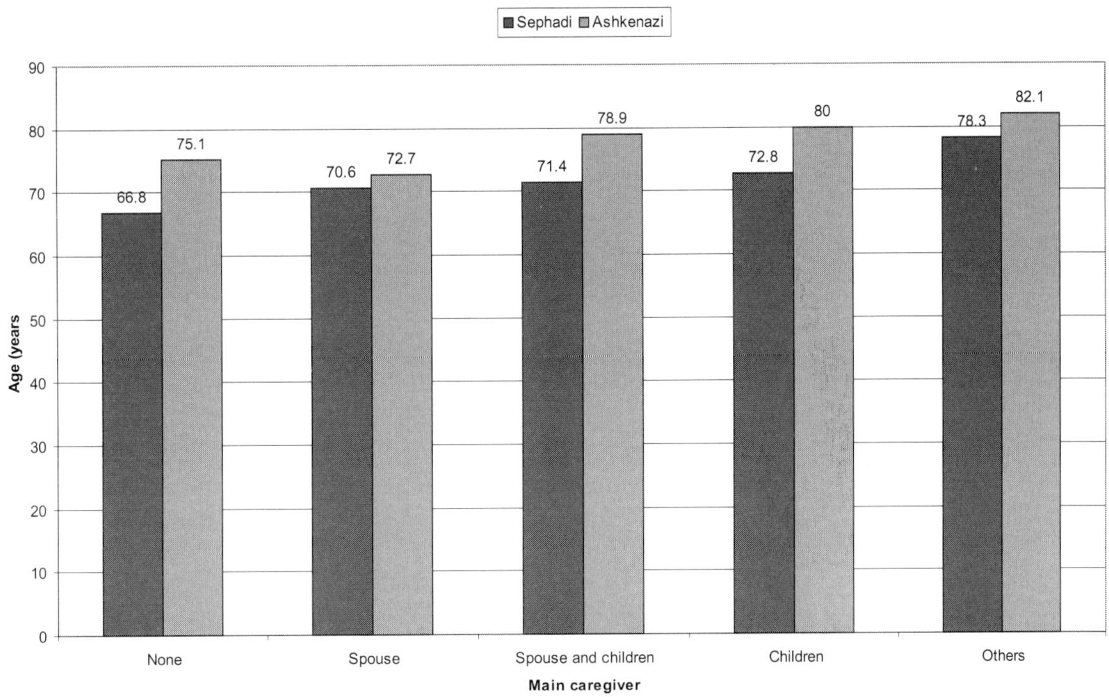

Figure 20.2: Mean age of the main caregiver by ethnicity

outside activities, but elderly Sephardi did display a high degree of involvement in religious activities (*Table 20.3*). Outside activities, while not related directly to ethnicity, were related to the subjects' age, profession, co-morbidity and related health problems.

Family instrumental support during hospitalisation

The second goal of the study was to determine the main factors that played a role in instrumental support for each ethnic group during the time of hospitalisation. The study also addressed the question of who played a key role in responding to the subjects' needs during hospitalisation.

Subjects in both ethnic groups almost always reported that it was a family member who was the main source of support. Some 44 subjects (13%) mentioned others as main visitor, but noted that they were not a stable source of support because they were not available all the time.

In general, the findings suggested that most of the elderly subjects had fairly extensive visits during hospitalisation and clearly were not isolated from family. Only 20 (6%) had no visitors. Furthermore, members of both ethnic groups spent a great deal of time with their elderly: 262 (78%) of the subjects had visits every day, 181 (54%) had visits during the daytime and 155 (46%) had day and night visits. Children were the most frequent source of support, and had a profound role in providing instrumental support. Of those who initially accompanied the subjects to the hospital, 134 (38%) were their children, and 138 (39%) of the main visitors who stayed with the elderly at the GRU were also their children.

Findings revealed that, for both ethnic groups, the higher the number of people who lived in the same household, the higher the number of family members serving as accompaniers.

Ethnicity, main visitors and subjects' age

Since the Sephardi were younger than their counterparts, one of the questions that emerged was the role played by the subject's age in accounting for the ethnic differences in relation to provision of instrumental support. Findings revealed that spouses and children together were the main visitors of the Ashkenazi subjects at the mean age of 73.7 years, while spouse and children together were the main visitors for Sephardi subjects at the mean age of 68 years (p<0.05). Findings suggested that the main visitors for younger subjects were more likely to be the subject's spouse and children together. At older ages, the main visitors at the GRU were children and others. It is important to mention that others were more likely to be younger than the subjects.

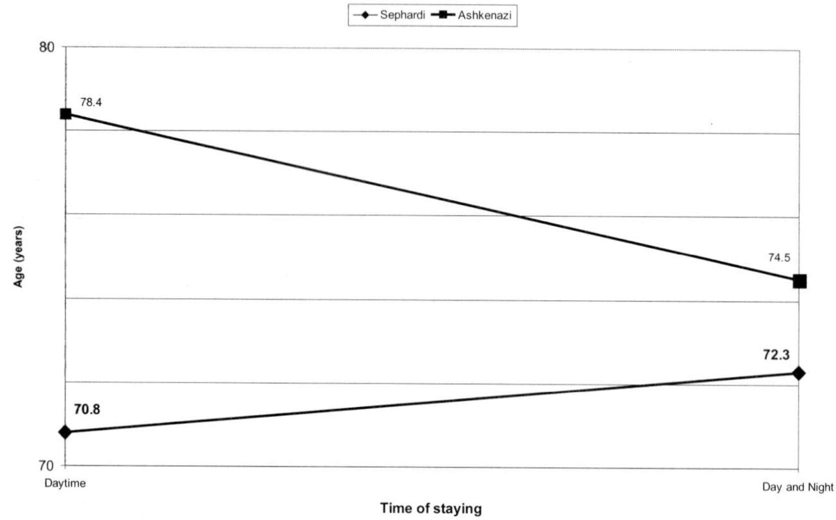

Figure 20.3: Length of stay in the GRU of ethnic groups by mean age

When two-way ANOVA was conducted — two ethnic groups and two categories of length of visits as independent variables, and age as the dependent variable — it was found that the pattern of length of visits differed between the two ethnic groups in relation to the age of the subjects. Findings revealed (*Figure 20.3*) that in the Ashkenazi group the older the subject, the more likely the main visitor stayed throughout daytime; the younger the subject, the more likely the main visitor stayed throughout both day and night times. In contrast, the pattern of the Sephardi group was that the older the subject, the more likely the main visitor stayed throughout both day and night times. In relation to chronological age, however, findings suggested that 'old' among Sephardi subjects was still younger than 'young' among the Ashkenazi.

Ethnicity, length of visit and social roles

Across both ethnic groups, findings revealed that subjects who had 'day and night' visits were more likely to approximate the mean score of 5.3 (±1.9) on the social roles scale than subjects who had visits during the day time, 4.3 (±1.9). In other words, the findings suggest the extent of performing social roles in the past tended to influence the frequency and extensiveness of visits.

Ethnicity and family relationship

The third goal of the study was to explore the variables that affected perceived family relationships. Good relations with their families were reported by 135 (83%) of the Ashkenazi and 117 (74%) of the Sephardi group (p=0.055). This suggested a trend for a significant difference related to ethnicity and family relationship. Across the two ethnic groups, those who had a higher level of education tended to evaluate their family relationships as 'good' more often than those who had a lower level of education (M=8.4±4.6 *vs* M=6.3±4.5, p<0.05, respectively); those subjects who lived in their own apartments rather than in 'other' arrangements (including nursing homes) evaluated their family relationship as 'good' (87% *vs* 65%, p<0.05, respectively); and subjects who were involved in more social roles were more likely to evaluate their relationships as 'good' than those with less social roles (M=5.14±1.8 *vs* ZM=3.06±2.1, p<0.001, respectively). Sixty-three percent of the married subjects, in contrast to 37% of the unmarried ones, evaluated their family relationships as good. The findings also suggested that family relationship was affected by the identity of the person providing instrumental support rather than the duration and length of visits.

Discussion

This study explored the differences among the first-time chronically ill elderly of two ethnic groups in relation to sociodemographic variables, instrumental support received during hospitalisation and perceived family relationships. Most subjects were characterised as low to moderate in socioeconomic class, with extensive instrumental support during hospitalisation, with considerable assistance from formal services prior to hospitalisation and with perceived good family relationships. Sephardi subjects were younger, more likely to be of lower socioeconomic status, to be less educated, to have less prestigious jobs, to have more dietary limitations and to have a larger family network. With a larger family network, it was found that more than one person accompanied the elderly relative through the hospital admission process. It was clear that the persons residing with the subjects assumed a wide range of responsibilities for the health of their elderly. Thus, one can conclude that, in the short-term, the Sephardi group had more available resources for greater support.

Marital status, living arrangements, performed social roles and level of education were found to significantly affect perception of family relationships as being 'good'.

During hospitalisation, subjects received extensive assistance from families. Most had small family networks that consisted mainly of spouse and children who performed most of the support required. Although 12% reported non-family persons as their main care-giver, they noted that these were not always available. This meant that the network was less stable than a family network might have been. Similar social network structure to that found in the present study have been described by Krause and Borawski-Clark (1995) and used to characterise the low-income class social support network. Antonucci (1985) called these a multiplex; that is, the same people exchanging a variety of different types of support.

This study emphasises that, while the family has traditional obligations to support its nuclear members, the age of the subjects and size of the family network significantly determined the source and amount of received support during hospitalisation. This is corroborated in a study by Penrod *et al* (1995).

Age was significant in determining the source and the pattern of the instrumental support provided. The two ethnic groups both exhibited the same visitation pattern. The younger the subject, the more likely it was that the main visitors would be the subject's spouse and children together. At older ages, the main visitors at the GRU were children and others. Sephardi subjects displayed this pattern at an overall earlier age than their counterparts.

In relation to visitation patterns, as shown in *Figure 20.3*, the main visitor of older Sephardi subjects was more likely to stay from morning until midnight; while it was the main visitor of the younger Ashkenazi subjects who stayed these long hours. One explanation may be that, since Ashkenazi patients were generally older, their spouses, who were generally their main visitors, were correspondingly older and often frail. This meant that the spouse did not have the physical energy to visit both day and night, nor to cope with the many needs of the patient in a hospital setting. The Sephardi patients, on the other hand, were generally younger, and their main visitors were either their spouses (who were correspondingly younger) or their children.

Social roles were found to be a personal resource for achieving extensive instrumental support and for perceived good relationships with family. It was found that, across ethnic differences, the more social roles performed by the subjects, the more instrumental support they received during their hospitalisation. Furthermore, the more social roles subjects' held, the more they perceived their family relationships as good. This finding calls for further attention since it emphasises on the one hand the dynamic quality of the family instrumental support process, and on the other hand the dynamic process of the exchange roles.

Chronic illness places elderly persons in a vulnerable and dependent situation. By being dependent, the elderly increase their risk of losing their power within their family and of being rejected. Previous social roles provide the elderly with a range of credits and obligations from family and friends. Social roles as an exchange product (Salisbury, 1991) give the aged meaningful, rewarding activities and relationships in their family context (Patric, 1993). Performed social roles in the past may seem to be a 'support reserve' (Antonucci, 1985) or an accumulated sense of 'helping others' (Krause and Borawski-Clark, 1995). This mutual relationship between family and the elderly describes a dynamic process of reciprocity and reward, resulting in perceived good family relationships (Phillips, 1991). It is a mechanism that can ease the position of being in need (Antonucci, 1985; Krause and Borawski-Clark, 1995; Phillips, 1991).

The role of children

Overall, children had a prominent role as main care-givers and providers of support. This finding has already been reported in the literature (Lieberman and Fisher, 1995; Mui, 1995; Penrod *et al*, 1995). However, there was a difference between the two ethnic groups in the order of a primary or secondary care-giver. Among the Sephardi group, children, as part of their traditional obligations, had major responsibilities for their elderly parents before and during hospitalisation, without any relation to their marital status. In the hospitalisation context, however, the prominent role of the children was perhaps more pronounced due to the fact that their parents had poor Hebrew language skills and sometimes could not understand the terminology of the rehabilitation setting. This may have made them more dependent on their children for translation of information related to their progress and rehabilitation. Among the Ashkenazi elderly, in contrast, the children usually played a secondary role in providing assistance. Ashkenazi subjects were more likely to live with their often equally frail spouses (who were their main care-givers) or by themselves.

From the social point of view, it is important to emphasise that, among the Sephardi elderly studied here, children entered the child-parent role much sooner than their counterparts — a reflection of cultural orientation; these findings are supported by the literature that deals with minorities in America (Perlmutter and Hall, 1992).

Although findings revealed that most of the subjects preferred to live independently with their spouse or by themselves, Sephardi subjects were more likely to live in multi-generational family groupings. This suggested that Sephardi subjects had more personal resources available, and were more likely to have a physically and numerically stronger and younger social network to provide support. In contrast, the majority of the Ashkenazi subjects had only small immediate family networks, mainly composed of their spouses, who were also frail and elderly, as main care-giver, and then, according to Cantor (1979), from their children. In the case of loss of spouse, Ashkenazi subjects lived by themselves and their children played the primary role in providing assistance and instrumental support during hospitalisation.

Findings suggested that the subjects did not differ in their instrumental support behaviour. Lack of substantial differences in instrumental support may be explained by the fact that, in Israel neither the Sephardi nor the Ashkenazi culture is homogenous; rather, each is an aggregate of the influences of several cultures that exhibit a wide range of values, behaviours and norms (eg. Sephardi Jews may come from Syria or Morocco while Ashkenazi Jews may come from Poland, Germany or even the United States).

Furthermore, in a melting pot like Israel, any uniqueness of a particular ethnic group may erode with time due to assimilation and acculturation (Perlmutter and Hall, 1992). After being in Israel an average of 36 years, individuals of any culture are likely to absorb influences of the dominant culture and the various subcultures with which they come in contact. We need to remember that most of the 'supporters' were the children, the second generation, who had been reared in Israel.

Conclusions

More research should be done to determine whether it is ethnic orientation that encouraged the Sephardi subjects to live within their extended families or economic imperatives. Multi-generational households could also have been a product of the fact that Sephardi subjects were younger and still had children living in their own homes who were not of the traditional age at which children move away from home.

In the two groups studied, Sephardi subjects were younger than Ashkenazi, and were more likely to face widowhood sooner. By contrast, the Ashkenazi had longer life expectancy and longer marital life. In addition, findings suggested that elderly Sephardi were more likely to have dietary limitations than their counterparts. These findings require additional exploration to rule out poverty variables that may affect cultural differences.

Because all the care burden during hospitalisation depends mainly on one person, it is highly recommended that his/her perceived family relationships be explored. It should be remembered that being the main care-giver, and/or the main visitor to his/her parent during hospitalisation may also take its toll in physical health and psychological well-being of those children who accept these responsibilities (Liberman and Fisher, 1995; Mui, 1995).

Limitations

Lack of substantial differences in instrumental support may be because the questions were very general. They focussed on identifying the person who accompanied and helped a patient in the process of admission to hospital, or the one who visited a patient and played a main role in providing assistance. The questions did not address themselves in describing particular and specific instrumental behaviour. Moreover, the questions allowed patients to indicate subjective perceptions about emotional or instrumental support, or affirmation.

Implications

Professionals recognise that social roles are a resource that enable subjects to maintain their family position in the face of social and physical losses and that engender a positive view of family relationships. It is, therefore, essential to educate the family about the importance of social roles, particularly for the elderly sick individual.

The ability of the family to respond or assist the elderly patient is a key factor determining recovery (Diehl, 1989; Given and Given, 1991). Therefore, professionals need to be aware that, when the social network is small and resources poor, the total burden of support may be distributed between children and a possibly frail, elderly spouse. The spouse, in particular, may require full institutional support, because he/she will not be able to carry the whole burden alone. Such a situation could easily strain family relationships both physically and emotionally when long-term care is necessary. Continued assistance by formal services is therefore strongly recommended.

References

Anderson R (1988) The contribution of informal care to the management of stroke. *International Disability Studies* **10**(3), 107–112

Antonucci TC (1985) Personal characteristics, social support and social behavior. In Binstok RH & Shanas E (eds.), *Handbook of againg and social sciences*, 2 edn. Van Nostrand Reinhold, New York: 94–128

Baich-Moray S, Zipkin A, Morginstin B (1994) *Assessment of dependency for long-term care benefits*. National Insurance Institute, Jerusalem

Barker JC (1991) Culture diversity changing the context of medical practice. *West J Med* **157**(3): 248–57

Ben-Sira Z (1991) *Regression, stress, and readjustment in aging: A structured bio-psycho-social perspective on coping and professional support*. Praeger, New York

Cantor M (1979) Neighbors and friends. *Res Aging* **1**: 434–63

Diehl LN (1989) Client and family learning in the rehabilitation setting. *Nurs Clin N Am* **24**: 257–61

Evans RV, Hendriecks RD, Haselkorn JK, Bishop DS, Baldwin D (1992) The family role in stroke rehabilitation. *Am J Phys Med Rehab* **71**: 135–9

Epstein L, Rishpon S, Bebtal E *et al* (1989) Incidence, mortality, and case-fatality rate of stroke in northern Israel. *Stroke* **20**: 725–9

Farzan DT (1991) Reintegration for stroke survivors. *Nurs Clin N Am* 26: 1037–47

Fong C (1985) Ethnicity and nursing practice. *Top Clin Nurs* **7**(3): 1–10

Friedland JF, McColl MA (1992) Social support intervention after stroke: Result of a randomized trial. *Arch Phys Med Rehab* **73**: 573–81

Friedman MM (1993) Social support sources and psychological well-being in older women with heart disease. *Res Nurs Health* **16**: 415–23

Gaines AD (1988) The contribution of informal care to the management of stroke. *Int Dis Stud* **10**(3): 107–11

Given BA, Given CW (1991) Family caregiving for the elderly. *Ann Rev Nurs Res* **9**: 77–101

Glass TA, Maddox GL (1992) The quality and quantity of social support: Stroke recovery as psycho-social transition. *Soc Sci Med* **34**: 1249–61

Glass TA, Matchar BD, Belyea M, Feussner RJ (1993) Impact of social support on outcome in first stroke. *Stroke* **24**: 64–70

Gulick EE (1994) Social support among persons with multiple sclerosis. *Res Nurs Health* **17**: 195–206

Helman CG (1990) Culture, health and illness: An introduction for health professionals, 2 edn. Butterworth-Heineman, Oxford

House JS, Kahn RL (1985) Measures and concepts of social support. In: Cohen S, Syme SL, eds. *Social Support and Health* Academic Press Orlando, FL: 83–108

IDC-Brookdale Institute (1989) *Final Report of an Interagency Committee for Coordinating the Care of the Elderly*. IDC Brookdale Institute of Gerontology and Adult Human Development in Israel, Jerusalem

Krause N (1987) Understanding the stress process: Linking soical support with locus of control beliefs. *J Gerontol* **42**: 589–93

Krause N, Borawski-Clark E (1995) Social class differences in social support among older adults. *Gerontol* **35**(4): 498–508

Lenz RE, Parks PL, Jenkins SL, Jarrett EG (1986) Life change and instrumental support as predictors of illness in mothers of 6-month-olds. *Res Nurs Health* **9**: 17–27

Lieberman MA, Fisher L (1995) The impact of chronic illness on the health and well-being of family members. *Gerontol* **35**(1): 94–102

Lindsey AM (1988) Social support: Conceptualizations and measurement instruments. In: Frank-Stromborg M, ed. *Instruments for Clinical Nursing Research*. Appleton and Lange, San Mateo, CA:108–119

McConnell ES (1988a) A conceptual framework for gerontological nursing practice. In: Matteson MA, McConnell ES, eds. *Gerontological Nursing Concepts and Practice*. W B Saunders, Philadelphia, PA: 5–31

McConnell ES (1988b) Nursing diagnosis related to psychosocial alterations. In: Matteson MA, McConnell ES, eds. *Gerontological Nursing Concepts and Practice*. W B Saunders, Philadelphia, PA: 529–77

McConnell ES, Matteson MA (1988a). Psychosocial aging changes. In: Matteson MA, McConnell ES, eds. *Gerontological Nursing Concepts and Practice*. W B Saunders, Philadelphia, PA: 431–79

McConnell ES, Matteson MA (1988b) Psychosocial problems associated with aging. In: Matteson MA, McConnell ES, eds. *Gerontological Nursing Concepts and Practice*. W B Saunders, Philadelphia, PA: 481–520

Mui AC (1995) Caring for frail elderly parents: A comparison of adult sons and daughters. *Gerontol* **35**(1): 86–93

Norbeck JS, Tilden VP (1988) International nursing research in social support: Theoretical and methodological issues. *J Adv Nurs* **13**: 173–8

Patric M (1993) Tasks of daily living associated with later life stages. In: Carnevali DL, Patrick M, eds. *Nursing Management for the Elderly*. 3 edn. J B Lippincott, Philadelphia, PA: 65–73

Penrod JD, Kane RA, Kane RL, Finch MD (1995) Who cares? The size, scope, and composition of the caregiver support system. *Gerontol* **35**(4): 489–97

Perlmutter M, Hall E (1992) Cross-cultural perspectives on adulthood and aging. In: Perlmutter M, Hall E, eds. *Adult Development and Aging*, 2 edn. John Wiley and Sons, New York: 467–90

Phillips, LR (1991) Social support of the older client. In: Cheinitz WC, Stone JT, Salisbury SA, eds. *Clinical Gerontological Nursing: A Guide to Advanced Practice*. W B Saunders, Philadelphia, PA: 535–44

Primomo J, Yates CB, Wood FN (1990) Social support for women during illness: The relationship among sources and types to adjustment. *Res Nurs Health* **13**: 153–62

Ragsdale D, Yarbrough S, Lasher AT (1993) Using social support theory to care for CVA patients. *Rehabil Nurs* **18**(3): 154–61

Reese DR, Gross AM, Smalley DL, Messer SC (1994) Caregiver of Alzheimer's disease and stroke patients: Immunological and psychological considerations. *Gerontol* **34**(4): 534–40

Salisbury AS (1991) Preventing excess disability. In: Cheinitz WC, Stone JT, Salisbury SA, eds. *Clinical Gerontological Nursing: A Guide to Advanced Practice*. W B Saunders, Philadelphia, PA: 391–421

Whall AL, Loveland-Cherry CJ (1993) Family unit-focus research: 1984–1991. *Ann Rev Nurs Res* **11**: 227–47

Wray LA (1992) Health policy and ethnic diversity in older Americans: Dissonance or harmony? *W J Med* **157**: 357–61

21

Woman care-givers for frail, aging parents in Taiwan

Shu-Yuan Chao and Patricia Roth

Due to ongoing improvements in health, living standards, and nutrition, and the science of medicine, the life expectancy of people in Taiwan has been greatly prolonged, increasing from 53.38 years in 1951 to 71.66 years in 1993 for men, and from 56.33 years to 77.52 years for women during the same period. As the older population continues to increase, the number of chronic illnesses will likewise increase, creating a need for more care. At the end of 1993, 7.09% of the total population in Taiwan was over 65 years (Department of Health, 1995). It is estimated that currently about 12% of persons over the age of 65 years in Taiwan are frail and/or have cognitive impairments, such as senile dementia, and cannot care for themselves (Department of Accounting and Statistics, 1990). Most of them live at home and are taken care of by a family member (Wu *et al*, 1991; Hu, 1994).

Sons in Taiwan traditionally have the responsibility and obligation of taking care of their aging parents. However, 72% to 80% of the elderly are actually cared for by their daughters-in-law (Hu, 1995), largely because of the influence of culturally based role expectations. Traditionally, in this patriarchal society, a woman is expected to devote herself to her husband, his parents and extended family, and this includes the care of her parents-in-law during their later years.

However, Taiwan is facing many transitions as economic and social forces affect family life. After 1945, when Taiwan was restored to China, Taiwanese women benefited by a constitutional change in their legal status. Subsequently, Taiwan established an independent political structure, but continued to have strong cultural ties to mainland China. Due to contemporary industrialisation and urbanisation, most women have joined the labour force (Tsui, 1987). Better opportunities for education and employment have helped women to gain more self-esteem and to broaden their degree of social and political involvement (Yao, 1983). As a result, Taiwanese women struggle with the internal conflict created by the demands of a career and the desire for greater independence, competing with the deeply imbedded cultural affinity for care of in-laws (Hu and Chen, 1992; Hu, 1995).

In addition to the altered status and roles of women, the structure and functions of families have also shifted. Employment and educational opportunities may separate extended families, and nuclear families have become prominent. Members of extended families may be unable to provide support to those members in need of assistance according to traditional patterns. For example, women may be faced with the competing roles of worker as well family care-giver for several generations (Tsui, 1987). As the multiple demands of child care, elder care, and career expectations increase, the impact on the health of care-givers and care receivers is more apparent (Wu *et al*, 1991; Ton *et al*, 1992).

The intent of this chapter is to explore from a cultural perspective, the experiences of women care-givers when parental care becomes necessary. Specifically, the reasons why women become care-givers are addressed, as well as care-giving practices and consequences. Care-giving experiences between the United States and Taiwan are compared and contrasted as a means of discovering shared stressors and solutions. An increasing ageing population and the demands of a modern socio-economic system necessitates creative approaches to healthcare delivery as Taiwan faces the future.

Why women become care-givers

Taiwan is a patriarchal society and descent and inheritance is through the male line, with the male maintaining legal authority over his wife and children in both domestic and religious functions (Hu, 1995). There is little research or documentation of women's lives and their care-giving responsibilities. Chao's (1997) research concerning women and the care of parents-in-law revealed that a parent-in-law's care would begin when a woman perceived there was a need for care and that it was her duty to provide it. There were many reasons described by these women for assuming care-giving responsibilities. They included meeting the expectations of filial piety as well as repaying the debt for the benevolence shown toward her husband. Some women suggested that care-giving of older relatives was an expectation of a woman's nurturing role, while others spoke of care-giving of frail family members in terms of simple human morality. Since all of these responses are deeply imbedded in the socio-cultural context of care-giving in Taiwan, it is important to understand the ethno-history of the Taiwanese people, family structure and values, woman's roles, and the concept of filial piety.

Ethno-history of the Taiwanese people

Taiwan is an island, located in the western Pacific Ocean, roughly 100 miles off the southeast coast of mainland China. Historically and culturally, Taiwan has been closely linked with the Chinese mainland. The island was settled by the Chinese in AD 239. During the seventeenth century, the island was subjected to a variety of foreigners, who occupied it, in whole or in part. They included the Dutch, Spanish, and French. In 1661, Cheng Cheng-Kung took Taiwan from the Dutch. Chinese people soon migrated to Taiwan and became the majority of the island's population. For the next 200 years, the island was a destination for emigrants from the provinces of Fukien and Kwangtung. Governed by Japan as a colony from 1895 to 1945, Taiwan reverted to Chinese administration at the end of World War II (Kuang Hwa, 1992; Lieu, Jor-Lin and Song-Youn, 1993). Thus, culturally, economically and politically, Taiwan has remained predominately Chinese, but influenced by foreign cultures.

Following Chinese culture, Taiwanese beliefs and ways of living were strongly influenced by the philosophy of Confucianism, Taoism, and Buddhism (Kleinman, 1980). Each of these philosophical perspectives and/or religious traditions has intricate belief structures and profound influences on patterns of life. Several key ideas are presented here to demonstrate how these views influence personal behaviour and relationships to others. The teachings of Confucius, which are principles for social interaction, emphasised loyalty and benevolence. It is expected that a person practice emotional restraint in order to attain a state of harmony with the surrounding environment. The notion of benevolence implies that one should help others to acquire the same things as one has or even to sacrifice the self. Confucian thought also implies that a person should accept his/her destiny, in other words, carry out the duties ascribed by fate.

'Tao' or 'Way' is the major concept of Taoism, which is the Taiwanese people's philosophy for interpreting the world-view. Taoism teaches that a person should be in harmony with nature or conform to the nature. The philosophical perspective of so-called 'fatalism' was also formulated from this concept. In Buddhist philosophy, 'Inn' and 'Ko' (cause and effect) are the principles that encourage people to do 'good' and to receive 'good' in return.

Based on these beliefs, delayed gratification and perseverance are practised when in unpleasant situations. Family members are expected to provide care for older, frail members even if this involves sacrifice. Shame and guilt are used to control an individual's behaviour, especially if a person should abandon a family member (Kuo and Kavanagh, 1994; Uba, 1994). These beliefs and values are very influential in formulating the dimensions of family relationships, care-giving roles and in coping with the constraints of care-giving (Chao, 1997). For example, women may strive to attain an inner harmony in spite of the harsh demands of a difficult care-giving situation based on religious or philosophical views of the meaning of life. They may view care-giving for the parents of their husband as their fate in life, reflecting a perspective of acceptance and serenity.

Family structure, values and filial piety

In the traditional Chinese family, the father maintains an unimpeachable authoritative relationship within the family, while the maternal role is to monitor the emotional well-being of the family. The family exerts a great deal of control and individuals are expected to be devoted to and rely on the family. Family solidarity is supported by the interdependence of the family members, hierarchical relationships in the family, and an orientation to the family as a whole rather than to the individuals within the family (Kuo and Kavangh, 1994; Uba, 1994). Thus, parents have an obligation to raise their children, while children have obligations to honour and assist their parents as a reflection of filial piety.

Traditionally, an authoritarian hierarchy based on generation, age, and gender has dominated life within the family. The oldest male had the highest status, and a woman's status is lower than that of any man (Gallin, 1994; Hu, 1995). Thus, the father has the highest rank, whereas the young daughter-in- law has the lowest rank in a family (Hu, 1995).

The roots anchoring the hierarchy within the Chinese society are the mores of filial piety, derived from the thoughts of Confucius. Filial piety is considered the basis of all moral behaviours. Ancient literature suggested that filial piety was the first priority among virtues (Huang, 1989). From the perspective of cultural ecology, the purpose of filial piety was to enhance or maintain family harmony, solidarity, and continuity. Therefore, it was expected that children would obey their parents and that sons carry the family name and take care of their parents (Yang, 1989). A further analysis of the concept of Chinese filial piety indicates that it requires taking care of parents, waiting on them; keeping them free from loneliness and worry; and, finally, burying and offering sacrifice with respect when the parents pass away (Yang, 1989). Thus the dimensions of family roles and deference to filial piety are inexplicably linked between generations across time.

Women's roles

Matrilineal clans were the basic social units prior to the Chou Dynasty (1100–120 BC) (Yao, 1983). However, the social status and rights of women deteriorated rapidly with the Chou Dynasty and the establishment of the patrilineal clan system (Chen, 1994; Lu, 1995). A feudal system was established to keep society in order and subsequently, the gap between the positions of men and women in the family widened (Lu, 1995; Yao, 1983). Woman's activities were restricted to their homes and their husbands were the core of their lives. Women were praised for being obedient, uncomplaining, and reserved, rather than being assertive and independent (Tsui, 1987). Females were taught to 'respect and obey' male family members. A woman was considered the property of the patrilineal family. Thus, she was expected to be devoted to the male and the family, with special emphasis on the care of parents-in-law. Deference to filial piety was necessary to fulfil these obligations (Uba, 1994).

Thus religious beliefs, social constructions of family life and political forces have influenced perceptions and enactment of women's roles. An enduring expectation of filial piety has influenced family dynamics and formed the underpinnings for care-giving roles and expectations. Although ideological, social, economic and environmental changes have influenced women's roles and offered alternatives, women's perceptions of providing care for parents-in-law are largely subjected to deeply imbedded cultural beliefs and values.

Care-giving practices in Taiwan

Although sons carry primary responsibility as care-givers for the elderly in contemporary Taiwan, this responsibility is frequently delegated to their wives as daughters-in-law. Wives generally have a longer life expectancy than their husbands in Taiwan, and daughters-in-law are obligated by cultural expectations to take care of the elderly. Very few elderly in Taiwan are cared for by their biological daughters, as these women are often taking care of their husband's parents (Hu, 1995).

There are many approaches used to care for the elderly, including home care, community care and institutional care (Yang, 1995). Only a few people live in nursing homes, but care provided by health professionals in home settings is very limited because these types of programmes are in their initial developmental stages.

Most elderly live at home with their sons/daughters-in-law, while a few live alone (Hsu, 1989; Shei, 1993; Hu, 1995). There are two major approaches to home care. They are referred to as 'meal rotation' and a 'federation family'. Meal rotation, which involves sons and their families taking turns in caring for their parents, is more popular in rural than in urban settings. Parents usually move from the home of one son to another in order to decrease the demands of care-giving on one family over a long period of time. The federation model involves providing financial support from a distance as opposed to engaging in day-to-day care-giving activities. Both models enable families to care for older members over long periods of time by diffusing the everyday demands of providing care and the financial responsibilities.

Most elderly people are unwilling to live in nursing homes. Because of traditional beliefs, they would feel discarded by their children if they had to live in such institutions (Chan, 1989). Not surprisingly, in Wu and Chiang's survey (1995), some elders had never heard of a 'nursing home'. Most members of the younger generation also prefer to keep their elders at home, because they do not trust the quality of nursing home care (Hu, 1994).

Although a government sponsored program for home care by health professionals was started in 1987, it is still in the early developmental stages. Some private 'geriatric home care' exists, but this is a costly alternative and there have been some reported incidences of abuse (Lee *et al*, 1990). In addition, inadequate medical insurance and a family's financial burdens often prevent patients from staying in hospitals for an extended period. The family may be the only provider for those who need extra care or rehabilitation after discharge from the hospital (Liu, 1991). Clearly, families continue to assume the major responsibility for frail parent's care in contemporary Taiwan (Wu *et al*, 1991). Because of increasing care needs and insufficient resources within the healthcare system, women in the family are expected to assume greater care-giving responsibilities. This may create a substantial burden, especially if they are employed outside of the home and/or involved in other roles within the families, such as caring for their own children.

Consequences of care-giving

Research on care-giving practices in Taiwan suggests that the experiences of care-giving not only influence the primary care-giver, but also family functions. Although most of the studies indicated that the care-givers were negatively impacted by care-giving tasks, some studies have found the care-giver satisfied with fulfilling the care-giving role. Overall, there are three major negative impacts or dimensions of stress associated with care-giving: physical, psychosocial, and financial.

In terms of physical stressors, several studies have suggested that care-givers of frail elders suffer from poor overall health and psychosomatic symptoms, such as headaches, weight change, and gastric disturbances (Lin, 1987; Ton *et al*, 1992; Wu *et al*, 1991). Care-givers may neglect their own health, and care-giving activities may disturb sleep and dietary patterns.

While physical stressors are clearly problematic, the most prominent effect on care-givers was in the psychosocial dimension (Die *et al*, 1990). Research consistently indicates that care-givers experience emotional distress, which includes, frustration, depression, fatigue, and feelings of burden (Lin, 1987; Chiu *et al*, 1988). Fulfilling the role of primary care-giver often interferes with personal lifestyle, social activities, and other obligations (Chiu *et al*, 1988). Some care-givers were forced to give up their jobs (Yui, 1989), and others noted that care-giving activities strained family relationships (Lin, 1987; Chiu *et al*, 1988).

Providing intimate aspects of care such as touching a father in-law's sexual organs during the process of care proved difficult and embarrassing for women care-givers (Hu, 1994). A daughter-in-law could also be criticised by other members of her husband's family if the in-law's condition became worse, a situation which is most stressful for women care-givers. Most women either tolerated the stress of providing care or accepted it as their fate. Some reflected their distress by displaying indifference to the care of the elderly, decreasing the quality and extent of their interaction (Hu, 1994; Chao, 1997).

Whereas the negative aspects of care-giving predominate in the literature, Chao's study suggested that women care-givers also achieved positive outcomes from the care-giving situation. For example, a woman achieved a feeling of peace or inner calm because she had carried out the expectations of filial piety, a value that is highly esteemed in this society. In addition, if a woman successfully fulfilled her care-giving responsibilities, her status in the family would be elevated and respected by other family members. A woman's husband could also recognise the value of her contribution to his family. Some women care-givers also expressed a sense of personal pride and emotional gratification that occured as a result of caring for parents-in-law (Chao, 1996; Chao, 1997).

Children in Taiwan take the major responsibility for the living and healthcare expenses of the elderly. Pensions for the older family members are so small that they offer little help (Shei, 1993) and government allowances for elderly people are not common. Therefore, clear evidence of financial burden in studies of care-giving exists (Lin, 1987; Ton *et al*, 1992; Shern and Chang, 1993). The situation becomes even more difficult if women care-givers must leave outside employment in order to provide care for aging relatives and total family income decreases.

Factors influencing the care-giving experience

Some factors were found to be related to the extent of stress experienced in care-giving reported in Taiwanese literature in the last decade. They include the degree of patients' deterioration (Hu, 1994; Tsai, 1995); the relationship with the elderly before they require care (Wu *et al*, 1991; Hu, 1994; Hu, 1995); the availability of resources and support (Wu *et al*, 1991; Ton *et al*, 1992; Wu, 1995), and personal coping behaviours (Ton *et al*, 1992; Shern and Chang, 1993; Wu, 1995; Tsai, 1995).

The care-giver's burden is significantly influenced by a patient's level of deterioration (Ton *et al*, 1992; Tsai, 1995; Hu, 1995). The more disturbing the behaviour of the elder, the less patient the care-giver becomes. The patient's deterioration or disability was seen as the most important indicator for choosing an appropriate setting or pattern of care-giving for a frail parent (Hu, 1994). While the patient's degree of dependency was one of the important factors relating to the care-giver's burden, the most difficult situation for the care-giver occurred when the physical condition changed unexpectedly and became very serious (Chao, 1997). Additional resources for support and care were difficult to mobilise when this type of situation occurred. The closer a care-giver's relationship with the elder and the greater the obligation for parental care they perceived, the larger the burden experienced (Wu *et al*, 1991; Hu, 1995). The relationship between elders and care-givers also influenced the quality of care provided. A close relationship would enhance a care-giver's willingness to provide care, but an alienated relationship would prevent the care-giver from becoming involved in the care-giving situation (Hu, 1994; Chao, 1997).

Further, available resources and adaptive coping strategies were identified as effective mediators to buffer care-giver strain (Ton *et al*, 1992; Shern and Chang, 1993; Chao, 1997). However, knowledge deficiency about effective coping strategies continues to be an important issue, and active involvement and availability of health care professionals in providing care for frail elders continues to be a challenge (Wu *et al*, 1991; Hu, 1994). In her research, Chao (1997), found that a family member's support, which gives the care-giver emotional satisfaction, could be more important and more effective than a formal support programme. Such support could be in the form of praise or encouragement, especially if it came from a woman care-giver's husband. Efforts to encourage and maintain family social support need to be fostered to enable care-givers to continue to provide care over time. Cultural influences such as religious beliefs, philosophical reflections on the meaning of life and prescribed role expectations deeply influenced a care-giver in accepting her care-giving role and balancing her inner mind to face the challenges of providing care (Ou, 1992; Chao, 1997). Such influences need to be explored with greater depth and shared with others who are experiencing similar situations.

Overall, the research on the care-giving experience in Taiwan has been somewhat limited. It has usually been identified within a subcategory of studies in a field of specific disease care, focussed primarily on care of stroke patients and patients with dementia. Limited samples have been generalised to include all family care-givers. Most of the studies have been quantitative in nature with factor analysis used to identify the dimensions of a care-giver's stress and to predict the risk factors. While very informative, these designs may limit the knowledge of the care-giving experience by eliciting responses that fit predetermined categories. Some studies have also been limited by the instrumentation that is inappropriate for the identified target population, or is culturally irrelevant.

There has been very little research exploring the experiences of daughters-in-law as primary care-givers, in spite of the prominence of this role in Taiwanese society. Currently, there are more qualitative studies being undertaken to explore the dimensions of care-giving, with greater attention being given to the cultural context. This approach may facilitate a greater understanding of the dimensions of the care-giving experience in Taiwan and suggest appropriate interventions for sustaining family care-givers when faced with long-term care responsibilities. At present, there is insufficient information to develop a complete model interpreting the care-giving experience.

Eastern traditions and western influences

Compared to care-giving experiences in western society, particularly in the United States, Chao (1997) found some similarities and some differences between the care-giving experiences of the Americans and Taiwanese worthy of consideration. For example, most of the Taiwanese daughters-in-law studied tended to be obedient and suppressed their personal feelings. They lived with the elders, providing care day and night, often without assistance. Their care-giving role tended to be that of a performer — they provided direct care, as well as managed many facets of the care that was required. In addition, Taiwanese daughters-in- law seldom had enough autonomy to control the environment. They were more subjected to cultural norms and tended to accept cultural expectations of the care-giving role. Furthermore, women in Taiwan provided care for the parents-in-law based on the idea of service of a younger generation to an older generation. Providing care was seldom seen as an act to bridge the relationship between their husbands and their husbands' parents, as was the case with American daughters-in-law. While the relationships between the daughters-in-law and the parents-in-law tend to be hierarchical in Taiwan, the relationships in the US tend to be more equitable. Although Taiwan is experiencing social and economic trends similar to other industrialised countries, clearly culturally induced beliefs and traditions continue to create differences in care-giving expectations and role enactment.

Challenges and opportunities

As life expectancy increases, the percentage of elderly people living among us will continue to grow, as will the need for healthcare and supportive services. Overall, this growth will also dramatically impact on family care-givers for the elderly. While Taiwan is rapidly changing in many social and economic areas, it remains a patriarchal society with the daughter-in-law delegated the primary responsibility for care of the elderly and the major financial responsibility allocated to the family. Therefore, strategies must be developed to support families and to enhance the well-being of elders as they age. Such efforts need to occur at the macro as well as the micro level of the social system.

Although children base their care-giving beliefs on the value of filial piety, social justice and human compassion demand a consideration of care-giving issues for frail elders in a broader socio-political context. Government needs to assume a greater degree of responsibility in further developing and implementing a comprehensive approach to elder care. Considering the realistic demands and the limited resources, there is an urgent need to develop a plan for quality long-term care and effective monitoring of the care provided. Currently, influenced by tradition and concern for parental well-being, institutional care is largely ignored or avoided by the younger generation and their families. However, it is also the family's only alternative if they are unable to provide for their ageing parents' care. To meet present and future needs, it is necessary to develop a continuum of care, that will enable acute care systems and community-based systems to interface, providing older persons and their families with a range of supportive services. To facilitate this effort, establishing a comprehensive nursing case management system is a high priority.

Effective nurse case management systems are based on an understanding of family dynamics. Since the family is the basic unit of community care, the healthcare team must get to know, not only the older adult client, but also the care-giver and extended family. This should include the family's organisation, coping strategies, and the impact of the illness or dependency on the family system. The assessment should include the relationship between the family care-giver and the older adult to discover unresolved issues and negative feelings, as well as sources of strength and resilience. Nursing interventions can be planned to offer support, provide information, mobilise resources, and strengthen families.

Nurses also need to develop increased sensitivity to the characteristics of traditional Taiwanese women, which could include inhibition of emotions in order to maintain a harmonious relationship with others in the family. In order to identify and recognise the overwhelming tasks of care-giving, a comprehensive assessment should include measures of how a woman experiences her role, the degree of stress she encounters and her ability to manage the care-giving situation effectively. Nurses and care-givers can then identify those approaches that may assist the care-giver in maintaining her own health and dealing with the issues at hand in a positive manner. For example, 'obligation' in terms of 'love' was found to empower a care-giver (Chao, 1997). Therefore, it is suggested that the role expectation of a care-giver for providing elders' care should be approached voluntarily and with respect for one another. Care-giving role expec- tations should be established by individuals with consideration of mutual responsibilities, not by obligations imposed by marriage contracts or forced altruism.

A deeper understanding of Taiwanese women's inner thoughts, feelings and communication within the family structure while assuming the care-giving role has been limited by quantitative methodologies and insufficient attention to culturally induced norms. Qualitative methods may be more fruitful in identifying strategies to enhance the coping abilities of families that are both valued and effective. Future researchers are also encouraged to pursue longitudinal studies of care-givers of aging parents in order to identify changes in the care-giving situation, as well as the tasks of care-giving. Clearly, enhanced understanding of the motivation of care-givers to provide care over long time periods for elderly relatives is essential for nurses to develop effective healthcare programs and to implement supportive interventions.

Today, Taiwan looks to the future filled with hope and the promise of a better life for all of its citizens. Hopefully, the traditional values of respect and concern for the elderly will lead to innovative care programs that will permit elders to remain in their homes with the necessary support systems to sustain them and their families. While the challenges are great, many opportunities exist for nurses to conduct research, facilitate policy development and participate in newly defined models of health care delivery.

References

Chan HS (1989) Taipei tu huei di chu lao jern fu li hsu chiu u chia ting chieh kou chien kuan si chih yen chiu [The research of the relationship between family structure and elderly people's welfare in Taipei urban area]. In: Ing CC, Chu SL, eds. *She Huei Hsien Hsiang de Fen Hsi*. Central Academy Sinica in Taiwan, Taipei, Taiwan: 57–88

Chao SY (1996) The Experiences of Middle-age Women Caregivers in Taiwan. Unpublished manuscript, University of San Diego

Chao SY (1997) *The Experiences of Taiwanese Woman Caregiving for Parents-in-law*. Doctoral dissertation, University of San Diego

Chen TY (1994) *The History of Chinese Women*. Shang Wu, Taipei, Taiwan

Chiu CZ, Lu SY, Shu YY, Ju Chen YJ, Liu LI (1988) The exploration of primary caregiver's burden and related factors among stroke patients. *J Nurs* **35**(1): 69–83

Department of Accounting and Statistics (1990) *The Survey of Status of Elderly Population in Taiwan, R.O.C.* Author, Taipei, Taiwan

Department of Health (1995) *Public Health in Republic of China*. Author, Taipei, Taiwan

Die YC, Yui YM, Lien YN (1990) Li huan chung feng tui chia ting te chung chi [The stroke patients impact on family]. *Kung Kung Wei Sheng* **17**(2): 171–80

Gallin RS (1994) The intersection of class and age: mother-in-law/daughter-in-law relations in rural Taiwan. *J Cross-Cult Gerontol* **9**: 127–40

Hsu LC (1989) *Lao Jern Wen ti u Tui Tsen* [Issues and strategies for the elderly]. Kuei-Kuang, Taipei, Taiwan

Hu YH (1994) *Home Care Choices Regarding the Chronically Ill Elderly: Cultural Constraints and Practical Need*. National Science Council report: #NSC 83-0301-H 010-002. National Science Council, Taiwan, R.O.C. Taipei

Hu YH (1995) *San Die Tung Tang* [Three generation — myth and trap]. Chu-Liu, Taipei, Taiwan

Hu YH, Chen CY (1992) The myth of social role and stress. *J Wom Gender Stud* **3**: 25–39

Huang GH (1989) Hsien die sheng huo chung hsiao te shih chien [Carry out filial piety in modern life]. In: Yang KS, ed. *Chung Kuo Jern te Hsin Li*. Kuei-Kuang, Taipei, Taiwan: 25–39

Kleinman A (1980) *Patients and Healers in the Context of Culture*. University of California, Berkeley

Kuang Hwa (1992) *Republic of China Year Book*. Author, Taipei, Taiwan

Kuo CL, Kavanagh KH (1994) Chinese perspectives on culture and mental health. *Iss Men Health Nurs* **15**: 551–67

Lee KE, Wang LT, Jou LC (1990) Pai-To te chu lao jern an yang chung shin ti ping ku [Evaluation of private geriatric nursing home in Pai-To district of Taipei city]. *Kung Kung Wei Sheng* **16**(4): 416–23

Lieu GC, Jor-Lin CJ, Song-Youn JY (1993) *Taiwan Pai Ker* [Taiwan Encyclopedia]. Ker-Ling, Taipei, Taiwan

Lin S (1987) *Problems and Crisis of the Family with Dementia Elderly*. National Science Council report # NSC 76-0301-H002-010-A. National Science Council, Taiwan, R.O.C, Taipei, Taiwan

Liu HE (1991) *Factors Related to the Quality of Life of Chinese Caregivers*. Doctoral dissertation, University of Illinois at Chicago

Lu SL (1995) *New Feminist*, 4 edn. Chien-Wei, Taipei, Taiwan

Ou M (1992) *A Study of the Related Factors and Relationships Among Stress Appraisal, Coping Style and Mental Health in the Female Spouses of Home-stay Stroke Patients*. Master's thesis, National Defense Medical College, Taipei, Taiwan

Shei MY (1993) *Lao jern Chang Chi Chao Hu te Hsiang Kuan Yi Ti* [Related issues to elderly people's long term care]. Kuei-Kuang, Taipei, Taiwan

Shern CJ, Chang SH (1993) Ching shen huan che chia shu te ya li yuan, ying tui tse lueh, chien kang chuang kuang [The stressors, coping strategies and health status among psychiatric patients' family]. *Chin J Men Health* **6**: 89–116

Ton LY, Mao GL, Chou JF, Chen JG, Liu SC (1992) Caregiver burden of demented elderly and related factors — an exploratory study. *J Nurs* **39**(3): 88–98

Tsai PL (1995) *The Burden and its Related Factors of Depressive Patients' Caregiver*. Master's thesis, National Taiwan University, Nursing School, Taipei, Taiwan

Tsui YL (1987) *Are Married Daughters "spoiled Water"? – A Study of Working Women in Urban Taiwan*. Population Studies Center National Taiwan University Taiwan, R.O.C, Taipei, Taiwan

Uba L (1994) *Asian Americans: Personality Patterns, Identity and Mental Health*. Guilford, New York

Wu CC (1995) Cross-cultural, cross-national study of family caregiver burden imposed by the mentally ill. *Chin J Men Health* **8**: 37–52

Wu SC, Chiang TL (1995) Long-term care in Taiwan: Issues and direction. *Chung Hua Wei Chih* **14**(3): 246–55

Wu SL, Hu SG, Yao KM (1991) Tai wan di chiu chu chia lao jern chao ku che fu ho ching hsing yen chiu [Primary caregiver's burden and needs for elderly people's home care in Taiwan area]. *Kung Kung Wei Sheng* **18**(3): 237–47

Yang HC (1995) *The Analysis of Policy for Long-term Care and Service System*. Department of Health, Taipei, Taiwan:

Yang KS (1989) Chung kuo jen hsia tao ti kai nien fen hsi [Concept analysis of filial piety among Chinese]. In Yang KS (ed.), *Chung Kuo Jern Te Hsin Li*. Kuei-Kuang, Taipei, Taiwan: 123–54

Yao ESL (1983) *Chinese Women: Past and Present*. Ide House, Inc, Mesquite, Texas

Yui PJ (1989) *Changes in Physical and Psychological Response, Social Support and Self-care Ability of Stroke Patients During Hospitalization*. Master's thesis, National Taiwan University, School of Nursing, Taipei, Taiwan

22

An exploratory study of attempted suicide by females in Taiwan

Yow-Hwey Hu, Shu-Chen Kuo and Jeffrey J H Tsai

Introduction

Epidemiologically speaking, 'attempted suicide' is predominantly a female phenomenon. However, as many feminist scholars have pointed out, the social causes of the high prevalence of women among attempted suicides has long been ignored. The 'gender-blind' social reactions are particularly severe in medical settings in terms of clinical diagnosis and treatment services (Barraclough and Hughes, 1987; Community Center, 1990; Hawton, 1986). Recently, the gender aspect has been the focus of research, and the findings provide an important base for developing prevention and rehabilitation programmes, including clinical services. For example, many western feminist scholars have started to discover the importance of 'family violence' as a cause of women's suicide attempts, and thus the conventional methods of preventing suicides in the field of mental health have been challenged, and the 'gender blind' practices in conventional medical treatment of female suicidal cases are also undergoing change.

In the earlier literature, the linkages between family violence and clinical medicine were usually confined to 'homicide' and 'battery injuries'; very few researchers linked battering of women to suicidal behaviour. When the question is raised, the findings are astonishing. For example, one study indicates that 35% to 40% of battered women have made suicide attempts (Walker, 1979). Another epidemiological study in the US reveals that among those females who attempted suicide, 36.5% had suffered family violence the same day, and 65.3% had suffered family violence within the last six months (Stark and Flitcraft, 1995).

The gender difference in suicide etiology has long been recognised in Chinese societies. For example, a written legal record in the Chin dynasty indicated that men's suicides were almost all attributed to political issues, and women's suicides were all due to oppression by family members (Hsieh and Jonathan, 1981; Rin and Tuan, 1983). In the past, most women who committed suicides were young women; however, the age pattern of women's suicide in Taiwan has undergone drastic changes — the young women's high suicide rate dropped, but older women's suicide rate rose to a peak (Hu, 1995; Wolf, 1975). Nevertheless, a number of studies indirectly indicate that attempted suicide in Taiwan is still a phenomenon of young women, and 'family problems' are still the main cause (Hu, 1988; 1990; Hu and Chen, 1992; Lin and Wu, 1988; Rin *et al*, 1975). Also, a few studies revealed that in Taiwan the clinical reactions to 'battered woman' cases are still confined to only 'medical treatment' (Chen, 1994a; 1994b; interview of a doctor in the emergency room of a teaching hospital), and no social interventions have been developed or referred in medical settings. Thus, it is of interest to determine the nature of clinical reactions to female attempted suicide cases, especially those with a history of family violence. In this study, we approached the issue through the records of emergency services and the follow-up psychiatric services in order to identify the specific problems in our medical system, and more broadly in our general socio-cultural system.

Method

Since there is no reporting system for attempted suicides, no statistical records can be found in any clinical settings. We must rely on qualitative methods to explore the issue. In this research, to gather enough information in a short period, we used a multifaceted method for the qualitative inquiry for reaching certain crucial insights in terms of how the system for treating attempted suicides operates. The multiple methods included:

1. key informant interviews;
2. preliminary content analysis of patients' records; and
3. in-depth text analysis of selected cases.

Each method was applied at different stages.

For the first step, three physicians in the emergency department of a teaching hospital in Taipei were our key informants, and were interviewed informally. The content of our interviews was focussed on the general rules for the hospital staff on how they deal with people who have attempted suicide in the emergency room. Based on this information, we were able to design the sampling frame for our data collection and primary content analysis from patients' emergency room records. The third step was to select cases for further investigation of the diagnosis and treatment during the follow-up psychiatric services. The text analysis focussed on the gender issue in the diagnosis and treatment processes and the related social-cultural systems in the medical setting.

Findings

The problem of identifying cases

Through the interviews with key informants, we were surprised to discover that in Taiwan's current medical system there is no such diagnosis as 'attempted suicide'. Consequently, hospitals have no record or statistics on attempted suicide, but also no such diagnosis on patients' record charts. However, our key informants assured us that cases of attempted suicide were fairly easy to recognise by the hospital health professionals, and most of these cases were formally diagnosed as 'poisoning by accident' or 'injuries'. According to the informants, suicide attempts were usually by young women, and swallowing pills or dangerous chemicals was the most common method.

Based on such information, we started to examine three months of hospital records of female 'poisoning' cases in the emergency room records, and these were the only records we were allowed to access. *Table 22.2* indicates that about 30 female cases were recorded as 'poisoning' per month in that hospital. The age distribution of these cases also indicates that about half of them were in the ages 25 to 44 years. Another quarter were 24 years or less.

To detect the 'exact' causes of such poisoning cases, we chose one month (September) as a sample for content analysis, and the original case report charts were examined. Based on our primary content analysis, 20 of the 39 poisoning cases (51.3%) could be clearly identified as attempted suicides. Their socio-demographic profiles are presented in *Table 22.1*. For example, 75% of them were under the age of 44 years, and 20% were under the age of 24. Thus, the figure still reflects the theme of a concentration among young women. In terms of marriage, we discovered that the marital status of those cases was not always recorded. However, among the 13 recorded cases, more than three-quarters were married.

Table 22.1: Demographic profile of females hospitalised after attempting suicide

		No	%	
Age				
	0–14	0	0.0	
	15–24	4	20.0	
	25–44	11	55.0	
	45–64	3	15.0	
	65+	2	10.0	
Marital status				
	married	10	50.0	(76.9)
	not married	3	15.0	(23.1)
	unknown	7	35.0	
Living near hospital				
	yes	9	45.0	
	no	11	55.0	
Referred from other hospital				
	yes	7	35.0	
	no	13	65.0	

In terms of residence, 45% (nine cases) were from the nearby community. Since this is an economically better-off community, and the cases were identified only through one form of suicide attempt (self-injury was not included), and since there are more than three general hospitals in the community to absorb suicidal patients, the figure of nine cases is an underestimate of the number of attempted suicides each month in this community.

Social etiology of attempted suicide by women and related medical intervention

Based on further inquiry into the social causes of these 20 attempted suicides, we could find little non-medical

Table 20.2: Age distribution of female poisoning cases during a three-month period in the emergency room of a Taipei general hospital

	July		August		September		Total	
Age (yrs)	**n**	**%**	**n**	**%**	**n**	**%**	**n**	**%**
0–14	0	0.0	3	6.7	5	12.8	8	6.7
15–24	7	19.4	8	17.8	6	15.4	21	17.5
25–44	21	58.3	14	31.1	17	43.6	52	43.3
45–64	5	13.9	13	28.9	8	20.5	26	21.7
65	3	8.4	7	15.5	3	7.7	13	10.8
Total	36	100.0	45	100.0	39	100.0	120	100.0

information. Through a thorough review of the record, we traced only certain clues from physicians' or nurses' notes. Based on such inadequate information, we can only identify six wife-battering cases. Also, five of the cases had repeated suicide attempts and five had received psychiatric treatments at the same hospital. Since five of the suspected family violence cases were also repeated suicide attempts who had received psychiatric interventions, the nature and history of their psychiatric intervention became the new focus of our inquiry.

History and nature of psychiatric interventions in cases of suspected family violence

By a detailed examination of these five selected cases of suicide attempts, we discovered that the frequencies of their psychiatric service visits varied from one to 80 times. Also, we found that almost all had looked for psychiatric help before and after their suicidal episodes.

Through text analysis of the psychiatrists' notes on all six cases, there are apparent problems in the so-called 'psychiatric services' in both diagnosis and treatment. These problems include over-medicalisation, over-routinisation, insensitivity to any social problems and sexism. For example, only psychiatric symptoms, such as depression, affective psychosis or neurosis were put into the notes. Also, only drugs were repeatedly prescribed. However, patients' complaints of family problems (including abuse and violence that were obvious to the authors) were ignored, and none of the patients received family therapy or were referred to any support screening for battered women. The problems of doctors' unresponsiveness to patients' needs for emotional and social support were especially severe for chronic cases.

From our review of chart notes, these problems (medicalisation, routinisation and sexism) identified in the hospital psychiatric services, were not just limited to suicidal cases, but also to other mental health problems prevalent among women, such as depression and anxiety. Since the hospital in our study is one of the more prestigious teaching hospitals in Taiwan and South-East Asia, notable achievements in medical technology is in cynical contrast to the backwardness of its practices in the area of social caring, especially for women's mental health services. Such a contrast may also reflect the polarised nature of the 'development' of healthcare in newly developed countries, such as Taiwan.

Conclusions

Attempted suicide as a unique gender feature has recently received the attention of feminist scholars. There is an urge for new directions in epidemiological inquiries and new service policies — including clinical services — in dealing with women's mental health issues in many developed countries. However, in many developing countries, this movement still lags far behind the advance of medical technology. Moreover, the danger of the emerging culture of medical dominance is increasing rapidly. Based on our qualitative inquiry into medical reactions to female suicide attempters at a prestigious teaching hospital in Taiwan, the specific problems of our medical system may be summarised as follows:

- there is no formal coding and reporting system in attempted suicides, so the problem of female suicide attempts is invisible and it is hard to conduct research into or develop policy for prevention and treatment
- based on our investigation, we estimated that at least 10 women tried to commit suicide each month in this community. In other words, the problem is severe and needs urgent social policy attention
- there are no known community service alternatives for women with family problems to look to for help; thus, the psychiatric service becomes the main service for women to rely on
- the clinical intervention, especially psychiatric services, are overly medicalised and gender-blind. This indicates that we have a great need for medical reform in order to make it more responsible to the emotional and social dimension of patients' needs, particularly in dealing with mental health problems that are important to women (including depression and attempted suicide).

The above problems are not limited to the medical field, but are entrenched in professions, family institutions and other social institutions. As feminist scholars, we not only need to do more critical research on the systemic impacts on women's mental health, but also on more local and international resources and support to advocate socio-cultural reforms. We believe that the most effective way to prevent suicides and promote mental health among women is to empower them.

References

Barraclough B, Hughes J (1987) *Suicide — Clinical and Epidemiological Studies*. Croom Helm, London

Chen R-R (1994a) The prevention of marital violence in clinical medicine (in Chinese). *The research Report for the Prevention of Marital Violence*. Awakening Foundation, Taipei: 40–9

Chen R-R (1994b) The prevention of marital violence in psychiatry services (in Chinese). *The Research Report for the Prevention of Marital Violence*. Awakening Foundation, Taipei: 61–8

Community Center (1990) *The Dictionary of Social Work* [in Chinese]. The Research Training Center of Community Development, Taipei

Hawton K (1986) Suicide in adolescents. In: Roy A, ed. *Suicide*. Williams and Wilkins, Baltimore, MD

Hsieh ACK, Jonathan DS (1981) Suicide and the family in premodern Chinese society. In Kleinman A, Lin T-Y, eds. *Normal and Abnormal Behavior in Chinese Culture*. D Reidel Publishing, London: 29–4

Hu Y-H (1988) Patterns and trends of suicide rates by marital status in Taiwan [in Chinese]. *Chin J Ment Health* **4**(1): 43–56

Hu Y-H (1990) Gender social roles, and depression symptoms [in Chinese]. *J Wom Gender Stud* **2**: 1–18

Hu Y-H (1995) Elderly suicide risk in family contexts: A critique of the Asian family care model. *J Cross-CultGerontol* 10: 199–217

Hu Y-H, Chen C-Y (1992) The myth of social role and stress. *J Wom Gender Stud* **3**: 25–39

Lin H, Wu YC (1988) A study of residents' psychological problems and their attitude toward psychiatric illness in Taiwan. In: Yang KS, Chu HY, eds. *The Changing Taiwan Society* [in Chinese]. Institute of Ethnology, Academic Sinica Taipei: 507–52

Rin H, Cheng LT, Shieh PH *et al* (1975) *Attempted Suicide: The Taipei Case*. Presented at the First Pacific Congress of Psychiatry, Melbourne, Australia, May 11–16

Rin H, Tuan C (1983) Suicide in Taiwan. In: Lee H, ed. *Suicide in Asia and Near East*. University of California Press, Berkeley, CA: 59–68

Stark E, Flitcraft A (1995) Killing the beast within: Woman battering and female suicidality. *Int J Health Serv* **25**(1): 43–64

Walker L (1979) *The Battered Woman*. Harper and Row, New York

Wolf M (1975) Women and suicide in China. In: Wolf M, Witke R, eds. *Women in Chinese Society*. Stanford University Press, Stanford, CA: 111–41

23

The role of knowledge generation, replication and reconstruction in nursing assistance to pregnant women

Delvair de Brito Alves, Ailema Cardoso Barbosa, Jussilene Jesus Souza and Valdemar de Almeida Rodrigues

Introduction

This chapter is a study of the effect of generation, replication and reconstruction of knowledge in nursing assistance. It is the result of a preoccupation with nursing as a predominantly feminine practice that is socially and historically determined. The specific focus of the study is the generation, replication and reconstruction of knowledge in the public health service at the sanitary district of Barra/Rio Vermelho in the city of Salvador, Bahia, Brazil. This district is where the teaching, research and extension activities of the Federal University of Bahia are integrated. Of the 12 sanitary districts in the city, this district is one of the largest, in terms of population served. It also has one of the highest concentrations of low, medium and high technology equipment. For this study, we asked the following questions:

- what effect does the process of production and reproduction of knowledge in nursing assistance have on pregnant women using the health service
- to what extent do questions of gender influence this process?

The study is part of a series of studies by the Group of Studies about Women's Health (GEM), Escola de Enfermagem, Federal University of Bahia, which organises health practices and research about women. Its objective is to determine how useful the process of research and education is for nursing assistants dealing with pregnant women, from the perspective of gender as well as the effect of the process on the pregnant women.

Theoretical basis

If we take knowledge in a general 'way of being in the world', then, as Alves (1995) indicates, 'if I only use knowledge, I am simply in the world (social dimension); if I make knowledge, I am creatively in the world (ideological dimension); if I take a position towards the knowledge, I am critically in the world (political dimension)'.

These categories are not isolated. Using, making and establishing are interfaces of the same reality, the reality of research, which works in an interrelated manner (*Figure 23.1*).

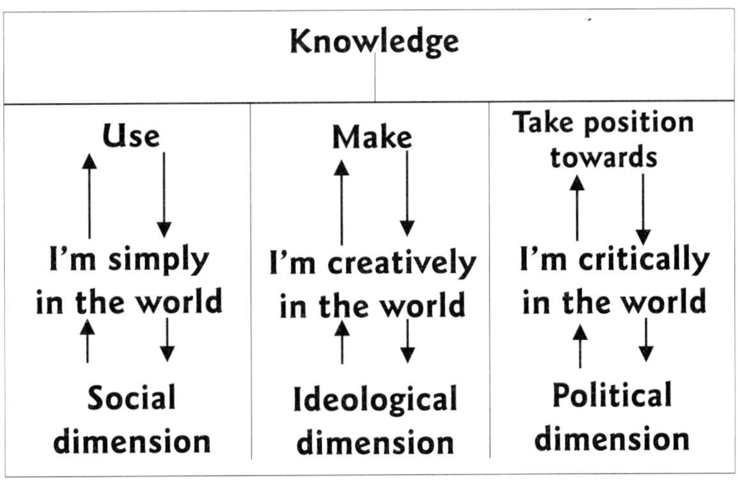

Figure 23.1: Knowledge as a form of being in the world (Source: Alves (1995))

We also take the common-sense approach that women's contribution to research must be acknowledged. We argue against the preconception that women cannot generate new knowledge or that the knowledge they produce is of lower quality. This preconception still has force in the scientific community, where men have dominated the generation of knowledge. Some scientific authors do not recognise the value of common-sense, seeing a threat to traditional scientific development. Acquired acumen or common-sense, however, is an inherent quality of women's research (Bachelard, 1990; Hühne, 1990). Science, philosophy and rational thought must all begin with common-sense, which is by its nature somewhat vague and undefined (Matallo Júnior, 1994; Popper, 1990; Solis, 1990).

Feminists also value research, but their approach is more all-inclusive and holistic, like that of a crafts person (Rose, 1983, cited in Gergen, 1993, p. 53). It goes beyond the masculine, industrialised work that is fragmented, and therefore mechanical, suppressing mental and emotional aspects. According to Gergen (1993), feminist scientists through history, and especially in recent decades, have tried to modify the way the academic world understands women's intellectual contributions. This has taken the form of starting up groups, courses and study programmes, or introducing feminist perspectives on academic research.

We need to look at the situation in nursing in order to overcome the empiricist-positivist view that prevails, retaining culture and addressing doubts that exist about knowledge produced in this area. In the process of scientific research, the fact that women are stigmatised by the expressions 'less intelligent' and 'less competent' must also be challenged.

This deprecation of women's knowledge is reflected in the assistance provided to pregnant women. Ferreira (1994) illustrated this point: 'To bring forth' was something women referred to as a natural mystery, ruled by fate. For centuries, knowledge about pregnancy, parturition and menses was the domain of the women who actually performed the roles of midwife, nurse and adviser. However, at the end of the eighteenth century, women's role as midwives was eliminated, removing their right to exercise their abilities in parturition The knowledge generation and replication was transferred to the masculine universe of medicine, as universities were forbidden to women until the end of the nineteenth century.

According to Hubbard (1993), women's absence from universities was a result of the view of nineteenth century physicians and biologists who thought that a woman's brain was smaller than a man's, and that the ovary and uterus required too much energy and rest to function appropriately. From this perspective, wasting energy in other activities would lead to atrophy of these organs, leading to extinction of the human race. Another example that demonstrates the intellectual limits imposed on women, and the discrimination as a result of the act of gestation, was the battle of physicians and biologists in the nineteenth century against political organisations fighting for gender equality; they maintained that women's reproductive organs disqualified them from any vocation except giving birth. Further to this, Hubbard pointed out that these authorities considered that:

> *'the capacity of a woman getting pregnant keeps her always incapable, in comparison to men. The scientific basis of those ideas were elaborated in the nineteenth century by white men above all higher classes, educated in universities that constituted mostly new professions such as obstetrics and gynaecology, biology, psychology, sociology and anthropology. These professionals used their own theories about the innate fragility of women with the purpose of disqualifying girls and women of their own race and class that could strive with them for education and professional status.*
>
> (Hubbard, 1993)

The feminine body was destined to maternity: 'the skeleton is shorter and less tough than a man's skeleton, the thorax is narrower and the basin wider, to hold the fetus' (Maldonado, 1985). Weakness and sensibility are the main characteristics of women and mothers. This definition predominates today, as does the nineteenth century argument that women should be confined to home, taking care of children and other similar activities.

In relation to the psychological aspects of pregnancy, Maldonado presents a historical retrospective of 'motherly love'. She refers to theories that emphasise the two basic figures of feminism and motherhood in Christian tradition: Eve and Mary. The first was a tempting and erotic woman who symbolises dangerous and sinful forces, and is rarely thought of as a maternity symbol, even though, as the first woman, she is the mother of us all. Mary symbolises virtue, and is even praised for her maternal image: she conceived without sin, without sex; so the purity, devotion, charity, humility and obedience attracted to the sexual life was a *sine qua non* of the possibility of redemption (Maldonado, 1985). Male ideology has two archetypes of woman, but one of man: the seductive Eve and motherly Mary, the first to enchant man and the second to beget his children; both to serve him (Noronha and Daltro, 1991).

> *'in biology, starting from the point that the capacity of pregnancy and having children is an exclusive appanage of females and women, therefore a universal law . . . [M]aternity is primarily a condemnation of a single human being, woman, that maintains through the familiar institution as a feminine oppression "locus".'*
>
> (Nascimento, 1996)

In a paper on reproductive ages, Barbieri takes a stand that values the female body:

> *'Women and men are indispensable to fecundation, but only women's body have guaranteed until now the survival of the embryo and therefore, the human being survival, in spite of huge efforts of certain science to avoid it . . . Up until today any man that wants to see his biological paternity possibility realized, has to meet a woman disposed to get pregnant, to give birth, and to take care of the conception fruit.'*
>
> (Barbieri, 1993)

Ziegel and Crantey (1985) maintain that, even though pregnancy is a biologically normal event, it is a special event in a woman's life that requires adaptations to promote her health and the health of the fetus. Consequently, the health professionals thought the prenatal attempt was an opportunity to maintain health and provide education for the client. The prenatal period constitutes 'a collection of clinical and educative proceedings with the object of promoting health and identifying early the problems that can result in risk to the pregnant woman's health and that of the child' (Brazil, 1986).

Fundamental to this assistance, according to Arkader (1992), is quality care; that is, meeting needs with humane adequate resources such as capable care-givers and a quality standard of available technology and pharmaceutical resources. It must include preventive action aimed not only at mother and fetus, but at the family and environment, since internment at a hospital is not necessarily required.

Nery (1991) notes that it is the obstetrical nurse who makes the actual consultation with the healthy pregnant woman and controls pregnancy risks through actions that, according to Ziegel and Crantey (1985), include: anamnesis (emphasising menses history, obstetric history, actual pregnancy, prior pathological history, and social history, including family and personal aspects); a general physical examination, including the collection of objective and subjective data required to form a complete picture of the pregnancy; and evaluation of the data, which permits the detection and evaluation of abnormalities, classification of risk and an outline of ongoing nursing diagnosis and care plans.

As complementary activities duties of obstetrical nurses include: conducting the patient to the physician, the nutritionist, social services, the dentist and other professionals as required; finding a residence for a woman who gives birth without family support; and giving courses on prenatal orientation, parturition, and postpartum care of mother and newborn (Nery, 1991).

Research method: the process of approximating reality

We visited 39 health services in the district and identified 22 that assist women. Most provided services to do with giving birth, especially services for prenatal women. From among these, we selected seven that used nurses for prenatal services.

At first we analysed the triage routines and protocols of departments where pregnant women were registered for assistance. This first encounter was for the purpose of gathering data about the type of assistance provided by the nurses in order to identify education and research carried out by nursing staff.

The data obtained, however, was mainly about anamnesis, physical exams and development of pregnancy. There was little about knowledge education, replication of knowledge and, in some instances, reconstruction of knowledge related to assistance to pregnant women. We also wanted to identify participants' perceptions of the relationship between being a woman, being married, having children and generating knowledge. We reviewed nurses' consultations and interviewed the pregnant women who had consulted them. The process occurred over a period of three months.

Knowing, knowledge: generation, replication and reconstruction in providing assistance to pregnant women — nurses' views

One of the nurses distinguished between knowing and knowledge as follows: the first applies to practice and the second to theory. Both were seen as something abstract, hard to express in words: academic concepts outside the working reality and belonging basically to the realm of research. To another nurse, knowledge was something that gave her power to occasionally affect care, to gratify the client. Knowledge was seen as something you apply. In the view of another nurse, knowledge was seen as information that could be gathered from the literature and from more experienced people through understanding. A nursing assistant saw knowledge as learning: learning things each day was learning the new, and led to self-actualisation.

With these perspectives, some nurses who were interviewed said that knowing and generating knowledge could be understood as 'something you learn and then from this point you add something new'; or a person's search of knowledge through study or from other more experienced professionals; or knowledge through daily practice with pregnant women to see what the possibilities are of sharing the theoretical baggage with them.

Knowing, knowledge and assistance for pregnant women

The people interviewed had difficulty relating the concepts of generation and replication of knowledge to pregnancy assistance. They did not believe they generated knowledge, nor were they cognisant of the replication of that knowledge in the actual process of caring for a woman in a precarious situation. What they saw, reflected directly in providing quality assistance, was that it was simply considered to be good or bad quality, depending on the actual standard for each service.

Some nurses consider themselves as mere replicators of knowledge, with even this level of application being difficult in view of precarious work conditions. The relationship between knowledge and actual practice was seen to be very complex for some, since the nurse 'has many tasks to perform and forgets to generate new ideas, since to generate new knowledge requires time and research'. Thus, to these nurses, replication of knowledge itself was more important than generation or transmitting the knowledge they acquired. This was the reason most of those interviewed gave for ignoring knowledge produced by nurses. One of the nurses said that nursing agents resist change. others revealed that the generation of knowledge was a reality: 'sometimes you retrain yourself and have to go beyond the books or other professionals'. They did not identify this retraining as generation of knowledge.

Thus, to these nurses, reproduction itself is more important than production, and this reproductive process consists of transmitting and applying the knowledge they acquire. When asked about principles they follow when modifying techniques or processes in assisting pregnant women, some of the nurses interviewed talked about the necessity of looking for new knowledge to make day-to-day assistance easier. Contact with the community and the scarcity of materials were the reasons cited for making changes in the nurses' techniques or processes. It is through such changes that nurses become acquainted with the ongoing process of improving knowledge (Alves, 1995).

Little knowledge by nurses was produced, recorded or published; the only knowledge that was recorded was what was performed during consultations for anamnesis, physical examinations or orientations. Thus, nurses thought that in the process of assisting pregnant women, they did not add anything new, they only applied or replicated knowledge they had received. Consider, however, that in the admissions record forms, in reports, protocols and specifically in books for the pregnant women, it was always important to evaluate the effect of treatment on the population being cared for and modify care as necessary. In the view of one nursing assistant, it 'is impossible to create new things; we always do things the same way and with great difficulty because the lack of material to work with here is very great, beyond the lack of incentive offered by low salaries'. In view of this, we believe that this professional does not relate improvement with merely making changes. The essence of producing special materials is tied to available financial resources.

Although some of the nurses interviewed had difficulties in applying the knowledge they acquired because of a lack of resources, others demonstrated how they increased and reconstructed their knowledge of the theoretical fundamentals. They used protocols to help them apply their knowledge with utmost care during daily practice, and modified these protocols to improve care. Some did not make this correlation between generation, replication and reconstruction of knowledge because they believed they could not apply much of what they learned under ideal conditions, to practice conditions that were less than favourable. Precarious practice conditions cited included a scarcity of human and material resources, insufficient physical space, the influence of politics (both internal and external) leading to a lack of feelings of self-fulfilment. Some of those interviewed attributed the difficulties to a lack of interest on the part of the institution to improve patient care.

The means that support for the generation of knowledge, such as journals, computers, books and networking, were not mentioned, possibly because the interviewees did not believe their acquisition was possible. This was another indication that none of those interviewed were involved in knowledge- generating scientific research.

The nurses saw prenatal care as attending to the mother and fetus, with a goal of detecting problems in advance. However, a nurse's role is divided the moment she distinguishes between her role of giving prenatal assistance to the pregnant woman and her role as a leader in referring the pregnant woman's problems to gynaecological, nutrition or social services. Prenatal care encompasses all these services. To many of those interviewed, the importance of this assistance is inherent in assistance to the mother and child. Its aim is to know about their health and detect any problems.

Knowing, knowledge, prenatal care and gender questions

The professionals interviewed had diverse answers to questions of being a woman (or man), being married, having children and involving themselves in knowledge-generation activities in the process of prenatal care. One nurse mentioned that one reason women generate less knowledge than men is that women are more worn out by excessive labour. One nurse argued that 'if you really want to [generate knowledge], you can, depending mainly on each one's interest. It's a question of time, a question of option . . . . If a person doesn't do anything, it's more a question of complaisance'. Another stated that:

> *'[I] left generating and growing professionally so that my husband could grow. However, I do not relate this matter to the fact of being a woman, but to [nursing] being a badly recognised profession and being badly rewarded. Nursing does not offer financial conditions needed to sustain a family and have a good life-style.'*

She also said that 'the fact that men produce more, does not mean that they have more capacity than women, but they have more chances in our society (including those given by women themselves)'. The nurse maintained that it was a very individual decision because it was her option to give space to her husband to grow and produce more than she, saying at the last that 'surely there are many women who have greater capacities than men'.

Another professional interviewed sees this dual relationship as something beneficial by the simple fact that as married women and nurses they were nearer to the actual reality of life. This could become a threat to traditional knowledge generation, which does not occur with men who are not responsible for domestic activities.

Clients' views

Clients have different views about knowing and knowledge. Some see it as a daily experience, others as what is learned in school where 'an individual is knowing something when learning and assimilating and when knowing about things deeply'. In the latter case, the individual rejected daily experience as a source of knowledge, and thus rejected common sense, which Solis (1990) considers the base for specific knowledge.

Some pregnant clients see prenatal assis- tance as assistance given from the beginning until the end of pregnancy, or in other words an opportunity to detect and to avoid risks and complications related to the perinatal period. Nursing assistance was seen as external assistance during pregnancy, which was more oriented to the pregnant woman's actual life. From this statement, it was possible to detect the gratitude of the clients for a professional who could identify with their human condition. This makes the nurse the professional person closest to the client. Another client saw the meaning of prenatal assistance as a learning experience, an apprenticeship period, related to knowledge of the body and fetal development. This intervention guides the mother to care for herself and not just automatically conform to another's prescriptive interventions.

According to those interviewed, the search for this kind of assistance when pregnancy is confirmed guarantees a good mother-fetus development during pregnancy, avoiding risks for the mother and the fetus, Many of these clients recognise the importance of this assistance, supporting early detection of problems and adopting actions that have a goal of resolving problems.

Of the professionals who deliver prenatal assistance, nurses and physicians are the ones most often mentioned by the clients. In some services, however, other professionals from the prenatal team were identified: psychologists, nursing assistants and nutrition technicians. We observed that some clients did not distinguish between these categories.

The norm used by clients to evaluate prenatal assistance was based on their treatment by some nurses in terms of their interpersonal relationships and the available resources used by nurses during consultations. Assistance was evaluated as:

- **excellent** when treatment by the nurse was humane, the client's clinical plan was correctly evaluated and the client was given clear directives
- **very good** when the nurse attended during the consultation, doubts were answered and directives given, and the consultation was complete
- **good** when treatment was good and advice was given by professionals
- **regular** if the obstetrical and clinical examination was incomplete or material resources were not available
- **very bad** if there was ill will during the consultation, indifference to the patient's problems and a scarcity of material resources.

Clients' learning in prenatal education began with the orientations given by the nurse during consultation. However, this education varied according to the professional and the institution they attended. In some cases, the pregnant client said she did not have any directions because the nursing assistance consisted mainly of asking about the patient's complaints and forwarding her to the physician. In other health units, the pregnant women displayed difficulties recalling the directives and the amount of information passed on to them. In general, the major elements emphasised during apprenticeship were care of the new- born, the breast-feeding period, the necessity to go for examinations, vaccination, medicinal care for teratogenic effects and, in some cases, the mother-fetus relationship.

Most of the women paid attention to the directions given, but some said they did not learn anything new because the information was exactly the same as they had received during previous pregnancies. Women who were pregnant for the first time thought it was all new. The new knowledge they emphasised included the importance of bonding between the mother and child, the rationale for structured directions and the procedure to follow in the event of certain symptoms. These directions were based on knowledge, common sense and the ever-present desire to complete a successful pregnancy. In some services, there was no education, even about essential aspects of pregnancy.

In terms of the most important knowledge acquired, respondents emphasised those relating to the necessity of successful completion of pregnancy, bodily health, proper diet, the reason for certain directives or instructions, and the necessity for making life changes to protect the fetus. The knowledge learned in the prenatal programme had been used in daily life for a more healthy pregnancy. The information transmitted during consultations on suckling, breast care and child care were the most important aspects of the instruction for the pregnant women. Some reported they taught close relatives, although others did not do so because of a lack of time or fear of teaching. Instead, they guided other pregnant women to look for the service just by briefly reporting what the prenatal consultation meant in their lives, assuring them of the safety this gave them in terms of reducing risks and ensuring an effective prenatal period.

Final considerations

Nursing agents (nurses and nursing assistants) do not think they generate knowledge with prenatal programmes. This is because they do not believe in their potential in relation to their commitment to their domestic activities, precarious labour conditions, lack of interest in generating new knowledge, scarcity of resources and gender questions. Thus, believing their function to be more replication and dissemination of information than generation of knowledge, they do not invest themselves in the process of producing knowledge, of contributing to dissemination or replication of nursing knowledge, and thus in the end fail to apply for assistance given to research.

This 'reductionist' position is argued by Alves (1995) in revealing possibilities of generating knowledge in nursing and showing how nurses are necessary to conducting and reporting research. A profession is recognised and respected for what it produces, the quality of what it produces, the usefulness of what it produces and, above all, the critical posture from which it is produced. The question is, how can we convince nurses that they are already part of the process of generating, replicating and reconstructing knowledge?

References

Arkader J (1992) *Pre-natal Assistance*. UNICEF, Rio de Janeiro

Alves D (1995) *Production/reproduction of Knowledge in Nursing Work*. PhD thesis, Faculty of Education, Federal University of Bahia

Bachelard G (1990) Epistemological obstacle notion. In: Hühne LM, ed. *Scientific Methodology. Texts, Notebooks and Techniques*, 4 edn.). Agir, Rio de Janeiro: 59–63

Barbieri T (1993) *Sobre la Categoria Gênero: Uma Introducion Teórico-meodológica* (trans. Lewinsky A) [About a gender category: A theoretical-methodological introduction]. SOS Body, Recife

Brazil, Minister of Health (1986) *Pré-natal of Low Risk*. Centrol de Documentaçao do Ministério da Saúde, Brasilia

Ferreira, SLF (1994) *The Woman and Public Health Services: Process Analysis of Work in Basic Units in Salvador*. PhD thesis, Escola de Enfermagem de Ribeirao Preto da Universidade de Sao Paulo

Gergen MM (1993) Direction to a feminist metatheory and methodology in social sciences. In: McCanney M, ed. *The Feminist Thought and Structure of Knowledge*. Rosa dos Tempos, Rio de Janeiro; EDUnB, Brasilia

Hubbard R (1993) Some ideas about masculinity of natural sciences. In: McCanney M, ed. *The Feminist Thought and Structure of Knowledge*. Rosa dos Tempos, Rio de Janeiro: 21–23; Brasilia: EDUnB

Hühne LM, ed (1990) *Scientific Methodology: Notebooks, Texts and Techniques*, 4 edn. Agir, Rio de Janeiro

Maldonado MTP (1985) *Psychology in Pregnancy, Parturition and Pre-natal*, 7 edn. Vozes, Petropolis

Nery IS (1991) *Nursing Consult to Pregnant: Interfering Factors*. These, Esocla de Enfermagem Alfredo Pinto da Universidade do Rio de Janeiro

Noronha CV, Daltro ME (1991) Is masculine violence directed to Eve or Mary? *Note Pub Health* **8**(2): 215–31

Mattalo Junior H (1994) The problematics of knowledge. In: Carvalho MCM, ed. *Building the Known: Scientific Methodology: Fundaments and Techniques*. Papins, Campinas: 13–27

Nascimento ER (1996) *Gender and Nursing*. Positiva, Salvador

Popper K (1990) The insecure starting point: Knowledge and critics. In: Hühne LM, ed. *Scientific Methodology: Notebooks, Texts and Techniques*, 4 edn. Agir, Rio de Janeiro: 57–8

Solis, DEN (1990) About common sense. In: Hühne LM, ed. *Scientific Methodology: Notebooks, Texts and Techniques*, 4 edn. Agir, Rio de Janeiro: 60–3

Ziegel EE, Crantey MS (1985) *Obstetric Nursing* 2 edn. Guanabara, Rio de Janeiro

24

An analysis of the experience of being physically challenged and a woman in Korean society

Margaret Storey and Sang Soon Choi

The purpose of this study was to begin to understand the experience of being a woman with a disability living in a society that is in a state of change, but remains patriarchal at its most basic level.

In Korea, Confucian ideals of appropriate behaviour are based on the assumption that a patriarchal society is best for preserving the nation (Chung, 1986a). In the latter part of the twentieth century, there have been many changes, but the underlying assumptions for many people are still patriarchal, and the role of women is to be good mothers and wives, and to manage the affairs of the household (Chung, 1986b). The end of the nineteenth and beginning of the twentieth century saw the beginning of the development of an active movement to advance the position of women. This, along with changes in the socioeconomic situation following the Korean War, and the increased number of women in the workplace, have led to many improvements for women (Kim, 1986). For example, there are greater opportunities for advanced education and opportunities within the university settings for young women to speak out and be heard, and for young men to be actively involved in child care and household tasks (Kim, 1994), but problems still remain, and women are underrepresented in most decision-making and policy formulating bodies.

As in many countries, physical wholeness and beauty are desirable characteristics in Korea. However, Koreans are considered to be a homogenous race where people who are different stand out. Within patriarchal societies, sons are preferred and receive many more benefits. Thus, men with disabilities have more educational and vocational opportunities than women with disabilities. The ratio of men to women in one vocational rehabilitation centre in Korea is four men to each woman. However, as a result of changes in society, daughters are becoming more acceptable, but only if they are perfectly normal. In this situation, what is the experience of women with disabilities?

Using a modified participant observer approach and an open question format, seven women were interviewed. They were asked to talk about things that were difficult for them as women with disabilities, to wonder what might be different if they were male, to talk about what they did when difficulties arose and to whom they turned for help, and to suggest ways in which healthcare professionals, particularly nurses, could help give care that is more accessible and acceptable.

The seven women's Korean names can be translated as Loving Respect, Bright Blessing, Gentle Motion, Beautiful Goodness, Gentle Flower, Hopeful Sight and Pure Brightness. They all live in the city of Wonju, a small city in the largely rural province of Kangwon. The authors had worked with all of them except Loving Respect in a nurse-client relationship. Bright Blessing, Beautiful Goodness, Gentle Flower, Hopeful Sight and Pure Brightness had been clients of nurses in a home care project; Gentle Motion was in a vocational rehabilitation project. Bright Blessing and Beautiful Goodness had been involved in both projects at different times. A nurse-client relationship with Loving Respect is anticipated when she is discharged from hospital. All the women are in their thirties.

Bright Blessing, Gentle Motion and Beautiful Goodness have had cerebral palsy since birth. Gentle Flower had a femur amputation at age 12 years due to osteomyelitis. Hopeful Sight had a history of being unable to walk because of leg weakness, present from birth, and then spinal tuberculosis as a teenager. Loving Respect and Pure Brightness had spinal cord injuries sustained in traffic accidents as adults.

Loving Respect, Beautiful Goodness, Gentle Flower and Hopeful Sight are married. Hopeful Sight has one daughter, Beautiful Goodness one son, Loving Respect a son and a daughter and Gentle Flower two daughters. Their educational levels ranged from no formal schooling for Hopeful Sight to community college graduation for Loving Respect. All the women are literate. None is presently employed in the regular workforce, but Gentle Motion is employed in a sheltered workshop, and Hopeful Sight and Beautiful Goodness have done piecework at home.

With the exception of Loving Respect, who was married before she suffered the spinal cord injury, the other three married women are married to men who are also disabled. All of the husbands are working. Loving Respect, Hopeful Sight and Beautiful Goodness live in a nuclear family; Gentle Flower lives with her husband's parents. Of those who are not married, Bright Blessing and Gentle Motion live in semi-independent group homes where they are both the manager of their respective homes. Pure Brightness lives with her brother's family, which also includes her mother. Hopeful Sight lives in a low-income apartment. Pure Brightness, Beautiful Goodness and Loving Respect live in moderately sized apartments. Gentle Flower lives in an apartment above the store where her husband works. The group home where Bright Blessing lives is a house built as a group home and is wheelchair accessible. The group home where Gentle Motion lives is a low-income apartment, and it, too, is wheelchair accessible.

Five of the women were interviewed at home. Loving Respect was interviewed in hospital. Gentle Motion was interviewed at her workplace. With the respondents' approvals, the interviews were taped and are being transcribed for further analysis. Notes were also taken during the interviews. To date, Gentle Motion and Bright Blessing have been interviewed twice. Hopeful Sight, Pure Brightness and Bright Blessing were interviewed with both researchers present. After the initial analysis was completed, the conclusions were discussed with Gentle Motion and Bright Blessing to verify that the analysis represented the actual reality as they experienced it.

The results of the study show that the experience of being a woman with a disability in Korea poses problems that are unique — problems that do not exist for women who are not disabled and problems that do not exist for men who are disabled. Some of the problems these women share with other women and some they share with men who are disabled. The categories that emerged from the data were 'being addressed', 'resource limitations', 'life at school and getting an education', 'being in hospital', 'looking one's best', 'getting married and having children', 'getting a job and having friends', 'driving a car' and 'receiving assistance and coping with disability'. Some of these women's experience were as follows.

Being addressed

The Korean language provides honorific forms of address that denote someone older and respected, but older children with disabilities are frequently called by their first name by younger siblings rather than being addressed using the respectful term for older brother or older sister, as they automatically would be if they were not disabled. Beautiful Goodness was not only addressed this way by her younger brother and sister, but they also addressed her as if she were a younger sibling. Fortunately, her grandmother heard them and scolded them for their lack of respect for their older sister and insisted they use the proper form of address. Bright Blessing and Beautiful Goodness had the experience of being shouted at, even though they have no hearing impairment. This was done by older women in the market who felt that people with cerebral palsy and the resulting speech impairment must also be deaf.

Bright Blessing, who has a severe speech impairment, has had the experience of being ignored when requesting directions or help. People just walk away, particularly other women and younger men. She finds it easier to get help from older people, but believes it is difficult to get people to help her because of her appearance and speech problems.

Beautiful Goodness, due to her limping gait, has had the experience of being asked if she was drunk when walking on the street at night. She felt that men would not be bothered because it is all right for a man to be drunk, but it is not all right for a woman to be drunk. She echoed the other women's opinion when she talked about being very aware of the negative remarks directed at her by young children on the street.

Resource limitations

Both financial and time resources presented problems for the respondents. Gentle Flower feels that going to hospital is very time-consuming and expensive since, not only is there the expense of the hospital charges, but she also feels a need to give something like a tip in thanks for service. She also had to make trips to Seoul, which is about three hours or 120 kilometres from Wonju, for rehabilitation; she found this even more time-consuming and expensive, but it was necessary because of a lack of facilities in Wonju.

Gentle Motion presented another reason for increased expense: the need to use taxis because public transportation is difficult or impossible. For example, buses in Korea are exited through the back door and getting to the back door of a moving bus while carrying something is difficult even for those who have good balance and coordination. While some bus drivers do ask other passengers to get up and give a seat to a disabled person, many are not very patient with older people who have some of the same coordination problems, and so Gentle Motion said she moved quickly to the back of the bus before the driver had an opportunity to say anything negative. However, she also found that taxi drivers could be a greater problem than bus drivers when the person with the disability has to be dependent on them. They can be rude when they think it is bad luck to have a passenger who is disabled and so they smoke even though they have a 'no smoking' sign in the taxi. The assumption is that they smoke because they are unhappy about having a disabled person in their cab. Sometimes taxi drivers will just drive right past and not stop when hailed by a disabled or older person.

Life at school and securing an education

Bright Blessing, Gentle Motion and Beautiful Goodness were all born with a disability and found acquiring an education a major problem. They felt that this would not have been the case for a disabled son. Bright Blessing and Gentle Motion were not encouraged to gain an education; in fact Gentle Motion's parents wondered what use an education would be. Both were allowed to miss school or not complete homework because of their disability and were not pressed by teachers or parents to finish assignments. Bright Blessing was able to go to primary school because she had the help of an older and then a younger sister, but when her sisters went to middle school it was too far away for her to be able to go. When Gentle Flower was unable to finish primary school and lost a year of middle school because of illness, catching up with her classmates seemed impossible, so she dropped out and went to work.

Because of her cerebral palsy, Gentle Motion was late starting school, so she was in the same grade as a younger brother. When the time came for them to go to high school, the parents saw no use her going to high school, and besides there was the younger brother who needed the family's resources for his schooling. The younger brother did not finish high school because of the bad influence of his friends. Beautiful Goodness, who did graduate from high school, was thankful to her parents for treating her the same as her brother and sister and making sure that she finished high school.

Gentle Motion and Beautiful Goodness felt that being allowed to miss physical education, in itself was all right if the class was engaged in an activity that was difficult to perform, but they did not like being completely excused from physical education classes. And when they were excused, they did not like having to spend the time alone in the classroom, where they experienced loneliness and fear. One day, Beautiful Goodness was accused of taking another student's money because she had been alone in the classroom, during a physical education class. With respect to going to university, the researchers are aware that several men with disabilities who live in Wonju have graduated from university or who are presently university students, but there were few, if any, women.

Relationships with other students were difficult, in that the students with the disabilities felt left out. Even in primary school, Bright Blessing was teased and called a 'cripple'. Other teasing included comments like, 'when I have a baby I am certainly not going to have one like you'. The students with disabilities were always the last to be chosen for any activity, and when the class had to be paired, a frequent occurrence in Korean schools, no one wanted to be paired with the student with a disability.

Being in hospital

All these women have had some experience with the healthcare delivery system. Generally the care they received was judged as being good, and nurses were seen as friendly. For example, Gentle Flower was allowed to wear her prosthesis, which she considers part of her, into the operating room when going for a caesarean section; she felt this was supportive of her. When Beautiful Goodness had to take her son to the hospital for immunisations or when he was sick, she reported that the nurses were very helpful in holding and lifting him, something she could not do by herself.

On the other hand, there were events in which nurses could have given more help. For example, Bright Blessing wondered why nurses did not make a greater attempt to understand people who have speech problems. Pure Brightness, one of the women with a spinal cord injury, was really upset when her complaints of pain were ignored because the nurse had seen it before and knew the outcome. Gentle Motion, who spent two months in hospital following a back injury, suggested that nurses could help people with disabilities feel more comfortable by offering to help them rather than waiting for requests for help. The women with cerebral palsy felt that medical personnel, in general, do not have enough knowledge about cerebral palsy, so they treat them as if they were mentally ill or mentally retarded. These women felt they should be able to expect more from healthcare professionals. When Beautiful Goodness and Gentle Flower had their children, they both had a caesarean section, and in both cases the decision was not made by the mother, but rather by the doctor in consultation with the woman's mother, for Beautiful Goodness, or her mother-in-law, for Gentle Flower.

Looking one's best

This involves personal hygiene and grooming as well as being able to dress appropriately. Being able to perform these tasks, which most people take for granted, presented real problems for these women. Bright Blessing and Pure Brightness mentioned the difficulties in taking care of menstrual hygiene. They also needed help with dressing and make-up. This help was given by someone at home, frequently their mothers, so was not such a problem. However, it was a major problem for Bright Blessing since she was able to go out in society and to go on trips by herself, but was not always able to meet these basic needs independently. Bright Blessing also found the use of public washrooms very difficult. The stalls are too narrow and the doors too flimsy, and there are no bars for support. In many public washrooms, the toilets are of a traditional type that requires women to squat; this can be very difficult when there is nothing to hang on to. There have been many improvements recently in providing wheelchair-accessible washrooms, but there are still many problems that need to be addressed. For Gentle Flower, who is also able to go out and be a part of society, but who wears a leg prosthesis, there is a lot of stress around the issue of what to do if something happens to the prosthesis, like a screw coming loose. If this happened, the only thing she could do would be to call a taxi and go home. This stress of wearing a prosthesis and being mobile has led to nervous problems.

Marrying and having children

This was a major concern for most of the women, but in many cases the parents do not believe this is possibility. In Korea, parents have a major responsibility for ensuring that their daughters marry. Since everyone who is married is expected to have children, Bright Blessing, whose disabilities include decreased muscle strength and coordination, decided that she did not have the physical ability to care for children, and, therefore, decided not to marry. She felt that it would certainly be easier for men because they do not have to worry so much about the direct day-to-day care of children nor, as Beautiful Goodness did, worry about carrying a child on her back when she had to take the child somewhere. The women also felt that it was easier for men with disabilities to marry and that sometimes they were even able to marry women who did not have a disability. They felt that women did not have such a wide range of options. On the positive side, marriage was seen as providing a person to share and talk with, and if that person is also disabled, providing a person who understands the problems.

However, not marrying has one other important implication for women in Korea. A woman who is not married remains officially the responsibility of her father, a part of her father's legal household, and he is her 'responsible' next of kin, even if she is living independently. So Bright Blessing found that when she went to the bank or other official agencies she was treated like a child and unable to do anything without her father's counter-signature. She also had a problem when her older brother planned to marry, because the future bride's family were not sure that she should marry a man who had a sister who was disabled.

When a Korean woman marries she becomes officially and legally part of her husband's family and the relationship to in-laws is very important and requires certain behaviour. For the three women who were married after they became disabled, their husbands also had a disability and the women received sympathy and understanding from the husbands' parents. But for both Beautiful Goodness and Hopeful Sight, when they visit their husbands' families, they are excused from all work and tend to be treated as women who can do nothing. This makes them feel sad because they are not allowed to do the household work or food preparation in the way a daughter-in-law should, even though there are things they could do. Not only is this true for the relationship between mother-in-law and daughter-in-law, but also for the relationship between the wives of brothers in the family. Each wife is expected to assist with the work required for any celebration or family event.

The women who were mothers had major concerns about caring for their children. Beautiful Goodness, whose son is five years old, expressed her concern about how to tell him about her disability, what to do when he asks why his mother is different, and what to do when other children say something about her being different. Visiting the school is something mothers are expected to do and is considered an important part of being a mother, but Hopeful Sight worried about reactions of students and teachers if she visits. Mothers, especially at the elementary school level, are supposed to take part at picnics in activities like singing and dancing, so this presented a problem for all of the mothers because they were not able to join in these activities.

Both Beautiful Goodness and Hopeful Sight found even the physical feat of going on a picnic was a problem if a lot of walking was involved, and Gentle Flower reported the problem of walking up to a third-storey classroom. Even though there were many difficulties, Gentle Flower and Beautiful Goodness found a certain amount of understanding from their children, even Beautiful Goodness's five-year-old, who was able and willing to help his mother.

Gaining employment and having friends

This is an important part of modern society, but was a major problem for most of these women. Even with a high school diploma, no job was available for Beautiful Goodness, so she felt bad for her parents, who had assured her a high school education and would be disappointed that she was unable to get a job. After three rejections, she was not angry but very sad, to the point of tears. Being unable to get a job also influenced her friendship with one friend who, with the same diploma, was able to get a job and earn some money. This friend felt sorry for Beautiful Goodness and if they went out for lunch, Beautiful Goodness felt bad because she was not able to treat her friends to lunch. Usually, in Korea, when friends go out to a restaurant or a movie theatre, one friend treats all the others. Among friends this rotates informally so that all have an obligation to treat on a fairly equal basis; thus it becomes a burden if someone is always unable to fulfil the obligation of treating friends.

Driving

Driving is an aid to mobility, but is not easily realised. Gentle Flower learned to drive but lost confidence after a minor accident. Gentle Motion has a driver's licence but cannot afford a car with hand controls. Loving Respect intends to drive after discharge from hospital, but needs a vehicle with hand controls. These are available in Korea, but expensive. Several men who are disabled, particularly those who have spinal cord injuries, drive in Korea, but there are very few, if any, women who drive.

Receiving assistance and coping with disability

All the women reported receiving help from members of their family, and in particular their own parents and siblings, who were considered the greatest source of help. For those who were married, there was help from in-laws, too. Only Loving Respect, who had not yet been discharged from hospital, felt that none of her family really understood the problems she faced. When it came to help with transportation, Pure

Brightness received help from her brother, Bright Blessing from her father and Gentle Flower from her brother-in-law and father-in-law. Bright Blessing received a lot of emotional support from her sisters. While Beautiful Goodness received help from her mother with child care and homemaking, particularly making kimchi, an important part of a Korean meal, Gentle Flower received a similar kind of help from her mother-in-law. Help with dressing and grooming for both Bright Blessing and Pure Brightness was given by their mothers. However, both Pure Brightness and Loving Respect felt that men who were disabled after they were married had a great advantage. They had wives who were expected to help them and who do, for the most part, help them. Although the women did report receiving emotional help from their families, many felt they really had no one to talk with about their problems. This was true for those who were injured, later in life, as well as for those who were born with a disability. For those who were injured, visits to the hospital by friends decreased over time and there were very few other women with similar injuries with whom they could share their difficulties and successes. Some of the women did find other friends who were disabled and with whom they could talk, but for both Gentle Motion and Beautiful Goodness a sheltered workshop was not considered the best place to be employed and have friends because these workshops are segregated from people without disabilities and there is no real privacy.

Life in society was described by Bright Blessing, whose disability is obvious, as 'difficult, because people tend to see the disability and not the person and to judge by outward appearances rather than waiting to see who the person really is'. But the women in this study did have some ways of coping in these situations. One solution to the problem of helping in school used successfully by Gentle Flower was to volunteer to do things that were possible before being asked to do things that were impossible. She also felt confident that she would be able to get help on the street if necessary. On the other hand, Pure Brightness, who uses a wheelchair, felt that it would be difficult for a woman to ask for help with the chair but it would be much easier for men to do so because men have been brought up to be more outgoing and in charge of seeking what they needed. For Hopeful Sight and Gentle Flower, an outgoing personality was a way to overcome these problems. Pure Brightness said that by being at home she developed a wisdom that allowed her to deal with life. She also found she could be helpful to other people with spinal cord injuries by talking and sharing with them over the telephone. This, in turn, contributed to her sense of well-being

Conclusions

Two major conclusions can be drawn from the experience of being a Korean woman with a disability. First, some problems they face are common to women in general, such as problems with menstruation and hygiene. Like other women, they also face the problem of their place in Korean society — a lack of emphasis on education for women, and the responsibilities they are expected to bear in relation to having and raising children, and becoming a part of their husband's family and in relation to their in-laws.

The other major problems they face are those they share to some degree with disabled men, but these are compounded because they are women. These can be summed up as problems of being left out of society — lack of opportunities for education and for meaningful jobs, not being able to obtain the assistance they need to dress and groom themselves appropriately in order to go out into society, not being able to use public facilities easily (washrooms, banks, post offices, buses, taxis), being limited in decision-making about major life events, such as marriage and childbirth, being limited in opportunities to make friends and finally being limited in the opportunity to do something even if it means hard work.

This study is limited and it is impossible to generalise the findings to all Korean society. It did not explore the problems of women in Korea who are either deaf or blind, and, further, the sample was of women living in a small city that has not had and still does not have a wide range of rehabilitation services available, but at the same time because of its rural atmosphere has been a more caring society. The women in the sample were from the lower middle-class or lower socioeconomic level, and do not represent women in the higher socioeconomic group.

Another limitation is in the description of violence. Literature from North America on women with disabilities indicates that a major problem is violence towards these women (Berkeley Planning Associates, 1997; Council of Canadians with Disabilities, 1997). In one study in Korea, violence by family members was reported at 71% for unmarried women and 63% for married women (Chai, 1996). Violence was defined as including assault, being ignored, being confined (to the house or one room) and verbal assault. While none of the women in the present study reported any physical violence against them, the results of the study show that there is violence even though it is not named as such.

In conclusion, over the past 10 to 15 years, there has been a major increase in welfare services available to people in Korea. These include universal health insurance, welfare care for the poor, more free education, an increasing number of wheel-chair-accessible buildings and more consumer goods. These have all benefited people with disabilities, but men more so than women. There is an urgent need for changes in attitudes that will lead to a breaking down of the barriers that marginalise women with disabilities, leave them open to abuse and preventing them from being included in the life of the community.

References

Berkeley Planning Associates (1997) *Service Needs of Women with Disabilities: Disabled Women Rate Caregivers' Abuse and Domestic Violence Number One Issue*. http://www.bpacal.com/pressrel.html

Chai U (1996) *An Analysis of Discrimination Against Women with Disabilities Within the Family in Korea*. Presented at the 1996 Women with Disabilities Conference, Seoul, October

Chung D (1986a) Women's liberation and the Korean ordinary language. In: Chung S, ed. *Challenges for Women: Women's Studies in Korea*. Ewha Woman's University Press, Seoul: 127–49

Chung S (1986b) Socialization and women in Korea from the perspectives of the family, school and social education. In: Chung S, ed. *Challenges for Women: Women's Studies in Korea*. Ewha Woman's University Press, Seoul: 173–91

Council of Canadians with Disabilities (1997) *Fact sheet: Women with Disabilities and Development*. http://www.pcs.mb.ca/~ccd/womefact.html

Kim M (1994) The gender division of labor within the worker's family — with special emphasis on male participation in child care. In: Cho H, Chang P, eds. *Gender Division of Labor in Korea*. Ewha Women's University Press, Seoul: 199–223

Kim Y (1986) Woman's movement in modern Korea. In: Chung S, ed. *Challenges for Women: Women's Studies in Korea*. Ewha Woman's University Press, Seoul: 75–102

Section V

Globalisation, corporate greed and their impact on women's image, health and work

The North American Free Trade Agreement (NAFTA), considered by governments and the corporate world to be progress, is in reality a free-investment agreement at the expense of human standards, national standards and equal partnership. Martha Lywak argues that women's health- care interests are adversely affected by NAFTA, since women are and continue to be the highest percentage of workers in the healthcare industry. The adverse effect of NAFTA on women, children and ordinary working people in Canada are set aside in the milieu of competition and profit-making within a global market economy. With NAFTA, healthcare services are being increasingly contracted out, and full-time employment is being reduced to part-time. The needs and rights of the majority of women, and especially women workers, are being sacrificed. Lywak's chapter exposes the various deleterious effects of NAFTA on Canadian women.

Perceptions of body size and beauty are often governed by society and culture. Most present-day media images of women are slender and thin; fat women are considered to be ugly and unattractive. If a woman does not fit the accepted image, she may feel ugly and undesirable. Obesity is a widespread problem in the industrially developed world. Although men and women are obese, fatness is generally denigrated more in women than in men and several negative stereotypes are attached to overweight women. Society often holds the obese person to be responsible for his or her condition. This social attitude is also held by many healthcare professionals. Dale Gietzelt investigated the impact of obesity and the difficulties obese individuals experience in Sydney, Australia. Her chapter discusses the attitudes and opinions people in general and obese people themselves have about obesity and obese people. She also presents interesting data on ethnic, age, gender and class differences in these attitudes.

Thalia Attié's chapter examines the phenomenon of drug addiction as we know it, which is a product of modern western society, and is expanding far beyond the frontiers of any one country. She attempts to see how we can learn from this phenomenon, for ourselves and for the society in which we live.

David Bullivent and Jacqueline Reeve discuss the results of their research project and the impact of caring. The goal of this study was to capture the ideas, attitudes, concerns and experiences of those who care for cancer patients via a phenomenological approach to data collection and detailed discussion of the study.

Poised on the edge of a new century, and with escalating hospital-based healthcare costs and the loss of hospital-based jobs, nurses are looking at other ways to care for people in need. Historically, preventing illness and promoting good health and care of the ill were carried out by nurses, often in collaboration with social workers, in homes and in the community. In their work of total care for people in need, nurses have collaborated with social workers since the beginning of the twentieth century. The two professions collaborated in providing healthcare in settlement houses, prenatal clinics, schools, factories, rural areas, homes and communities, and created new models of care delivery. At the end of the twentieth century, once again the primary setting for care moves into the homes and community. Joellen Hawkins *et al* propose a relevant model of collaborative care by nursing and social workers. Their model was derived from their interview data from several social workers and nurses. They discuss the usefulness of the Biopsychosocial Individual and Systems Intervention Model of Nurse-Social-Worker Collaboration at a time when healthcare has become beyond the reach of many poor and disadvantage people in society.

25

Losing ground: The impact of NAFTA on Canadian women's health and welfare

Martha Marie Lywak

Introduction

This chapter addresses how the Canada-US Free Trade Agreement (FTA) and the North American Free Trade Agreement (NAFTA), which are products of globalisation, affect Canadian women's health and welfare. It discusses how the social community continues to be guided by corporate interest, resulting in loss of ground for Canadian women. Finally, it outlines solutions for Canadian women that could help achieve a rightful representation of Canadian women's health and welfare needs during policy formation and trade negotiation.

Globalisation

We have all been told that globalisation is a natural phenomenon, something that we cannot control or amend. However, contrary to popular belief, globalisation is carefully planned, shaped and guided by a series of international agreements (Nova and Sforza-Roderick, 1997). The term *globalisation* has become a popular explanation for the changes in the global economic setting that began before the introduction of NAFTA. According to McBride and Shields, authors of *Dismantling a Nation: Canada and the New World Order*, globalisation is characterised by three main features:

> *'The first is the creation of larger markets — the nation-state can no longer satisfy the needs of multinational corporations, so big business is demanding larger trading areas; second, in this new environment capital has become increasingly mobile; and third, there has been greater global specialisation of production.*
>
> (McBride and Shields, 1993)

They assert that these economic forces have pushed the issue of market liberalisation to the forefront of internal and external government policy. The dismantling of trade barriers is requiring that nations radically alter their institutions to accommodate the changes in world trade. Governments are entering into agreements with other nations, such as NAFTA, in accommodation to this process of globalisation.

Social impacts of NAFTA

NAFTA, which came into effect January 1, 1994, is a trilateral agreement between Canada, the United States and Mexico, expanding the US-Canada Free Trade Agreement implemented in 1988. The negotiation and signing of the agreement was accompanied by assurances from the Canadian government that the Canadian healthcare system and social welfare net would be protected in NAFTA and protected from the aggressive global strategies of the corporate community (Fuller, 1996). Unfortunately, this has not been the case. The strong social welfare net and labour protection in Canada previously enabled Canadian women to compete equally within society. However, the creation of NAFTA has served to limit state autonomy and enhance corporate interest at the expense of Canadian women's health and welfare needs. NAFTA does not follow the intentions of the General Agreement on Tariffs and Trade (GATT) to liberalise trade, for NAFTA is not a free trade agreement but a free investment agreement. This free investment is at the expense of human standards, national standards and equal partnership. This means NAFTA, 'contrary to conventional wisdom, is protectionist: it is designed to protect corporate interests' (Grinspun, 1993).

The liberalisation and deregulation of trade and investment has had major social repercussions within Canada. Through the pressures for harmonisation between the three countries under NAFTA, the Canadian government is now restricted from certain interventions into its own economy. As a result, many Canadian standards are dropping. One of the most important areas being affected is social programs, including healthcare. With the destruction of universal healthcare in Canada, corporations will gain access to a $52 billion healthcare market (Clark, 1997).

Since the creation of NAFTA, there has been a parallel pressure on the Canadian government to not only resist creating new social policies for Canadians, but also to dismantle social policies already in existence. In both the FTA and NAFTA, management services fall under 'national treatment' rights. National treatment means that rules governing management services cannot discriminate against US or Mexican firms. Therefore, this may create greater pressure to privatise social services, since the governments in both Mexico and the US are not as involved in protecting labour through social policies as is the Canadian government. In the case of creating new public services, such as national child care, under both the FTA and NAFTA, foreign corporations have the right to claim compensation for loss of potential earnings (McBride and Shields, 1993). Therefore, despite years of political promises, Canadian women will not see nationally subsidised child care in this country because it will be too expensive to pay off the big American corporations who have an interest in this market.

Canadian women's health and welfare

Women are, and continue to be, the primary losers in this new economic arrangement. Canadian women's employment is concentrated in the service sector. Further, about 80% of those working in medicine and healthcare services are women (Canadian Labour Congress, 1997). As a result of NAFTA, these services, which are traditionally publicly owned, are being pressured to harmonise with the lower standards south of the Canadian border. For example, health services are increasingly being contracted out and full-time employment is being reduced to part-time employment. In 1996, women constituted 45% of the workforce, but 69% of part-time workers (ECEJ Report, 1996). These new conditions have had an impact on women's wages, working conditions and the control women have over their performance as healthcare providers. This economic crisis is part of a political reorganisation in which the needs and rights of the majority — women — are being abandoned in favour of corporate demands.

The corporate demands have proved to be insensitive to women's health needs. For example, in 1991, officials from Health and Welfare Canada and from Consumer and Corporate Affairs Canada advised the Infant Feeding Action Coalition that the Canadian government cannot bring in legislation to comply with the World Health Organization (WHO) code protecting breast milk and breast-feeding from aggressive corporate advertising of infant formula. This was because the WHO code is superseded by the Free Trade Agreement. Considering that mortality rate of infants who are bottle-fed is 14 times higher than that of breast-fed infants in developing nations, the Canadian government should pay particular attention to the fact that Canadian women are saturated with advertisements that push baby formula (Campbell, 1992).

In addition, Canada is being pressured to dismantle its healthcare policies in order to compete within the North American marketplace. For example, Canada has extended patent protection on brand-name drugs, which falls right in line with NAFTA's call for strict protection of intellectual property rights. The virtual elimination of Canada's generic drug industry will cost Canadian women billions of dollars in increased prescription drug prices (Woman to Woman, 1993). Pharmaceutical companies are now guaranteed 20 years of patent protection. As a result, since 1989 drugs have become the fastest growing expenditure of provincial health plans. From 1987 to 1993 the average cost of a drug claim increased 93%, far above the rise in the consumer price index of 23.1%. Between 1993 and 1995, claim costs rose 25.6%, while the actual manufacturing price per drug fell 2%. This discrepancy was caused by the prescription of costly patented medicines.

> *'It is predicted that, by the end of the decade, Canada will have increased spending on drugs by up to $1 billion per year. Not surprisingly, provincial health plans are beginning to eliminate coverage for many drugs, leaving low-income earners, including senior citizens, to fend for themselves.'*
>
> (CCPA, 1995)

This dismantling of Canada's healthcare system will place greater responsibility on women to be the primary caregivers of the young, sick and elderly within society. NAFTA will push women deeper and deeper into poverty. With accelerated job loss, lower wages, lack of full-time employment and increased demands on them as caregivers, women are going to find it increasingly difficult to cope within our deregulated and corporate-oriented society. As a result, 75% of Canadian women can expect to live out their retirement below the poverty line. This situation will worsen as continental free trade progresses (ECEJ, 1994).

The corporate interest and the social community

Provincial governments, who administer healthcare, are also feeling the effects of NAFTA. Federal cutbacks in transfer payments to the provinces have decreased to about 10% of provincial healthcare expenditures. The cumulative loss of revenue to the provinces as a result of Ottawa's unilateral funding cuts to health between 1985 and 1996 totalled $30 billion (Fuller, 1996). This has led to large-scale decentralisation of medical services, with hospital closures, the contracting out of medical services and referring to patients as customers, which reinforces a corporate slant on healthcare. In addition, the federal government's power to obtain provincial compliance with the Canada Health Act has been impaired (Clark, 1997). A recent survey of Canadian nurses showed that these factors have led to understaffing that has been endangering patient care (CCPA, 1995).

The nurses surveyed who work in acute-care hospitals said they would need 50% more time than they are now given to provide adequate care to their patients. In addition, 'in acute-care hospitals, nurses attribute nearly two-thirds of reported accidents and errors to inadequate staffing on their units' (CCPA, 1996). Provinces have moved to contain costs in the hospital sector by implementing US-style treatment guidelines designed to discharge patients earlier than previously done in Canada. One Canadian nurse, who has been in practice for the past 25 years, illustrated the dangers of this system:

> *'Mothers and their newborns are being discharged six hours after delivery. We have four mothers going through one bed in a day . . . New mothers are not trained to notice some of the signs, like jaundice, for instance. By the time we get them back, they are in such bad shape. We end up having the babies back in the emergency room.'*
>
> (CLC, 1996)

The US model of for-profit healthcare and private insurance is much admired by entrepreneurs. However, it is also expensive, corrupt, inefficient and hazardous to public health. Whether measured in absolute dollars or as a percentage of the national economy, the US has the world's most expensive healthcare system. In addition, 'despite this enormous expenditure, the US lags behind most developed nations on the most basic measures of health, health coverage, and economic efficiency' (Meech and Askin, 1996). Unfortunately, the Canadian healthcare system is moving toward this system as NAFTA progresses. NAFTA was not designed to shield healthcare or other social services, but was designed to open up the Canadian economy to multinational corporations. As Canada harm- onises its standards with those south of the border, it should be remembered that in the US 40 million people, many of them children, have no healthcare insurance, and 30 million more are grossly underinsured (Nader, 1996).

At the international level, according to the Canadian International Development Agency, more than 1 billion people world-wide still live in a state of absolute poverty, meaning they are unable to meet their own essential needs. This situation affects women in particular, who represent 60% of these people. On average, women have less access than men to resources, education and healthcare. They single-handedly shoulder a large part of the task of providing basic care and maintaining life within families — a task whose economic value is still not recognised (CIDA, 1996). With this being the case in most developing nations, harmonisation as a result of NAFTA should be avoided. However, Canadian women appear to be losing ground. The poverty rate for single women under 65 years of age rose from 40% in 1993 to 45% in 1994 (ECEJ, 1997).

The content of NAFTA is clear in illustrating the vulnerability of Canada's healthcare system under this agreement:

- Article 1102 places all Canadian health services under the agreement
- Articles 1102 and 1202 require Canada and its provinces to accord US health service providers the same treatment as Canadian providers, without exception
- Chapter 15 erects insurmountable barriers to returning privatised health services to public ownership. For example, once a service like home-care is privatised, it will be almost impossible to reclaim these services under universal healthcare. This will limit elderly women's access to home-care, because these services will be profit-driven under privatisation
- Article 1029(b) in effect obliges Canada to progressively remove restrictions that prevent US health service providers from operating in Canada on the same basis as Canadian providers. (Clark, 1997)

Conclusions

The advancement of NAFTA has jeopardised Canadian women's health and welfare to the benefit of corporate interest. When commenting on NAFTA, a veteran trade negotiator, Mel Clark, stated, 'During 26 years as a civil servant and trade negotiator, I never witnessed such a complete accommodation of corporate interest, with such lethal consequences for Canada and its citizens' (Clark, 1997). As already stated, this is not a free trade agreement but a corporate investment agreement that elevates the advantage of the few with the largest concentration of wealth by taking advantage of cheaper labour and non-existent labour protection laws at the expense of workers.

However, there are solutions. Women can gain ground. Canadian women can demand that the government not relinquish its right to regulate trade at their expense, but should represent women's interests at the bargaining table and ensure that their health and welfare is protected under any trade agreement upon which Canada embarks. They must hold the current Canadian government accountable to their election platform promise to protect and promote women's health. Canadian women can align with non-governmental organisations, healthcare unions and other healthcare advocacy groups who research issues resulting from globalisation and trade agreements that affect women's health and welfare. A lack of information in this area is obvious. Information needs to be improved through publications and presentations on this and related topics. By increasing awareness and knowledge, women can unite and place pressure on governments to ensure the representation of their interests. This pressure can increase accountability of governments that will have an impact on both internal and external policies regarding their health and welfare needs. As a result, globalisation will be guided by women who advocate for the protection of their healthcare and other social rights.

References

Campbell B (1992) *Canada Under Siege: Three Years into the Free Trade Era*. Candian Centre for Policy Alternatives, Ottawa

[CCPA] Canadian Centre for Policy Alternatives (1995) *CCPA Monitor* March

[CCPA] Canadian Centre for Policy Alternatives (1996) *CCPA Monitor* July/August

[CIDA] Canadian International Development Agency (1996) *Strategy for Health*

Clark M (1997) NAFTA fails to protect Canada's healthcare system. *CCPA Monitor* May: 12–13

[CLC] Canadian Labour Congress (1997) *Women's work: A report*

[CLC] Canadian Labour Congress (1996)

[ECEJ] Ecumenical Coalition for Economic Justice (1994)

[ECEJ] Ecumenical Coalition for Economic Justice (1996) *Economic Justice Report*, **7**(4)

[ECEJ] Ecumenical Coalition for Economic Justice (1997)

Fuller C (1996) Doctoring to NAFTA. *Can For* June: 14–18

Fuller C (1996b) The Monitor, **4**(5).Canadian Center for Policy Alternative, Ottawa, Canada: 18

Grinspun R (1993) NAFTA and neoconservative transformation: The impact on Canada and Mexico. *Rev Rad Pol Econ* **25**(4): 14–29

McBride S, Shields J (1993) *Dismantling a Nation: Canada and the New World Order*. Fernwood Publishing, Halifax

Meech C, Askin S (1996,) US firms push healthcare privatization. *CCPA Monitor* November: 1, 6

Nader R (1996) Stop Americanizing Medicare, Nader warns us. *CCPA Monitor* February: 16–17

Nova S, Sforza-Roderick M (1997) After FTA, NAFTA, brace yourself for the MAI. *CCPA Monitor* April: 1, 5

Woman to Woman Global Strategies (1993) *Changing economies: Free trade and the global agenda: Bringing women into the picture*. Correspondencia, Toronto

26

'Why don't you stay inside?': The stigma of obesity and its effects on women's health

Dale Gietzelt

According to Allon (1975), of all conditions for which a person may be stigmatised in the west (ie. race/ethnicity, religion, physical disability or sexual preference), the stigma of overweight may be the most debilitating. Its immediate visibility has the potential to affect most social interactions, not only because it is perceived as unaesthetic and ugly, but also because the obese person is held responsible for her or his own state.

The attitude shines through in the results of my ongoing research into the stigma of obesity in Sydney, Australia. Some 300 randomly selected householders in six geographically, ethnically and socioeconomically diverse areas of Sydney were asked questions about their perceptions and attitudes toward obesity. The survey used open-ended questions, a five-point Likert scale of agreement for 56 questions and a section examining the social acceptability of different body sizes for women and men aged about 30 and girls and boys aged 10. In Phase 2, obese women were recruited from Phase 1 to discuss on a one-to-one basis their feelings and experiences. Phase 3 will survey selected health professionals about their attitudes.

When respondents[1] were asked to describe their thoughts when they first saw an obese person in the street, some took on a **belligerent** tone: 'I am very much against obesity'; 'if they want to lose weight, they could'; 'why don't they do something about it?'; their condition is 'easily rectified'; and 'they don't like to work'.

> *A lot are not trying to lose weight — you see them eating the wrong food.*
>
> *Depends on the circumstances. If they're walking out of McDonald's, it's one thing. . .*
>
> *I have to make way for them.*
>
> *They don't push themselves away from the table.*

Others are just **rude**: 'if they're too big, I feel sick'; 'I don't like it'; 'you fat bastard'; 'gross'; 'grotesque'; 'abnormal'; and 'smelly'.

> *Huge — wow! Can't see a bone! Are humans like that?*
>
> *Oh God, look how fat they are!*

The other responses reveal a rich diversity of attitudes toward the obese. First, there were some **neutral** comments ('I have no particular conception' and 'as long as they're happy') and **positive** comments ('I feel respect for them').

> *I treat obese people just the same as the rest of the population.*
>
> *I feel strongly about people abusing or making rude comments about obese people.*
>
> *We shouldn't judge people.*

Some **sympathise**: 'must be hard to find nice clothes'; 'they need help' 'some look unhappy with the way they are'; 'must get tired easily' 'they're not obese by choice'; 'maybe they can't help it, even though they try'; and 'it's not their fault'. There are also those who **seek a reason** to explain what seems to be perceived as an anomaly: 'medication can cause you to put on weight'; 'must be diseased' or 'sick'; 'a health/ medical/glandular/thyroid/hormonal/ metabolic problem'; 'could be an environmental problem'; 'could be a genetic/inherited problem'; 'could be cultural'; and 'maybe they've been ill'.

> *People are not always overweight because they eat too much. They could have a sickness that we don't know about.*
>
> *Is it glandular? If it is, then I feel very sorry.*

Most responses, however, fit into the various stereotypes for obesity: ugly, fat, lonely, lazy or idle, overeats, huge, eats fatty foods/takeaways (take-outs), happy or jolly, slow, lack of self-esteem, greedy, self-indulgent and inactive.

I differentiate between obese men and women. With an obese man, I have no real reaction. Being heterosexual, I see things differently, eg. at a party, the last person I'd spend time with is a really overweight woman. I'd talk to an overweight man and not worry. I think [obese] men are more visually attractive.

If you are in a shopping centre the bigger people are the ones eating cream buns, chips and ice creams.

Others took on a **dictatorial** tone: obese people '**should** lose weight', '**should** cut down a bit', '**should** go on a diet', '**should** stop eating the things they like most', '**should** exercise', '**should** dress to suit their shape', '**should** go to 'Gloria Marshall'[2] (emphasis added).

I think they should close fast food shops — they're not for the young, the old or the obese. There should be scales at the door. [Should ban] cars too, they don't get enough exercise. Too much good things [sic] too early.

Some people lose weight and then put it on again. They should stop eating fatty food.

Some were somewhat **condescending:** 'often they look very attractive in the face'; 'some are warm-hearted' or 'nice-natured'; 'some are intelligent'; 'a bit stupid'; 'poor person' and 'they lose their looks'. Some took a **pitying** tone: what a waste!'; 'how unnecessary'; 'I feel sorry for them'; and 'what a pity'.

If they're ***abnormally*** *obese, I would feel very sorry for them. [emphasis added]*

Finally, there were those who revealed a **double standard**:

I have great sympathy for people who have a medical condition — my comments only really apply to people who let themselves go.

It's terrible but I was thinking, 'Why do you present yourself? Why don't you stay inside?'

Obese people were characterised as slow, pleasant, insecure, clean, unhappy, invariable, calm, weak, heavy, delicate, modest, optimistic, capable, passive, large, extroverted, relaxed, willing, likeable, static, prudent, intelligent, warm, kind and brave. However, different subgroups held comparatively more negative or more positive positions than the average. For instance, men were more negative than women at a rate of 2:1; younger (under 35s) were more negative than their older counterparts, as were the so-called 'normal' — and overweight, high- income earners compared with low-income earners (though only two-thirds of respondents provided their annual household income), those with postgraduate qualifications compared with those with only a primary, trade certificate or school certificate education; and those from central Europe and Israel (although this must be viewed with caution, since sample sizes were small), compared to the more positive Aboriginal and South American respondents (again, with small sample sizes).

Many of these subgroups continued to express similar attitudes in the next section of the questionnaire, which dealt less with characteristics of the obese and more with overall attitudes. Again, males expressed more negative opinions than females, the overweight and, this time, the obese themselves showed more negativity, as did those with postgraduate qualifications (especially those with master's degrees), while university students were the most positive subgroup, followed by those with only a primary school education. Respondents from the Indian subcontinent, southeast Asia, southern Europe and eastern Asia expressed the most negative attitudes, while the South American, Fijian Indians (interestingly), Aboriginal and eastern European were the most positive. Middle-income earners ($A40,000 to $A70,000) were more positive than either low- or high-income earners.

In the next section, respondents were asked to peruse four cards with eight silhouette figures on each, signifying a smaller and larger underweight, normal weight, overweight and obese person for women and men aged 30 years and girls and boys aged 10 years. The results, as seen in *Figure 26.1*, indicated that there was greater social acceptability in the Sydney sample for:

- an overweight woman than an overweight man (though the difference between obese men and women is negligible)
- for a larger boy than girl.

This latter result coincides with data from another Australian study. In a focus group of mothers of obese children in Melbourne, differences in how the stigma of obesity affected children of each sex surfaced:

'All mothers of girls in the programme reported them as being sensitive about their weight and fearful of teasing and ostracization. Mothers of boys thought their sons were not

embarrassed and were accepted by society. Most of the group felt that there was cultural disapproval of fat girls in Australian society but that fat boys were tolerated as long as they were physically fit and outgoing'.

(Court *et al*, 1977)

This could in part be due to how girls and boys have been traditionally socialised: females deriving their value and status from how they look, and males from what they achieve. But this does not explain the surprising results of overweight women being more accepted than overweight men. This can to some extent be explained by the fact that, not only did women comprise some two-thirds of the sample, but males once again showed themselves as less tolerant of larger sizes than women, who may possibly have greater empathy for other women struggling to control their weight.

From the data presented here, it is clear that obesity carries with it a value judgement: few people are neutral toward obesity. Stigmatisation and negative evaluation exist, and it is important to ascertain both the extent of their stigmatisation and the impact it has on the stigmatised, not least because stigmatisation can result in a variety of harms to people (Gilmore and Somerville, 1994). Stigma often imposes constraints on an individual's lifestyle. Lost social opportunities may mean reduced life chances. At its most practical level, the exclusion, marginalisation and disempowerment engendered through stigmatisation (even through fear of ridicule or a look of repulsion on the faces of health professionals) can impede access to preventive services, such as pap smears and breast examinations.

Plain (1978), who undertook her research in Canberra, Australia's capital, found that most women in her study led socially isolated lives. She suggested that social isolation leads to obesity, but it could be argued that obesity leads to social isolation. Various studies have highlighted how obesity and poor body image (Allon, 1979; Fuller and Groce, 1991), low self-esteem (Manus and Killeen, 1995; Martin *et al*, 1988), self-deprecation (Cahnman, 1968; Crocker *et al*, 1993), depression (Ross, 1994), loneliness (Elder, 1969; Fuller and Groce, 1991; Schumacker *et al*, 1985; Vener *et al*, 1982; Walster *et al*, 1966), lack of confidence in social encounters (Hill and Silver, 1995;

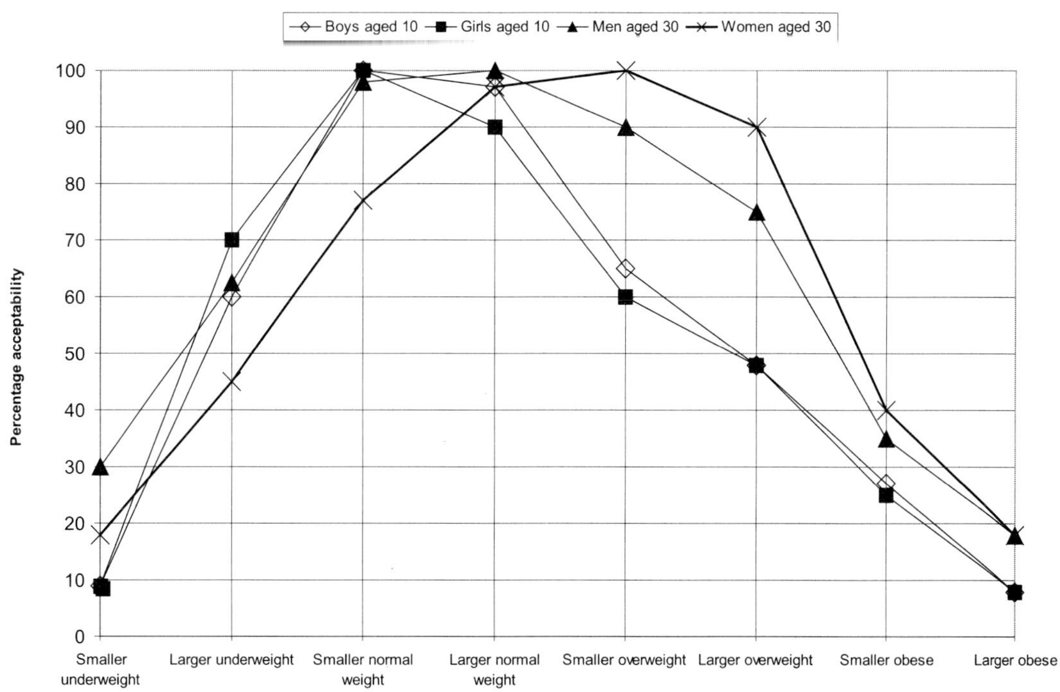

Figure 26.1: Social acceptability of body size, according to gender and age

Miller *et al*, 1990) and being made to feel at odds with one's surrounding space (what English (1993) calls a 'violation of territory') often, but not always, go hand-in-hand. Fear of territory violation forces the obese into avoiding certain social situations, thereby contributing significantly, along with public ridicule, to their sense of social isolation (English, 1993).

These psychosocial issues frequently influence the obese person's sense of identity, especially for women. If obese people are constantly under the gaze of others, being judged harshly if they are seen eating an ice cream or coming out of a fast-food outlet, then obese women are doubly burdened, since other women scrutinise and judge them; their competency in playing the game for male approval by abandoning what is both acceptable and aesthetic is called into question and their social identity corrupted. An informant stated:

> *'People can't stand the thought that some people don't conform to their ideas of 'normal' and [they] do everything they can to bring [those] people down. It's sort of an inverse Tall Poppy Syndrome. It's not trying to drag the high achievers down to an . . . egalitarian level; it's more . . . trying to drag others down from an egalitarian level to something even lower. I mean, what's their problem? Are they threatened by big people?[3]'*

Stigmatisation can also occur through its potential to harm by dehumanising the obese person. An example of depersonalisation was related to me by a middle-aged female, obese informant:

> *'I was walking down a city street about 9 or 10'clock at night with my husband. A group of three drunken males approached us, and said as they passed us, 'You're not fucking that, are you, mate? She's like Jabba the Hutt' [from the Star Wars movie — a great behemoth]. That showed . . . the total rejection of [me as] a fat, ugly woman. But it was more than that: I was an alien, dehumanised to something not even animal-like, but out of this world. I think from that moment onwards, my husband has been uncomfortable being seen in public with me, believe it or not.'*

This latter is what Goffman (1968) refers to as 'courtesy stigma', whereby a person is stigmatised or devalued based on her or his association with a a stigmatised person. Fear of courtesy stigma towards 'normals' probably leads to their avoiding stigmatised individuals, thereby contributing to the obese person's social isolation and, presumably sometimes, shame.

Not all obese people are affected similarly. Some are severely affected in the ways outlined above; others, however, take the negativity in their stride and do not let it hamper the way they carry out their lives. Why the distinction? Fuller and Groce (1991) may have the answer. They found two types of obese female informants. The first emerged from a childhood fraught with castigation and ostracisation, with low or negative self-esteem. Such women described themselves negatively, defining themselves as 'overweight' rather than 'obese'. They were the group most aware of their size and were constantly embarking on weight reduction techniques. The second type also emerged from an alienated childhood, but their identities were not engulfed by their body size. 'They [seemed] to see themselves and their lives in a holistic sense which [enabled] them to take pride in their educational and professional accomplishments' (Fuller and Groce, 1991). Such women have been able to dissociate themselves from the prevailing cultural standards of appearance and find satisfaction and a strong sense of self-worth through their achievements.

The latter group appear to accept their size as just one aspect of their being, and for the most part seem to embrace life fully, even when it comes to going to the doctor. However, this is not the case with all obese women.

Despite the possibility of being trained **not** to discriminate against any patient, evidence from around the western world suggests that the attitudes of doctors often reflect and correspond to the attitudes of the general community, that is, with negativity. An example of this can be seen in a letter to the major daily newspaper, *The Sydney Morning Herald* (16 May 1981), by a doctor from the city's eastern suburbs:

> *'It is high time that those who choose through gluttony and sloth to burden their bodies with excess fat were made to bear the costs in terms of higher insurance premiums, excess weight charges on airlines and other such direct measures'.*

Uniformly negative reactions of doctors toward obese patients have been found in various studies (Adams *et al*, 1993; Maddox and Liederman, 1969; Najman *et al*, 1982; Price *et al*, 1987). Third-year American medical students also demonstrated almost uniformly negative responses toward the so-called morbidly obese, and their negative feelings did not change after contact with such patients (Blumberg and Mellis, 1985).

First-year Australian medical students showed the strongest negative reactions toward obese patients compared to others, such as alcoholics or those with heart disease (Najman and Arnold, 1984).

Anecdotal evidence enriches the findings of these studies. For example, as proof that some doctors take their stereotypes of obese people into the consulting room with them, an obese American woman stated:

> *'I went to this gynaecologist, and she was taking down the questions, and she goes 'And you're not sexually active now, are you?' And I said, 'Well, yes, I am sexually active.' 'Oh, are you?' 'Yes, I am.' So she's examining me and she's talking about this, that, and the other thing, and then she says again, 'You know, if you were sexually active, I'd do this, or that, or whatever,' and I said, 'Well, I am sexually active. I'm very active now, sexually.' [Then] she was talking about my period, and how I didn't need it unless I wanted to get pregnant, but I'm probably not sexually active. And I couldn't believe it. [Finally on] my paper work, she wrote something about 'sexual activity — none.'*
>
> [Anonymous, 1994]

A similar incident occurred with one of my own informants who was attending a new gynaecologist to discuss a certain treatment, a side effect of which would be sterility. This obese married woman was hoping to conceive and did not want to undertake any treatment that would impede a possible pregnancy. Although she had written on her card that she was married, the gynaecologist said:

> *'Let's be realistic here. You're 43 years old. First you have to find a man and then you have to try to have a baby with him.' That doctor [said the informant] just assumed that because I'm fat, nobody would want to be in a relationship with me. Fat equals ugly which equals unloved and unlovable. She shouldn't have assumed I was single; she could've easily asked if I was in a relationship!'*

An obese Sydney woman (Mrs S), who had been hospitalised with what was later diagnosed as the relatively unknown Idiopathic Odema Syndrome, could not get the doctors to take her pain seriously:

> *'A specialist Doctor K operated at King George V Hospital [in Sydney] . . . and put a sling on my bladder. He didn't listen to me when I tried to tell him about my syndrome. Or how I develop infections easily because of my illness. He thought I was just fat. I should have had intravenous antibiotics before my operation, but he gave me two pills instead. The result was a massive infection, heart complaints, and I ended up in intensive care. I was in hospital for eight weeks instead of ten days. Because he would not listen to me, I now need surgery every twelve months to keep a passage open for urine. I feel that doctors do not believe me, and they make me feel like a stupid woman.'*
>
> (Connolly, 1995)

Mrs S stressed that 'doctors make comments without knowing your background or problems. They assume that I eat too much.' One incident that occurred about 10 or 11 years ago highlighted the distress she has been forced to suffer through stigmatised attitudes of doctors.

> *'Well they think they are God! One time when I was in Westmead Outpatients [in Sydney], and was having trouble with my veins, a doctor saw me through an open door, and both my husband and I heard him say to his interns, 'Don't waste my time, look at her size!' This doctor took my dignity away.'*
>
> (Connolly, 1995)

It should come as no surprise then, that studies in North America and Europe have shown a reluctance on the part of obese people to visit their primary care providers (Adams *et al*, 1993; De Waard *et al*, 1984; Torgerson *et al*, 1994), owing at least in part to the reactions to their obesity, and also to the fact that furniture and equipment often fail to cater to their special needs (Anonymous, 1992). Furthermore, reluctance on the part of heavyweight people to attend clinics for health checks has been found in several studies. A study of non-attenders to a health promotion clinic aimed at reducing cardiovascular disease showed they were heavier in weight than those who did attend (Waller *et al*, 1990). Non-attenders at an osteoporosis clinic in Britain weighed more than attenders, even after controlling for social class (Torgerson *et al*, 1994). A Dutch breast-screening programme also revealed a higher body weight for non-attenders than for attenders (De Waard *et al*, 1984). Another study (Adams *et al*, 1993) found reluctance on the part of both physicians and obese women to undertake pelvic examinations. Such unwillingness to initiate an encounter with health professionals is potentially very serious and life-threatening.

'I've gone to doctors for minor complaints and come out suicidal because of what the doctor said to me. You know . . . a doctor really has the ability to make you want to die in a lot of ways that are direct and indirect. It certainly makes you want to never come back, and ultimately, if you happen to have some disease process, that can kill you.'

(Anonymous, 1994)

However, I believe we need to reconsider whether obesity and overweight are actually unhealthy states *per se*. It is certainly commonly thought so. Almost 70% of my respondents agreed or strongly agreed with the statement, 'A person who is very overweight is not a healthy person'. I would first like to suggest that we start to view obesity in much the same way we do old age. Old age is a risk factor for cardiovascular disease, breast cancer and prostate cancer, among others; but just because one is old does not mean one has these illnesses; one is just **more prone** to them. Similarly, obesity is a risk factor for cardiovascular disease, hypertension and diabetes; but just because a person is obese does not automatically mean he/she has these illnesses or conditions; he/she is just **more prone** to them. In other words, you can be a healthy older person and you can be a healthy obese person (though chances are you may be **unfit**, which is a different matter entirely). While obesity is a risk factor for certain conditions and diseases, it is not unhealthy in its own right, and is actually beneficial in some conditions like osteoporosis, something not publicised by the medical profession or public health workers. We must ask ourselves why the negatives of obesity are highly propagated and the positives hushed up.

Biomedicine tends to treat all people presenting the same symptoms in the same manner, ignoring any individualised causality or social factors impinging on the person. This holds true for the 'problem' of obesity, too. Since the 1950s, biomedicine has increasingly defined obesity as a medical problem (Turner, 1987). Treatment under the biomedical model generally centres on curbing excessive eating and exercise, and any psychosocial elements at the root of this 'abnormal' eating pattern are neglected.

If physicians place emphasis on the conduct of the individual, in terms of their lifestyle, then some larger individuals may feel too ashamed to visit their health practitioners unless their weight reduction has been both 'properly treated' and 'successful', despite the overall lack of success of such programs (Garner and Wooley, 1991). While obese people continue to be blamed for not adhering to weight-reduction techniques, they continue to be held responsible for their 'deviant' condition, and this may well have adverse effects on their seeking healthcare.

This is where our health promotion campaigns are failing. One way of improving the overall health of obese women is to educate the public in general, and the health professions in particular, into size acceptance. If an obese woman feels accepted and not pitied or judged critically, she is more likely to seek medical attention and participate in health checks prior to a symptom proceeding to something serious. To achieve this, one thing we need to be careful of is the apportioning of blame and moral deficiency for the state of obesity. The data presented here go some way towards targeting particular sectors or groups in Australian society that hold less tolerant views. The findings also show that there is a tendency to differentiate the reasons behind a person's obesity into those whose own actions (such as overeating, eating the wrong foods or failing to exercise) incur their weight 'problems' and those who are big through no fault of their own (genetics, glandular or hormonal problems, or thorough certain medications). This coincides with popular attitudes towards AIDS: the blameless versus the others who brought it on themselves.

References

Adams CH, Smith NJ, Wilbur DC, Grady KE (1993) The relationship of obesity to the frequency of pelvic examinations: Do physician and patient attitudes make a difference? *Women Health* 20(2): 45–57

Allon N (1975) The stigma of overweight in everyday life. In: Bray G, ed. *Obesity in Perspective*. US Government Printing Office, Washington, DC: 130–74

Allon N (1979) Self-perceptions of the stigma of overweight in relationship to weight-losing patterns. *Am J Clin Nut* **32**: 470–80

Anonymous (1992) Dealing with large patients in health care. *Obes Health*, Sept/Oct: 93

Anonymous (1994) Overweight: Dr Fat-Attack. *Psychol Today* **27**(2): 10

Blumberg P, Mellis LP (1985) Medical students' attitudes toward the obese and the morbidly obese. *Int J Eat Disord* **4**(2): 169–75

Cahnman WJ (1968) The stigma of obesity. *Sociol Q* Summer: 283–99

Connolly D (1995) Personal communication (transcript of interview with an obese Sydney woman)

Court JM, Johns N, Wilson M (1977) Obese children and thier families: A study of a discussion group. *Aus Paed J* **13**: 170–5

Crocker J, Cornwell E, Major B (1993) The stigma of overweight: Affective consequences of attributional ambiguity. *J Personal Soc Psychol* **64**(1): 60–70

De Waard F, *et al* (1984) The Dom project for the early detection of breast cancer. *J Chron Dis* **37**: 1–44

Elder GH (1969) Appearance and education in marriage mobility. *Am Sociol Rev* **34**: 519–33

English C (1993) Gaining and losing weight: Identity transformation. *Deviant Behav Interdis J* 14: 227–41

Fuller ML, Groce SB (1991) Obese women's responses to appearance norms. *Free Inq Creat Sociol* **19**(2): 167–74

Garner DM, Wooley SC (1991) Confronting the failure of behavioral and dietary treatments for obesity. *Clin Psychol Rev* **11**: 729–80

Gilmore N, Somerville MA (1994) Stigmatization, scapegoating and discrimination in sexually transmitted diseases: Overcoming "Them" and "Us." *Soc Sci Med* **39**(9): 1339–58

Goffman E (1968) *Stigma: Notes on the Management of Spoiled Identiy*. Penguin/Pelican, Harmondsworth

Hill AJ, Silver EK (1995) Fat, friendless and unhealthy: 9-year-old children's perception of body shape stereotypes. *Int J Obes* **19**: 423–30

Maddox GL, Liederman V (1969) Overweight as a social disability with medical implications. *J Med Educ* **44**: 214–20

Manus H, Killeen M (1995) Maintenance of self-esteem by obese children. ??*JCAPN*?? in full. Journal not listed under this shortform?? **8**: 17–27

Martin S, Housley K, McCoy H *et al* (1988) Self-esteem of adolescent girls as related to weight. *Percept Mot Skills* **67**: 879–84

Miller CT, Rothblum ED, Barbour L, Brand PA, Felicio D (1990) Social interactions of obese and nonobese women. *J Pers* **58**(2): 365–80

Najman JM, Arnold L (1984) An initial explanatory model of medical students' preferences for patient types. *Med Educ* **18**: 249–54

Najman JM, Klein D, Monro C (1982) Patient characteristics negatively stereotyped by doctors. *Soc Sci Med* **16**: 1781–9

Plain JM (1978) Obesity: A product of isolation in society. *Women's Health in a Changing Society*. Proceedings of a Conference on All Aspects of Women's Health, Commonwealth Department of Health. Australian Government Printing Service, Canberra: 141–7

Price JH, Desmond SM, Krol RA, Snyder FF, O'Connor JK (1987) Family practice physicians' beliefs, attitudes, and practices regarding obesity. *Am J Prev Med* **3**(6): 339–45

Ross CE (1994) Overweight and depression. *J Health Soc Behav* **35**: 63–78

Schumacker JF, Krejci RC, Small L, Sargent RG (1985) Experience of loneliness by obese individuals. *Psychol Rep* **57**: 1147–54

Torgerson DJ, *et al* (1994) Population screening for osteoporosis: Do non-attenders have a lower risk of osteoporosis? *Osteopor Int* **4**: 149–53

Turner BS (1987) *Medical Power and Social Knowledge* Sage, London

Vener AM, Krupka LR, Gerard RJ (1982) Overweight/obese patients: An overview. *Practit* **226**: 1102–9

Waller D, *et al* (1990) Health checks in general practice: Another example of inverse care? *Br Med J* **300**: 1115–18

Walster E, Aronson V, Abrahams D, Ratlmann L (1966) Importance of physical attractveness in dating behavior. *J Personal Soc Psychol* **4**: 508–16

Notes

1. Just over two-thirds of respondents were female, and over two-thirds were aged from 18 to 44 years. Fifty percent were Australian-born; a sixth came from Europe, an eighth from Asia and slightly less from Oceania. Aboriginal descent accounted for one percent. A total of 27.3% lived in a nuclear family with children under 14 years of age, while a sixth lived as a couple without children. More than a sixth had matriculation as their highest educational level, with 27.6% having tertiary qualifications, 46% having not finished high school and a tenth still studying. Self-reporting both height and weight; 8.3% were obese, 22% were overweight, almost 60% were normal weight and 10% were underweight.
2. Catering to women only, 'Gloria Marshall Figure Salons' are a weight-reducing company in Australia specialising in calorie-controlled diets and exercise centres.
3. In Australia, the Tall Poppy Syndrome occurs when a successful and pre-eminent person is criticised mercilessly by the public and the media, as if they have become 'too big for their boots'. This is how the 'tall poppy', which has struggled to raise its head above the other 'poppies', gets cut back down to size.

27

Drug addiction: Can we learn something about ourselves and about the society we live in?

Thalia Attié

The phenomenon of drug addiction as we know it is a product of our modern occidental society, and is expanding far beyond the frontiers of any one country. This chapter attempts to see what we can learn from this phenomenon, for ourselves and for the society in which we live.

What has changed in the conditions of drug addiction or toxicomania?

We are obliged to recognise that the conditions of drug addiction or toxicomania have changed since the mid-twentieth century. The phenomenon has been expanding from the societies of scarcity to the societies of abundance. We can raise the question: abundance of what? An abundance of goods? Elder writes that after the economic crisis of the 1930s, and then the Second World War, even if parents tried to transmit the values and hopes of a better world to their children, the unconscious message was the failure of the hope of progress; the end of faith in science and in the fundamental goodness of social nature; and the loss of the security of knowing where humanity was aiming (Elder, quoted in Roussel, 1989). A gap opened. Public gratifications were devalued relative to private ones; this was reflected in the family. Some years later, these were partly abandoned to the benefit of individual gratifications, as we shall see, from the 1970s on. It could be that the generations following those of the 1930s and 1940s resented this lack of hope and the collapse of the beliefs in human values dictated by society, and this led in large part to the movements of the 'communities' in the 1960s. Abundance and economic welfare were not enough to give a sense of meaning to a person's life.

A second turning point occurred in the 1970s because of the way that drugs were ingested. While the 1960s were the era of 'H', and marijuana sustained the ideology of 'peace and love', from the 1970s onwards there were major changes in the consumption of drugs:

1. Ideology no longer supported drug-taking — it became a personal matter;
2. At the same time, the products lacked 'fidelity'. In part, this can be explained by the number of products that could be found in the market, but as we question the expansion of the drug phenomenon, so may we question this fact. Does it reflect a lack of 'constance of object', experienced in the early years of existence, and reaffirmed by the use of disposable objects, or to put it another way, by a society of 'waste-makers' (Packard, 1963), or does it reflect a search for something 'more', due as much to personal experiences as to a mass media society?
3. The number of consumers is increasing while the age of the first ingestion of the product is decreasing;
4. During the last decade, other changes have occurred that affect drug addiction or toxicomania. Rhythm, rite and social control have disappeared in drug use. This may be partly explained by what we said earlier, ie. the vanishing of rite and social control could reflect the loss of credibility in social values and ideology. However, these factors also reveal the changes of notions of time and space that constitute the body image of the person and are consequently an essential part of identity. It seems that time and space are no longer ruled by society as an anchor for the individual in the world, but rather as tools to be used efficiently. We shall discuss body image further below.
5. Finally, what addicts usually search for is the 'flash' stimulation, violent sensations, the oblivion

or stupefaction. As one searcher wrote, they search to fill the emptiness they feel, or to get rid of the over-stimulation they receive.

What is happening in our society that pushes adults, adolescents and even children to look for external, artificial magic ways of reinforcing feelings that they wholly exist, or to try to forget their living condition?

By analysing the changes of conditions of drug addiction, we became aware of some facets or some changes in our society. Before answering the question asked, we shall analyse the characteristics of the drug addict and what conditions are needed to be a toxicomaniac.

Drug addicts

The four types of addict:

1. Recreational addicts consume drugs occasionally. They can generally be found in specific circles.
2. There are those who use drugs regularly for physical or psychological reasons.
3. There are also occasional or temporary drug addicts. In some conditions, people can use heavy drugs, but they stop when conditions change. The best example of this phenomenon are the heroin consumers of Vietnam who stopped using the drug once they were back home.
4. Finally, there are the real toxicomaniacs.

These four categories should be dealt with separately, although they are frequently treated without any distinction in most cases. This includes: by legal authorities (penalties, jail, etc), families, the media and medical/scientific authorities, where we find a lack of precision in terms of vocabulary: addictions include love addiction, television addiction, work addiction, etc. This reveals another phenomenon in our society at the end of the twentieth century: the inflation of language, or what could be called the unbearable lightness of the language (Attié, 1993), which deprives individuals of another essential reference in their lives.

Factors needed to become an addict

To become a drug consumer, several factors need to be identified:

1. some kind of constitution or some neuro-biological conditions;
2. some elements or experiences that, joined together during infancy, form a special combination of family and social history;
3. a certain type of society.

Two other factors that cannot be forgotten, to which Olievenstein (1983) draws attention, are:

1. the 'hazard' or the 'encounter' with the product at a specific moment;
2. the 'voluntariness' or the will to decide whether to continue or to try to stop taking the drug.

All these conditions are necessary, but not sufficient, for a person to become an addict. Some people possess all these characteristic but do not become drug addicts.

The drug addict's personality

The recurring characteristics of the majority of drug addicts are:

1. A profound affective 'failure' due to the relationship with the mother. This does not mean that the mother is guilty, but that something went wrong in this relationship at an unconscious level. This could be due to the mother's infant history, to her later experiences, to the state of the actual family, to her conjugal history, etc;
2. dysfunction in the family: an absent father, physically or symbolically, ie. as a representative figure of the law (Lacan, 1966); or merely a parent's affective immaturity that prevents satisfactory identification with parental images;
3. Above all, in adulthood, a failure to find stable and satisfactory identification figures in the outside world.

These factors help develop:

- a dependent, auto-aggressive personality that challenges authority, searching at the same time for an identity at different levels
- relationships with one's own body that are more at a behavioural level than at an appraised symbolic authentic one
- relationships with others that are constrained by distance and a lack of profound affective implication
- some diffuse culpability.

We can see how our society tends to create individuals of this type who are not necessarily drug addicts. Nevertheless, to become a toxicomaniac, other factors are necessary. The 'failure' or trauma of the possible future toxicomaniac had to happen before the infant could integrate the notion of time. This means that a mother's absence represented for him a definitive loss since he could not conceive a future where she could come back. Furthermore, according to Olievenstein (1983), this failure occurred during the mirror stage (cf. Lacan, 1966), in which the infant sees his own image in the mirror, becomes conscious of his unity, his identity and consequently becomes aware of his differentiation from the other. Olievenstein says that the toxicomaniac catches only a glimpse of his own image. The mirror fell apart. From then, his need is to regress to this stage and gain control of his unity through the drug.

This theory helps explain the toxicomaniac's need for recourse to 'magic' means that operate instantaneously and give him back sensations and body changes, together with feelings of power, and of the ability to change reality, even if it only lasts for the 'trip'.

The toxicomaniac's family

Again, there are differences between the family of the toxicomaniac and that of the drug addict. In general, the mother of the toxicomaniac is a person who did not desire her child, or if she did, her desire was different, to fill a gap: for example, to take the place of a dead child. In this way, the toxicomaniac-to-be finds himself filling a place that does not belong to him, a place out of phase with his own. Furthermore, in many cases, there is a mother's unconscious desire to 'devour' her child in order to stay young and not die — a mother who fights her own mortal anxiety (Olievenstein, 1983). In this context, the father is no longer a masculine virile figure, but is viewed as a weak person, 'unable to give sexual enjoyment to the mother' (Olievenstein, 1983).

In this type of family, not only the child's difficulty in establishing a stable sexual identity can be seen, but also an atmosphere of death anxiety, due to unelaborated griefs. This is combined with a gigantic ego ideal and its corollary of diffuse culpabilities. This atmosphere or 'melody' (Olievenstein, 1983) is experienced by the subject and, perhaps, by other family members as an impossibility of life.

Due as much to the failures in the infant's development as to the family conditions, traumas will repeat themselves throughout the person's history, and he may become a drug addict or a toxicomaniac. We are aware that, in any human life, positive 'repairing' (cf. Klein, 1968) experiences occur that can prevent the child, adolescent or adult, whose life characteristics follow the above pattern, from a fatal evolution to drugs.

The toxicomaniac's social surroundings and the world we are living in

At present, there is much discussion about the phenomenon of drug addiction and toxicomania. Is it that the toxicomaniac is the visible iceberg of other phenomena we do not want to see? Is he the caricature of our modern world, as Bergeret (1982) describes?

We shall briefly reiterate our previous descripton of the drug addict in general: a passive, dependent person who cannot bear a delay, and who feels thwarted: he is waiting for a reward that will never come. Auto-aggressive, defying authority, but, above all, in search of an identity.

What are the characteristics of our society of abundance that causes the development of such a personality?

1. As viewed by the author, the technological world in which we live, rather than the industrial society, radically changed the relationship of **time-space** to the human being, a relationship that is problematic for drug addicts. Indeed, to have a stable and coherent space for an infant nowadays seems to be an unattainable luxury. When he is not trailed about at a month old, or before, he is put in day nurseries before he is one year old. If he is unlucky, in these institutions or at home, the person who takes care of him changes. From childhood on, he learns that effortlessly, by just pushing a button, he is conveyed, not by imagination, but by a maniacal magic act to countless spaces and times that do not correspond with his. Casually, if he is taken out for a drive or to travel abroad, the child or pre-adolescent realises that reality is not the ideal portrayed on the television screen, unless he finds a mall, a McDonald's, the last soft drink of the moment, etc. in the place he is visiting. There is no space for sharing time

with adults or even with his peers in this conception of time and space. Even for adults who have some specific space-time conception, the new means of communication, both transport or telecommunications, have seriously shaken the scheme of things.

From this perspective, it is not surprising that the **body image** is weakened. This is further reinforced by our throwaway society, as from infancy onwards, diapers and milk bottles are labelled 'disposable'. Later, advertisements and even medical care view the body as separate parts, not as a valuable part of the person, but as a means of efficient performance.

3. **The development of language:** even language no longer fulfils its function; it is no longer a stable reference point. The development of language is vital if the ability to conceptualise what one thinks is not lost. This allows individuals to hold on to reality, to develop some critical sense and allows them to access their feelings.

   In the family, as at school, the child and then the adolescent learns the uselessness of personal communication unless he expresses what the adult wants him to say (Attié, 1989). Furthermore, it is well known that nobody is really interested in producing thinking human beings, since countless people think for them, nor feeling persons, since feelings are something dangerous that obstruct the rational functioning of matters (Attié, 1993). The result is people 'lacking in imagery' (Anatrella, 1990), diminished in their feelings, functionally illiterate, who interpret at a behavioural level, as toxicomaniacs do, what they cannot express verbally.

4. **Human references or possible images with which to identify.** We all collaborate in the development of the predominance of competition and the enthroning of the 'Money God' (Olievenstein, 1987). We accept a father's desertion and the subsequent loss of credibility in masculine values. The crisis of the institutions, of values and of ideologies, combined with the ego, social inflation and the urge to remain young, cause adults to offer a weakened or immature image, who lack the ability to compromise with their peers or with the society in which they live.

Our discussion of these points highlights the fact that our modern society lacks the ability to offer solid referents to children, adolescents or adults, at a time-space level, at a bodily integration level, at a conceptual level and at a deep human level.

Conclusion

Our technological society exacerbates needs, promotes the artificial at all levels, establishes no real sexual or individual level, drives us to develop an ill-focused aggressiveness that leads to violence and provokes a diffuse anxiety, even towards mere existence, anxiety in the face of which the person feels impotent.

This chapter has tried to identify some of the social characteristics that help to create personalities, whether toxicomaniac or not, which are dependent, impotent, passive, auto-aggressive, affectively immature, fearing human relationships. However, it is the toxicomaniac personality that reflects, in all its splendour, the society that produced it, its failures and its stumbling blocks, because it could not find in it a mirror, a guiding reflection that could orient it, in its search of another kind of identity.

References

Anatrella T (1990) *Interminables adolescences*. Paris: Cerf/Cujas

Attié T (1993) Violencia social silenciosa. *Psiquis* **2**(5): 111–15

Attié T (1989) Apprentissage de la lecture, apprentissage à la démobilisation? *Réel* **27**: 30

Bergeret J (1982) *Toxicomanie et personnalité*. PUF, Paris

Klein M. (1968) *Essais de psychanalyse (1921–1968)*. Payot, Paris

Lacan J (1966) *Ecrits*. Seuil, Paris

Olievenstein C (1983) *Destin du toxicomane*. Fayard, Paris

Olievenstein C (1987) *Le non-dit des émotions*. Odile Jacob, Paris

Packard V (1963) *The Waste Makers*. Pocket Book, New York

Roussel L (1989) *La famille incertaine*. Odile Jacob, Paris

28

Focussed services: Perceptions for care-givers in cancer in the UK

David Bullivent and Jacqueline Reeve

Literature review

With the implementation of various community policies and strategies in the United Kingdom, the needs of informal carers has supposedly been articulated, in that services have to be available and responsive to recipients' needs (Challis and Barton, 1990; Department of Health, 1989). As a part of this ongoing implementation of policies, and recognising the fact that deliberations in the UK have concentrated on institutional provision (Ebrahim *et al*, 1993), Plymouth Acute (NHS) Trust strove to continue to strengthen its relationship of mutual support with the informal carers within the local community, aimed at providing a better service for its patients and their carers. This was a natural step for a state organisation still pursuing the spirit of the Griffiths recommendations of innovation and commitment (Department of Health and Social Security, 1988).

Due to factors, such as advanced scientific technology and better living conditions, people are living longer, with a particular increase in those people aged 80 years and over (OPCS, 1991). Carers can be defined as those who 'are looking after, or providing some regular service for, someone who was sick, elderly or handicapped' (Green, 1988). Often, caring is assumed to be a natural event, and community care policies depend on contribution from informal carers. Such dependence has been viewed as an exploitative relationship that has been studied by theorists, such as Wilson (1982), Land and Rose (1985) and Dalley (1988).

Whether the relationship can be seen as exploitative or not, caring in a family unit is generally a private affair and we, as outsiders, can never know all that goes on (Boss, 1988; Biegel *et al*, 1991). This is because caring transcends both public and private lives, and thus the complex experiences and motivations involved in the role may be misunderstood (Biegel *et al*, 1991). It appears that caring requires a shift in relationship, for example, turning a normal father-daughter relationship to one where both members have to involve themselves in highly intimate activities. Such relationships depend on the concept of 'caring about', which Green's earlier, instrumental definition failed to take into account. Adams (1987) found 'caring about' is central to care-givers' perceptions of their role, and theorists such as Levin *et al* (1989) argue that affection and obligation are precursors to the care-giving role. Hirschfield (1983) also describes the relationship as a 'love for another', and it seems reciprocity is central in that the care-giver gains affection from the dependant and vice versa.

Despite this romantic view, caring is time-consuming and demanding, since it may involve two types of work. The first involves practical non-intimate assistance such as cleaning or shopping for someone. The second incorporates personal intimate care. The latter is more likely to be performed by relatives, due to its intimate nature (Henwood, 1990) and usually involves participating in activities such as comforting, dressing and washing another person. Such activities are not only time- consuming and intensely personal, but helping someone on and off the toilet or helping them mobilise can also be physically demanding (Twigg *et al*, 1990).

Equally demanding is the comforting role (Parker, 1981). Carers experience greater difficulties with this role if it is conducted over a long time and the receiver does not get better. They frequently feel tied down, suffer from lack of personal free time and develop feelings of resentment, hopelessness and guilt as a direct consequence of caring (Hirschfield, 1983; Levin *et al*, 1989). Despite this, carers usually remain in the care-giving relationship longer than they are able to cope with it (Pitkeathley, 1989). Similarly, others argue that carers try to protect the person they are caring for, by anticipating the need for future care and preventing the former coming to either physical or psychological harm. This is probably related to the concept of the family and their responsibilities to it and the person being cared for. Additionally, Sainsbury and Grad de Alarcon (1970) identified emotional disturbances in carers, with many suffering from headaches and depression and severe effects on family dynamics. The General Household Survey of Carers (Green, 1988) identified that nine-tenths of carers suffered with at least one persistent or recurring health problem.

Braithwaite (1990) found that carers experience increased levels of stress or emotional strain as a result of their caring responsibilities. Until carers realise they are in a stressful situation, it is difficult to do anything about it, and even when they do recognise it, the nature of the carers' relationship may have become ingrained (Graham, 1983). Consequently, the carer will not necessarily seek hospice care or professional help. Carers may even deny the extent of deterioration and suffering experienced by the person for whom they are caring (Adams, 1987), and this can act as a cognitive coping strategy. Additionally, the extent to which a family succumbs to stress will be dependent on that family's resources in terms of previous learning, finance and individual intrinsic strengths (Adams, 1987). On a more pragmatic point, if carers are stressed, they are less likely to be able to perform care and thus are more likely to seek professional help and thus resources.

It may seem to be natural to take on the informal role of care-giver and a person may be engaging in the role before even recognising it as such. However, theories of motivation in becoming a care-giver exist. One school centres on the fact that care-giving gives the carer an egotistical, self-serving motive, while the other is motivated by altruism and empathy (Bannister and Fransella, 1980). Finch and Mason (1990) identify guilt and indebtedness as reasons for becoming a carer. Other egotistical motives include the anticipation of reward, such as gaining social approval, or a fear of anticipated loneliness if the relationship is terminated.

If the motivation to care is empathy or altruism, then the benefit to the person to be cared for is uppermost. Motivation to care probably resulted in the well-known phrase 'labour of love', and Finch and Groves (1983) state that both labour and love are required in order to 'care'. Such care may result from filial obligations and duty, with Dawson (1987) showing that carers often cite their marriage vows as the reason for caring for their spouse. This is supported by Green's (1988) work, which found that out of all the different types of caring relationships, spouse carers are the least likely to have outside help. Similarly, Levin *et al* (1989) reported kinship and duty, the honouring of promises and lack of acceptable alternative options as other reasons for caring. Despite the rationale, it is important for service providers not to make assumptions about the easy extension of marital intimacy into other forms of physical intimacy (Parker, 1992).

Carers may also suffer from the social isolation imposed on them as a normal result of caring. For example, Henwood and Wicks (1984) found that a carer looking after an elderly person spent up to 50 hours a week caring. Carers also report feeling sad and bereft at having no one to share their personal confidences with, a role that was normally undertaken by the person for whom they were caring. Even if the carer is not spending time caring, he or she still faces a limited social life as a consequence of caring (Parker, 1992). This is perhaps confounded by the work of Levin *et al* (1989), which showed that, although relatives and friends may initially be carers, as time goes on, this input and support gradually lessens. The same study stated that carers believe that such people should provide them with more social support. This becomes difficult, however, if the person with cancer is very ill, and other family members are reluctant to bring their friends around.

The purpose of this study was to examine, in depth, the experiences of lay people caring for people with cancer. Because the research sought to reveal the essence of a complex and uniquely human lived experience, it was conducted within the interpretive paradigm using a phenomenological approach. As Patton (1990) recognises, this approach is naturalistic and inductive, and seeks to understand the human experience within the context it occurs. The study aimed at describing and interpreting the experience of caring for someone with cancer as a basis for assisting the service provider to plan and implement appropriate cancer care services.

Sample

The sample was drawn from volunteers who responded to either an article in the local press or an appeal through local radio stations. In both methods, the need for an awareness of carers' needs and the purpose of the workshop were addressed. Inclusion criteria for participants included geographical location (south-west England), and either a current or recent involvement in caring from someone with cancer. The sample had 42 women and 13 men, a total of 51. Ages ranged from 29 to 75 years. All were Caucasian and most from business and professional occupational backgrounds. The period of time they had been caring for someone with cancer ranged from two months to eight years. Some 65% of participants experienced the death of the person with cancer for whom they had been caring.

Procedure

In the afternoon of the workshop, participants were broken down into small groups in order to be able to conduct group interviews. The nature and purpose of the study was explained to all participants and all participants were assured that they could refuse to participate or withdraw from the study at any time. As the workshop involved group work to glean attitudes and experiences from the participants, it was impossible to ensure total anonymity and confidentiality. However, confidentiality of authorship of statements by participants was assured. In addition, reassurance was given that information could not result in their personal identification. All participants were willing to participate in the workshop and they consented in writing to be contacted at a later date to confirm aspects of data analysis and interpretation. All semi-structured interviews were conducted during the workshop, and each began with the question: 'Could you tell me in your own words about the experience of caring for someone with cancer?'

Interviews were taped, and during these, prompts were used to encourage people to discuss their feelings about, and perceptions of, the experience of caring for someone with cancer. The objective of the analysis was to describe the essence of the phenomenon in the fullest breadth and depth possible without preconception and presuppositions (Spielberg, 1975). Data was transcribed into hard copy in preparation for the analysis that was conducted.

Analysis

Central to the phenomenological approach, the analysis included bracketing out personal assumptions; comparing, interpreting and extrapolating meanings from the data; then engaging in a process of continuous reflection and intuition to identify and clarify emergent themes (Munhall, 1994).

Consistent with the research process, interview responses were categorised by examining the transcripts and identifying significant themes and meanings. This was performed at the manifest level, as recommended by Fox (1982), wherein classifications were made to what the participant actually said, rather than attempting to interpret the response. Additionally, field notes enhanced the data by allowing observations and reflections to be made that were contrasted and compared with the data. By using this process, unique and common emergent significant themes were identified and comparisons were made. As themes recurred, it was easy to identify commonalities between them and as themes evolved, they were collapsed into fewer themes.

After collapsing of themes, three clusters were identified. As the phenomenon of caring for someone with cancer was analysed, we were trying to determine the structures that make up this experience (ie. the theme). Although repeated words, phrases and beliefs were identifiable and repeated, it was not easy to place all statements easily into one particular theme, and in some instances overlapping occurred. These were placed in miscellaneous themes, which are not acknowledged in this discussion.

Themes were validated by referring back to the transcripts to check that none of the data had been ignored or discarded. All themes were kept and no contradictions in the data were evident. After each interview, interview schedules were compared within the research team in order to facilitate consistency in analysis. Once significant themes were identified, these were presented in written form and mailed to subjects in order for them to validate the formulated descriptions. This was in accordance with Guba and

Lincoln's (1981) recommendation that researchers should return to their sample population in order to ascertain whether the representation of answers was correct and if they wish to add further information, as a source of data credibility.

Findings

At the interviews, most participants were extremely open and frank about their experiences, and many commented on the value of the workshop as a forum for enabling them to share common experiences. Due to the number of participants involved and their willingness to share their experiences, vast amounts of data were generated. A plethora of significant statements were identified, and as such cannot be detailed in full in this chapter. A selection of descriptions from the three emergent theme categories follow, since space limitations prevent inclusion of the whole data.

Professional caring

All participants referred to the roles of the professionals. Many of these statements referred to the positive aspects of the role.

> *'As a carer I had a great admiration for the ward team. It really made my life easier to know I was valued, and actually seen as someone who could help my husband in this dreadful situation.'*

> *'The nurses and doctors explained everything to us, not as if we were stupid; they were just being friendly really, trying to make us at ease, I think.'*

> *'Whether it was the district sister, the Macmillan nurse or an auxiliary, it was such a comfort and relief for them to come round to the house, even if it was for five minutes, just to see how we were getting on. It just helped us from the intensity of being together constantly.'*

At other times, carers felt they were being disempowered by healthcare professionals and comments revolved around the way they were treated, the quality of support they were given, and the amount and quality of information that was offered to them. One woman was distressed by the way she had been told of her father's illness.

> *'When asking to speak to someone about my father's progress, the nurse told me she didn't feel happy talking about that type of information to me. She would prefer for a doctor to tell me the news, as she couldn't be sure of the time scale involved. I can remember her saying that I was obviously aware of the outcome of his illness, and the word 'obviously' came into this short conversation numerous times. I think she only realised it wasn't obvious to me, when I sat down, and she realised I was totally shell-shocked by this news. When I told her we'd been reassured over and over again that my father was 'clear' and his problems were with the wound site, she started back-peddling as fast as she could.'*

> *'Nothing was ever explained to us. It was if this was something so separate, something that we weren't to be part of. The charts, the temperature recording etc, all of it was never part of the life we knew, and because it was never explained to either my husband or us, we felt so isolated. It was if how we normally lived, our relationship just wasn't significant enough for them.'*

> *'I know it sounds daft, but the most important thing I can remember about the ins and outs of 3 years of hospitals, is the time he'd just been diagnosed as terminally ill, and he looked absolutely awful. I'd worked in intensive care, so when the dynamap read 67/39 mmhg [blood pressure reading], I was amazed that no medical treatment was ordered. When talking to a nurse about this, she quickly went to find his chart. The nurse who had taken his Bp and recorded it, had put it down as 80/60 mmhg. I actually felt like killing this nurse, when I found this out. I was absolutely enraged, it felt that she couldn't be interested with him, and us, just because he was dying. That nurse did more harm to us than you could imagine.'*

These extracts not only tell us of the disempowering nature of professional caring, but also of the insensitivity of some healthcare professionals.

Physical changes

The nature of caring for some participants had necessitated a major life change. This was relevant to those who were caring for people who had undergone either major surgery or long periods of chemotherapy/radiotherapy, or alternatively had cared for someone who had subsequently died. In these instances, the nature of active caring had not only become a necessity, but also a priority, and participants recognised that many aspects of their life had been put 'on hold'. This does not necessarily have to be construed negatively, since no participant explicitly stated an unwillingness or resentment, but they did identify changes in their physical being.

> *'The amount of headaches and migraines I was getting was incredible, I just felt I had no way of controlling them — all my energies seemed focussed on helping her to get better, how I was feeling was irrelevant really.'*
>
> *'Because he felt nauseated and sick because of the chemo, I couldn't be bothered to get myself meals either. Fortunately, he got over this as soon as the treatment stopped and we both began eating then. I'd probably faded away otherwise.* [Laughing] *. . . I even thought that when we went to out-patients that people probably thought it was me that had got the cancer, 'cause the weight had dropped off both of us, but I'm sure I looked the most worried and haggard.'*
>
> *'I felt as if I was in a different world, I know it was the psychological impact, but it affected my health as well, sometimes I'd be going around in a daze, I'd drop things, bump into things and the amount of mistakes, stupid mistakes, I made at work was frightening.'*

Psychological changes

As seen in the above statement, the psychological impact affected carers, and in many instances manifested themselves in physical symptoms. Many carers commented on the transformation of their general emotional well- being. Emotional responses identified by the participants included: depression, sorrow, inadequacy, guilt, frustration and anger. One woman articulated the transformations she had experienced as a result of the experience of caring.

> *'Nothing could have ever prepared me for the emotions I felt, and still do, I guess. I experienced everything people tell you you're going to, but you never believe until you've been there yourself. The usual things that used to stress me out, just meant nothing. At work, I used to find myself like being detached when others were winging on about something irrelevant. I kept thinking 'you know nothing, nothing at all.' On retrospect, I think I felt like no-one else had ever been through anything like this before. I know it's stupid, 'cause billions have been through it, yet in so many other ways, it is unique, 'cause no-one else has got that unique relationship with him.'*
>
> *'It was a continual roller-coaster of emotions. One minute I'd be on an all-time low, then this would be superseded by intense anger, frustration and futility at the whole thing . . . At times, I could have easily hit someone who could have done the smallest thing to annoy me. Then of course, I'd feel guilty that I'd be getting wound up about something irrelevant, when she'd be facing chemo which would make her feel sick and lifeless. . . . I'd also feel fed up that I was having to take her everywhere, do all the jobs round the house, look after the kids etc. It made me realise how much she actually did for us.'*

There were also ramifications upon the carer's health status due to the nature of uncertainty of disease progression and the treatment.

> *'. . . it was, it was a continual roller coaster. We used to say to ourselves that it couldn't get any worse, but of course it did. My sister and I had full-time jobs, and she's got children as well. The stress on us seemed unbelievable; we'd never experienced anything like it really. God help that we never do again.'*

Discussion

Other studies adopting attempts to explain the processes involved with being a carer, include small sample sizes due to the time-consuming nature of this kind of research (Field and Morse, 1985), and have adopted either a grounded theory or an ethnographic approach. Although acknowledging the limitations of being unable to generalise from qualitative studies that identify a certain section of the community, the results provide more detailed insight into the real nature of care-giving than more quantitative studies (Kuhlman *et al*, 1991). Subsequently, the findings from this study suggest that caring for someone with cancer is a profound experience that affects all facets of the carer's life. The findings of the current study concur with previous research in concluding that carers readily enter the caring relationship. Many forgo other activities in order to provide care, but, in doing so, experience detrimental physical and psychological changes.

Informal carers increasingly provide care with no financial recompense (Henwood, 1992). The strategic paper 'Caring for People' (Department of Health/ DSS/Welsh Office/Scottish HHD, 1989) reinforced economic reasoning as the dictate for new policies, since the cost of residential and hospital care was unacceptably high. Consequently, it appears that community care has become synonymous with family care, and health and social services rely on providing a back-up to family care rather than acting as first-line providers (Sinclair, 1990). In fact, it is reported that up to 80% of long-term care is provided by informal family carers (BMA, 1995). This is perhaps recognised by the recommendation that 'a key responsibility of statutory service providers should be to do all they can to assist and support carers' (Department of Health, 1989). Paragraph 3.2.6 also emphasises the need to include consideration of the wishes and requirements of both the carer and the people cared for, and the provision of flexibility in order for carers to exercise choice. Clearly, the importance of carers cannot be underestimated when service providers are planning and implementing cancer care services.

To see carers as a discrete group of people, however, would be underestimating the uniqueness of each individual, human relationship. Department of Health/Social Services Inspectorate Guidance (DOH/SSI, 1996), which accompanied the *Carers (Recognition and Services) Act, 1995*, supports the fact that each caring situation should be seen as unique. It further confirms that willingness to care should not be assumed and offers the statutory right to a separate assessment of their needs. It is then seen as a powerful tool for nurses who are genuinely concerned about improving the position of family carers (Nolan, 1996). It should be recognised, however, that people can dip in and out of the caring relationship, which should be recognised as a continuum, requiring professional support at some times but not at others. To see it otherwise would assume that there is a universal understanding of the concept of care-giving that is, in fact, open to different understandings and interpretations (Twigg *et al*, 1990). This uniqueness was apparent throughout this study, so, even though the data provided rich, common themes, the actual relationships and experiences were unique to each participant.

Statements reflected that some carers experienced disempowerment by professional carers, and in some instances were not offered information and support relating to their situation. These findings were in direct contrast to *The Declaration of Rights of People with Cancer* (Cancerlink, 1993). This stated the importance of people with cancer having correct information about their condition and treatment. It is assumed that their carers (with their agreement) should also be party to this information. Such inadequacies may be attributed to the failings and actions or inaction of professional carers, but also to the structure and organisation of healthcare systems (James and Field, 1996). For instance, task orientation and competency-based nursing can be viewed as impeding the establishment and maintenance of trusting relationships between staff and patients, which are necessary for this type of information-giving. Another structural factor that can be seen as affecting information-giving is the plethora of services involved in supporting the patient with cancer, which makes the use of effective communication between different levels of staff and different occupations essential. Within such a system, it is easy to ignore the patients' and their carers' needs; however, in order to provide a better service, these should be seen as influencing factors, and not as excuses.

An important factor within the theme 'professional caring' seemed to be the amount of control professionals facilitated. Decreasing the amount of control a person has results in helplessness, apathy and even death. The lack of control acts as a major psychological stress (Weinberg and Levine, 1980). Connell and Wellborn (1990) think that humans have a basic psychological need to be effective in their interactions, and this theme is a major representative theme in the theory of psychology: for example, Bandura's (1977) theory of self-efficacy, theories of learned helplessness (Abramson *et al*, 1978) and Weiner's (1979) attribution theory.

Bandura's work has been very influential in terms of self-efficacy theory, and it is felt that it contributes theoretically to the experiences of participants in this study. Self-efficacy shapes how people think, feel and act, and refers to personal control or agency. This means that an efficacious individual will exercise control over events that affect their lives, while, conversely, an inefficacious person will be incapable of doing so. Unfortunately, carers usually do not choose to be carers as part of their life trajectory, and thus they do not actively seek this environment. However, a highly efficacious person will readily undertake the challenging role of caring, regardless of the environment. What is of concern is the inefficacious carer, who may experience the negative effects of low self-efficacy.

The professional caring environment appeared to be uncontrollable to some participants and support for carers appeared to be diminished. As a result of being part of a caring relationship for a long time, some carers reported very limited social networks (Atkin, 1992), which suggests that loneliness can be a severe problem for carers if the care receiver either dies or is admitted to a residential or nursing home. Social support acts as a protective function against stress, and, although it is not a fixed entity, it can encourage people to seek help for themselves (Bandura, 1996). Seemingly, many carers do not seek this help, and carers frequently feel tied down, suffer from a lack of personal time and develop feelings of resentment, hopelessness and guilt (Hirschfield, 1983). Carers may feel the care receiver has become a burden and, in the long-term, it is likely they may become exhausted (Biegel *et al*, 1991).

Some participants experienced both physical and psychological changes due to the experience of caring. This is not surprising, given the amount of perceived stress evident. Physical problems that have been reported include headaches, obesity and cardiovascular disease associated with stress (Hirschfield, 1983). In the study by Levin *et al* (1989), nearly two-fifths of carers reported having recurring physical health problems, the most common being arthritis or rheumatism. In addition, 40% reported recurring backache or lumbago that may be a result of the heavy physical tasks involved with care-giving.

Caring is seen as a critical or stressful event that some saw as worsening their personal circumstances, despite the original acceptance of the role. Such events are generally seen as risk factors for depression, and, indeed, emotions such as sadness, hopelessness and alienation are evident in some statements. Brandstadter (1996) found that people afflicted by personal illness showed a significantly greater increase in depressive tendency and an associated decrease in life satisfaction. This significance was found in comparison to a complementary sample of people not experiencing such an event. The emotional impact an individual experiences as a result of caring appears to exert a stronger influence on depressive episodes than the ability to control personal events. Thus, healthcare workers should be aware of the higher occurrence of these symptoms in some carers and be able to offer the appropriate support, skills and advice in order to combat these symptoms.

In conclusion, carers of individuals with cancer will differ in their experiences due to the nature of the cancer. However, for the terminally ill, their carers will have to cope with physical and behavioural problems experienced by the sufferer, and the role is almost invariably intense. At the same time, the care relationship will depend on the prognosis, thus recognising the changing nature of the caring relationship. Healthcare professionals should recognise that the costs of care-giving are immense and can be summarised into four categories: economic, physical, psychological and social, and that potentially the most influential nursing contribution will be the support of these individuals (Nolan, 1996).

Recommendations

Recommendations relating to further work have been categorised into two distinct areas. One is related to the immediate service needs that have become so apparent in the pursuit of the study, and the other is related to the need for further research work that inevitably is revealed in a phenomenological study of this type. The former has received the greater attention to date.

A network of healthcare professional services should be developed to mirror the non-clinical services offered to people with cancer, but with the carer as the focus. Services covering information, counselling, befriending, respite, relaxation and stress management should be made available, together with access to other provision of social and welfare supportive care.

At the same time, strategies will need to be developed to identify those who are most at risk in the caring episode in order for a proactive, interventionist approach to be pursued if appropriate and welcomed by the individual.

From the research point of view, further work in the role of self-efficacy and the role of health care workers in promoting efficacy, eg. guided mastery, vicarious experiences, is seen to be a useful way forward. At the same time, it is clear that the study was narrow in its sample population, and there is some evidence of bias and confounding. Two approaches may provide further insight, subject to funding being identified for this next stage.

Conscious of the fact that the caring experience changes over the episode and is unique, the authors think that a cohort study of a number of carers would be useful, using ongoing individual interviews over entire episodes from diagnosis to death. At the same time, a larger quantitative study is planned, based on issues that have been revealed from the work to date.

References

Abramson LY, Seligman MEP & Teasdale JD (1978) Learned helplessness in humans: Critique and reformulation. *J Abnorm Psychol* **87**: 49–74

Adams T (1987) How does it feel to be a caregiver? *Commun Psychiatr Nurs J* June: 11–17

Atkin K (1992) Similarities and differences between informal carers. In: Twigg J, ed. *Carers, Research and Practice*. HMSO, London: 30–58

Bannister D, Fransella F (1980) *Inquiring Man: The Theory of Personal Constructs*. Penguin, London

Bandura A (1977) Self-efficacy: Toward a unifying theory of behavioural change. *Psychol Rev* **84**:191–215

Bandura A (1996) Exercise of personal agency through the self-efficacy mechanism. In: Schwarzer R, ed. *Self-efficacy: Thought control of action*. Taylor and Francis, London

Biegel D, Sales S, Shulz L (1991) *Family caregiving in chronic illness*. Sage Publications, Newbury Park

Boss P (1988) *Family Stress Management: Family Studies Text Series*. Sage Publications Inc, California

Braithwaite VA (1990) *Bound to Care*. Allen and Unwin, Sydney

Brandstadter J (1996) Personal control over development: Some developmental implications of self-efficacy. In: Schwarzer R, ed. *Self-efficacy: Thought Control of Action*. Taylor and Francis, London

British Medical Association (1995) *Taking Care of Carers*. BMA, London

Cancerlink (1993) *Declaration of Rights of People with Cancer*. Cancerlink, London

Challis D, Barton R (1990) Evaluation research and experiment in social gerontology. In: Peace SM, ed. *Researching Social Gerontology Concepts, Methods and Issues*. Sage Publications Inc, London: 75–100

Connell JP, Wellborn JG (1990) Competence, autonomy, and relatedness: A motivational analysis of self-system processes. In: Gunnar M, Sroufe LA, eds. *Minnesota Symposium on Child Psychology, No. 22*. University of Minnesota Press, Minneapolis: 43–77

Dalley G (1988) The ideological foundations of informal care. In: Kitson A, ed. *Nursing Art and Science*. Chapman Hall, London: 11–24

Dawson T (1987) Evaluation of a community based night sitter service. In: Fielding P, ed. *Research in the Nursing Care of Elderly People*. John Wiley and Sons, Chichester: 87–106

Department of Health/DSS/Welsh Office/Scottish HHD (1989) *Caring for People: Community Care in the Next Decade and Beyond*. HMSO, London

Department of Health (1989) *Working for Patients: Medical Audit*. Working Paper No. 6. HMSO, London

DOH/SSI (1996) *Carers (Recognition and Services) Act, 1995: Practice Guide*. Department of Health, London

DHSS (1988) *Community Care: Agenda for Action*. Report to the Secretary of State for Social Services (chair Sir R Griffiths). HMSO, London

Ebrahim S, Wallis C, Brittis S, Harwood R, Graham N (1993) Long-term care for elderly people. *Qual Health Care* **2**: 198–203

Field PA, Morse JM (1985) *Nursing Research: The Application of Qualitative Approaches*. Croom Helm, London

Finch J, Groves D, eds (1983) *Labour of Love: Women, Work and Caring*. Routledge and Kegan Paul, London

Finch J, Mason J (1990) Filial obligations and kin support for elderly people. *Ageing Soc* 10: 151–75

Fox DJ (1982) *Fundamentals of Research in Nursing*, 4 ed. Appleton-Century Crofts, New York

Graham H (1983) Caring: A labour of love. In: Finch J, Groves D, eds. *Labour of Love: Women, Work and Caring*. Routledge and Kegan Paul, London:13–30

Green H (1988) General household survey: Informal carers. HMSO Office of Population Censuses and Surveys. *Social Survey Division series GH5*, No. 15, Supplement A

Guba E, Lincoln Y (1981) *Effective Evaluation*. Jossey-Bass Publishers, London

Henwood M (1990) *Community Care and Elderly People*. Family Policy Studies Centre

Henwood M (1992) Through a glass darkly: Community care and elderly people. *Kings Fund Institute Report*, No. 14. Kings Fund, London

Henwood M, Wicks M (1984) *The Forgotten Army: Family Care and Elderly People*. Witley Press for Family Policy Studies Centre

Hirschfield MJ (1983) Homecare versus institutional action: Family caregiving and senile brain disease. *Int J Nurs Stud* **20**(1): 23–32

James V, Field D (1996) Who has the power? Some problems and issues affecting the nursing care of dying patients. *Eur J Cancer Care* **5**: 73–80

Kuhlman G, Skodal Wilson H, Hutchinson SA, Wallhagen M (1991) Alzheimer's disease and family caregiving: Critical synthesis of the literature and research agenda. *Nurs Res* **40**(6): 331–7

Land H, Rose A (1985) Compulsory altruism for some or an altruistic society for all. In: Bean P, Ferris J, Whynes D, eds. *Defence of Welfare*. Tavistock, London

Levin E, Sinclair I, Gorbach P (1989) *Families, Services and Confusion in Old Age*. Avebury Gower Publishing, Aldershot

Munhall P (1994) *Revisioning Phenomenology: Nursing and Health Service Research*. National League for Nursing Press, New York

Nolan M (1996) Supporting family carers: The key to successful long term care? *Br J Nurs* **5**(14): 836

OPCS (1991) *Social Trends, 21*. HMSO, London

Parker R (1981) Tending and social policy. In: Goldberg EM, Hatch S, eds. *A New Look at the Personal Social Services*. Policy Studies Institute, London

Parker R (1992) Counting care: Numbers and type of informal carers. In: Twigg J, ed. *Carers, Research and Practice*. HMSO, London: 6–29

Patton MQ (1990) *Qualitative evaluation and research methods*, 2 edn. Sage Publications, Newbury Park, CA

Pitkeathley J (1989) *It's My Duty, Isn't It?* Souvenir Press, London

Sainsbury P, Grad de Alarcon J (1970) The effects of community care on the family of the geriatric patient. *J Ger Psychiatry* **4**: 23–41

Sinclair I (1990) Carers: Their contribution and quality of life. In: Sinclair I, Parker R, Leat D, Williams J, eds. *The Kaleidoscope of Care: A Review of Research of Welfare Provision for Elderly People*. HMSO, London: 32–64

Spielberg H (1975) *Doing Phenomenology: Essays on and in Phenomenology*. Martinus Nijhoff, The Hague

Twigg J, Atkin K, Perring C (1990) *Carers and Services: A Review of Research*. HMSO, London

Weinberg J, Levine S (1980) Psychobiology of coping in animals: The effects of unpredictability. In: Levine S, Ursin H, eds. *Coping and Health*. Plenum, New York

Weiner B (1979) A theory of motivation for some classroom experiences. *J Educ Psychol* **71**: 3–25

Wilson E (1982) Women, the community and the family. In: Walker A, ed. *Community Care: The Family and Social Policy*. Blackwell, Oxford

29

Lessons from the past, models for the future: Social workers and nurses collaborating in the community

Joellen W Hawkins, Carole W Pearce, Nancy W Veeder and Peggy S Matteson, with Valerie A Hamel, Carol J McMahon-Morin, Ellen Trabka and Susan L Williams

Historical background for collaboration

At the end of the nineteenth century, there were few positions in hospitals for graduate nurses, since hospitals with training schools 'found a cheap labour source in the **pupil nurse**' (Lewenson, 1993). So graduate nurses teamed up with social workers in the community. In rural areas and in cities across America, social workers and nurses created new models for care by founding baby tents, prenatal care clinics, settlement houses in tenement neighbourhoods and rural health centres, and by bringing health and social services to migrant labour camps, to school children and to workers. An early example of this collaboration was cited by Carolyn Van Blarcom, a maternity nurse, in her book on prenatal care: social workers were part of the team for maternity and infancy work under the Sheppard-Towner Act of 1921 (1929). Laura Gamble, Director of Nursing for the Cattaraugus County New York Board of Health, and Josephine Brown, Associate Field Director for the American Association for Organizing Family Social Work, wrote in 1926 about the work of nurses and social workers in rural districts: social workers and nurses were needed to provide 'family health supervision' and 'family case work'.

This collaboration was helpful to each of the neophyte professions. And the shared goal of caring for the unfortunate fitted with a feminine approach to social reform. Co-founder of Hull–House in Chicago, Jane Addams, a founding mother of social work, believed in a feminine perspective in addressing the social problems of America's cities. Her contemporary in New York City, Lillian Wald, a graduate of New York Hospital Training School for Nurses and founder of the Nurses' Settlement, later renamed Henry Street Settlement, urged women who had the advantages of an education, to embrace opportunities to serve humankind. In cities, besieged by hundreds of new immigrants, the settlement house was the answer to urban problems and to Lillian Wald's challenge.

Settlement houses were laboratories for social reform characterised by consensus building and co-operation. Such an approach has been ascribed to a woman's world view. The alliance between social workers and nurses probably evolved because virtually all members of both professions were women at the beginning of these professions. The social settlements literally brought nurses and social workers together, for one of the principles of the settlement house was that the workers would live in the tenement neighbourhood it served. However, such collaboration was not unique to the United States.

Social settlements and district nursing had their origins in Great Britain in the nineteenth century (Brainard, 1922; Holden, 1922). And in the early decades of the twentieth century, in Germany, Austria, France, Belgium, Spain, Rumania and Italy, public health work grew out of tuberculosis and child welfare programs, blending social work and nursing in the community with a focus on the general welfare of families and their children, rather than on bedside care. Some European training schools include both social work and nursing in a programme comprising one year of nursing and two years in social work.

With the decline in settlement houses in the United States, social workers and nurses were deprived of their most important setting for collaboration. Hospitals employed many nurses and social workers, but the departments were separate and opportunities for collaboration had to be deliberately sought out rather than occurring naturally. Many important models of collaboration were created as social workers and nurses tackled new problems together. It was not until the war on poverty of the late

1960s and early 1970s, however, that the two professions were united once more in neighbourhood health centres (NHC). These were offshoots of settlement houses that had survived the decades, or the result of either zealous healthcare professionals or neighbourhood activists. In NHC, collaboration was in a way reborn in settings not unlike those where it first began.

The decade of the 1990s has challenged social work and nursing in ways reminiscent of a century ago. With a perspective of 100 years of collaboration to draw on, we became curious about collaboration in a managed care environment.

Background for the study

We were guided in designing our study by the work of Reinharz (1979; 1981; 1992). In her literature review on interviewing (1992), she explored the positive attributes of semi-structured or open-ended interviews, concluding that this method allows feminist researchers to create 'important new ways of seeing the world. By listening to women speak, understanding women's membership in particular social systems, and establishing the distribution of phenomena accessible only through sensitive interviewing, feminist interview researchers have uncovered previously neglected or misunderstood worlds of experience'.

Our work was also guided by that of other feminist researchers, including Belenky *et al* (1986), Finch (1984), Fornow and Cook, (1991); Gilligan (1982); Gilligan *et al* (1989), Gilligan *et al* (1988), Graham (1984), Harding (1987), Nielsen (1990), Riessman (1990), Roberts (1990), Stern and Pyles (1985) and Tuana (1989). We wanted our participants to tell their stories, sharing their perspectives on the challenges to collaboration posed by managed care. We considered ourselves, in Reinharz's words, 'involved [and had a] sense of commitment, participation, and sharing of fate' with the participants (1979). The major questions we chose to explore were:

1. What is the history of collaboration between social workers and nursing in a variety of agencies and institutions?
2. What are the pluses and minuses in the ways in which social workers and nurses interact; how can social workers and nurses evaluate the outcomes of their practices or interventions?
3. What might an ideal system of collaboration look like?
4. What opportunities might managed care or a system of capitation offer for nurses, social workers, and their clients for access to care, a holistic approach to care, health promotion and disease prevention, and integration of alternative or complementary therapies?
5. What new opportunities might there be for collaboration between these two professions?

In this chapter, we will address only the first and third of these questions.[1]

The most appropriate method to answer these questions was feminist interview research. We anticipated that most of our participants would be women and recognised the congruence between this method and achieving 'the active involvement of their [feminists]' respondents in the construction of data about their lives (Graham, 1984).

We interviewed our participants in their places of work, audio-taped the interview with permission of the participants, and wrote field notes to capture the context and nonverbal content that would be lost on the tapes.

Our participants came from large teaching institutions, community agencies, those offering primarily inpatient care, those totally community based, and those with a continuum of care. These agencies and institutions offered specialty and generalist healthcare services, ambulatory care, home care, acute, subacute and long-term care, and multidimensional services for special groups, such as women using substances during pregnancy and children with developmental delays. Our participants were directors of social services or social work and vice presidents, clinical directors, or directors of nursing or patient care services. Each of these persons were credentialed as a social worker or nurse. The sample consisted of 16 nurses, 16 social workers, and one person who is a social worker and a nurse, from 16 different agencies. Most were women, reflecting not only current but historical perspectives.

Findings

In the context of significant changes and challenges to social workers and nurses, our participants shared their concerns. They also expressed confidence that collaboration will thrive as a principal means for refocusing our collective professional energies in the community.

History of collaboration

We first asked our participants to describe the history of collaboration between nurses and social workers in their practice settings. In the words of one social worker in an agency with nearly a century of such collaborations: 'It is not a power play about control, but it is that in fact that patients have needs and if we are both very good about what we do then that's the model'. One nurse commented:

> *'It's always been there. I don't even remember working without a social worker on that component . . . We're together all the time. We refer as many people to social workers as they refer to us in the clinic, whether it be a social worker calling with an AIDS patient that needs intervention for IV therapy or us meeting an AIDS patient that's just coming home from New York to his family to die and we need their help in looking for services for the family or in supporting the family.'*

Her social worker colleague added:

> *'The relationship between social workers and nurses goes way back. Social work has been part of this institution since the 1920s — shortly after the role of social workers in healthcare evolved, when it really started at* [the hospital] *in the early 1990s . . . Historically . . .* [this hospital] *was formed by a local group as a charitable organization in the late 1800s; it started as child care for sick kids for mill workers and then kids were abandoned so it became an orphanage . . . There was always a common focus.'*

The nurse leader in a community hospital that was among the first to implement a nurse/social worker team approach (almost 15 years ago) described a triad of nurses, social workers and physicians working together in the inpatient, subacute, homecare, and community services.

In the view of a social worker in a mental health specialty facility, nurses and social workers come from different orientations (that is why one chooses one or the other profession), but share a similar core. Collaboration can be exciting, she said, when both professions give up turf guarding.

The nurse leader in an urban teaching hospital described her nursing department as a closed system, misusing power and alienating social workers. In her view, nurses there suffer a lack of role models. Believing they were under siege, nurses got kicked, so they kicked other departments, creating strained relationships. The result was that nurses and social workers engage in parallel activities; each discipline lacks role clarification. She did note some positive examples of collaboration in the AIDS group practice, the haematology/oncology multidisciplinary team, and in paediatrics.

We interviewed two social worker/nurse dyads involved in collaborative models. One model was designed to assist pregnant women with substance abuse problems and the second focussed on families enrolled in an early intervention program. The nurses and social workers characterised their collaboration as a holistic approach to care and perceived their relationship as supportive to one another and as helping each other out.

We heard many stories of long-term collaboration: it [collaboration] has 'always been there'; 12 years of collaboration, working closely together; over a 100 year history of collaboration; collaboration in case management. One nurse participant described collaboration thus: 'Now we've got these two experts . . . two pairs of eyes looking at one family and giving each other the missing parts of the puzzle'. Both nurses and social workers seemed to agree that together they provide a holistic approach; a 'natural collaboration'; 'the best of both worlds — people with training in emotional and mental health and people with training in physical health'. In the words of a social worker: 'When you're able to use both [social work and nursing], you really rally the forces, and come up with a good package to get the person home and we've seen that work pretty well'. These social workers and nurses seemed to value their past successes in collaboration and were excited by challenges of this decade.

Ideal system of collaboration[2]

We asked our participants to imagine the ideal in collaboration. One suggested that nurses and social workers could create a system of case management for a broad community of patients. Case managers could protect the quality of and access to care, addressing food and transportation needs of elders, housing and social concerns, consolidating these and other healthcare needs. Roles of social workers and nurses could run across the care continuum in home care setting, acting as resource co-ordinators. Nurses and social workers could contract directly with managed care systems and physician groups to provide services to their enrollees.

The focus in an ideal model of care would be on patient needs instead of what a particular healthcare provider is trained to do. The case manager or healthcare manager would evaluate the needs of a patient at any point in time and co-ordinate services; the caregiver assuming the role of case manager might change as the patient's needs changed. The role would be assumed by whoever offers the needed skills and knowledge based on assessment of the patient, her/his capacity for activities of daily living, and so on. Both professions could offer coordination of care among settings, creating a circle of care.

These participants, all social workers and nurses in leadership positions, shared their energy and enthusiasm for imagined ideals of collaboration, reminding us of their foremothers and forefathers of the late nineteenth century who dared to dream a new profession (social work), new models for care when there were no jobs in hospitals (nurses), and new specialties (medical social work, public health nursing). One nurse participant urged that we stop whining about what managed care is doing to us, stop reeling under managed care, and begin to say, 'let's all take charge', embracing the power we have together. In her opinion, the collaboration forced on us under managed care and capitation schemes could create equal opportunities for both professions.

A proposed model for collaboration

From our data and from the literature on collaboration, a model emerged, the Biopsychosocial Individual and Systems Intervention Model of Nurse-Social Worker Collaboration (BISIM). The characteristics of this proposed collaborative nurse/social worker case management service delivery model are as follows:

1. **Both client-focussed and system-focussed.** The National Association of Social Workers defined case management, as it is to be practised by professional social workers, as 'a method of providing services whereby a professional social worker assesses the needs of the client and the client's family, when appropriate, and arranges, coordinates, monitors, evaluates, and advocates for a package of multiple services to meet the specific client's complex needs' (NASW, 1992). The tasks performed by both social workers and nurses under this model are both client-level **and** system-level interventions, acknowledging that considerable variation may exist in these tasks, and in the role responsibilities assumed by either profession.
2. **Advanced case management by advanced systems practitioners.** Under our proposed model, advanced level nurses and social workers would provide direction and supervision to bachelor's prepared social workers, registered nurses with various educational preparation, paraprofessional staff, and, where appropriate, volunteer individuals and families. These professionals would be considered to be, by their education and experience, advanced level practitioners. In the home healthcare area, for example, social workers must have a master's degree, whereas nurses can have a minimum of a baccalaureate degree.
3. **Clinical case management.** In the words of Raiff and Shore, clinical case management has 'a two-pronged thrust: it is more focused on the changes, options, and pacing of relationships than 'broker' models, and it weaves clinical understandings throughout the process of disposition planning, service referral, advocacy, and follow-up. Some view this as an advanced, more expert modality. It builds on an infrastructure of the generic skills of assessment, planning, linking, monitoring, and advocacy and weds this to client engagement, consultation, and collaboration to other treating clinicians, individual psychotherapy, psychoeducation, and crisis intervention. 'A clinically informed practise is manifested through the conduct of skilled biopsychosocial assessments, demonstrated understanding of different personality types and their needs, skill in tailoring the client's physical and social environment, and being able to intervene appropriately as the client's need for support and structure changes' (1993).

4. **Holistic view of the biopsychosocial person-in-situation.** Integral to this model is an approach by which caregivers address the many factors germane to problem resolution.
5. **Life model, strengths, client competency enhancement conceptual framework.** The conceptual framework will be an integration of the Life Model of Germain and Gitterman (1980), the competence-oriented model of Maluccio (1981), and the strengths perspective model of Kisthardt and Rapp (1992) and Saleeby (1996).
6. **Interdisciplinary team case management: the transdisciplinary model.** We recommend consideration of the relatively new transdisciplinary model borrowed from early education (McGonigel and Garland, 1988; Woodruff and McGonigel, 1987). This approach reduces many interdisciplinary collaboration issues, especially 'professionally fragmented, pluralistic theories of individual behaviour and how to best meet needs' (Raiff and Shore, 1993).
7. **Roles differentiated between nurse and social worker** on the team according to those tasks for which each is clearly best trained, and those tasks that may be undertaken by either one or both professions.
8. **Flexible** in assessing community needs and responding to changes in individuals, groups, communities, and organisations.
9. **Strong community health education** and physical and mental illness prevention component.
10. Strong **advocacy** component.
11. **Available as needed** in the community throughout the life span.
12. **Strong qualitative and quantitative monitoring** and outcome evaluation accountability component.

Concluding thoughts, a common vision

The proposed BISIM intervention model is neither linked to an institution nor in any way restricted in its usefulness as a conceptual base from which social workers and nurses can create or revise existing care delivery systems in response to the needs of individuals, families, groups and communities. At the end of the nineteenth century, social workers and nurses created preventative education programmes for new immigrants, school children, factory and quarry workers, pregnant women, their infants and young children, giving birth to public health nursing, medical social work, settlement houses, and neighbourhood health centres. Surely, as the inheritors of this legacy, we of the late twentieth century can create new models of care to meet the social welfare and healthcare needs of all citizens for the twenty-first century. We can design and implement studies to measure outcomes of our care,[3] and then revise care based on our findings.

> *'Social workers and nurses should take the helm in developing the new leadership skills needed to implement major change, and the management of process, and how not only to help each other fit into the new delivery system but assist the patient[s] to also know what changed and how and where they access the system'*
>
> (study participant, 1996).

References

Belenky MF, Clinchy B, Goldberger NR, Tarule JM (1986) *Women's Ways of Knowing: The Development of Self, Voice, and Mind*. Basic Books, New York

Brainard AM (1922) *The Evolution of Public Health Nursing*. WB Saunders, Philadelphia

Finch J (1984) 'It's great to have someone to talk to': The ethics and politics of interviewing women. In: Bell C, Roberts H, eds. *Social Researching: Politics, Problems, Practice*. Routledge and Kegan Paul, London: 70–87

Fornow MM, Cook JA, eds (1991) *Beyond Methodology: Feminist Scholarship as lived Research*. Indiana University Press, Indianapolis, IN

Gamble LA, Brown JC (1926) Ask a question. *Survey* May 15: 276–7

Germain CB, Gitterman A (1980) *The Life Model of Social Work Practice*. Columbia University Press, New York

Gilligan C (!982) *In a Different Voice: Psychological Theory and Women's Development*. Harvard University Press, Cambridge, MA

Gilligan C, Lyons N, Hanmer TJ (1989) *Making Connections: The Relational Worlds of Adolescent Girls at Emma Willard School*. Emma Willard School, Troy, NY

Gilligan C, Ward JV, Taylor JM, eds (1988) *Mapping the Moral Domain*. Harvard University Press, Cambridge, MA

Graham H (1984) Surveying through stories. In: Bell C, Roberts H, eds. *Social Researching: Politics, Problems, Practice*. Routledge and Kegan Paul, London: 104–24

Harding S, ed (1987) *Feminism and Methodology*. Indiana University Press, Indianapolis, IN

Hawkins JW, Veeder NW, Pearce CW (1998) *Nurse-social Worker Collaboration under Managed Care: A Model for Case Management in the Community*. Springer, New York

Holden AC (1922) *The Settlement Idea: A Vision of Social Justice*. Macmillan, New York

Kisthardt WE, Rapp CA (1992) Bridging the gap between principles and practice. Implementing a strengths perspective in case management. In: Rose SM, ed. *Case Management and Social Work Practice*. Longman, White Plains, NY: 112–25

Lewenson SB (1993) *Taking Charge*. Garland, New York

Maluccio AN, ed (1981) *Promoting Competence in Clients. A New/old Approach to Social Work Practice*. Free Press, New York

McGonigel MJ, Garland C (1988) The individualized family service plan and the early intervention plan: Team and family issues and recommended practices. *Infants Young Child* **1**(1): 10–21

[NASW] National Association of Social Workers (1992) *Standards for Social Work Case Managment*. NASW Press, Washington, DC

Nielsen JM, ed (1990) *Feminist Research Methods*. Westview Press, Boulder, CO

Raiff NR with Shore BK (1993) Advanced case management. In: *New Strategies for the Nineties*. Sage, Newbury Park, CA

Reinharz S (1979) *On Becoming a Social Scientist*. Jossey-Bass, San Francisco

Reinharz S (1981) Implementing new paradigm research: A model for training and practice. In: Reason P, Rowan J, eds. *A Sourcebook of New Paradigm Research*. John Wiley New York: 415–36

Reinharz S (1992) *Feminist Methods in Social Research*. Oxford University Press, New York

Riessman CK (1990) *Divorce Talk: Women and Men Make Sense Of Personal Relationships*. Rutgers University Press, New Brunswick, NJ

Roberts H, ed (1990) *Doing Feminist Research*. Routledge, New York

Saleeby D (1996) The strengths perspective in social work practice: Extensions and cautions. *Soc Work* **41**(3): 296–305

Stern P, Pyles SH (1985) Using grounded theory methodology to study women's culturally based decisions about health. *Health Care Women Int* **6**(1–3): 1–24

Tuana N (1989) *Feminism and Science*. Indiana University Press, Bloomington, IN

Van Blarcom CC (1929) *Obstetrical Nursing*. 2 edn. Macmillan, New York

Woodruff G, McGonigel MJ (1987) Early intervention team approaches: The transdisciplinary model. In: Jordan J, Gallagher J, Huntinger P, Karns M, eds. *Early Childhood Special Education: Birth to Three*. Council for Exceptional Children, Reston, VA: 163–182

Notes

1. For a complete report of this study, please see: Hawkins, Veeder, Pearche (1998).

2. One social work director pointed out that no one wants to be a case and no one wants to be managed, so maybe we need different language.

3. Mary Breckinridge, founder of the Frontier Nursing Service, Lillian Wald and Lina Rogers the founders of school nursing and pioneers in settlement house work, Jane Addams, and many more of our foremothers and forefathers in nursing and social work collected data and demonstrated that the models of care delivery they had created made a difference in outcomes.